Tutorials in Paediatric Differential Diagnosis

For Elsevier:

Commissioning Editor: Ellen Green
Project Development Manager: Helen Leng
Project Manager: Frances Affleck
Design Direction: George Ajayi

Tutorials in Paediatric Differential Diagnosis

SECOND EDITION

Edited by

David Field MBBS(Hons) DCH FRCPCH FRCP(Ed) DM

Professor of Neonatal Medicine, Department of Health Science, University of Leicester Leicester, UK

David Isaacs MD FRCPCH FRACP

Clinical Professor in Paediatric Infectious Diseases, The Children's Hospital at Westmead and University of Sydney, Sydney, Australia

John Stroobant FRCP FRCPCH

Consultant Paediatrician, Honorary Senior Lecturer, Children's Hospital Lewisham, London, UK

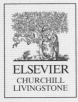

ELSEVIER
CHURCHILL
LIVINGSTONE

EDINBURGH LONDON NEW YORK OXFORD PHILADELPHIA ST LOUIS SYDNEY TORONTO 2005

ELSEVIER
CHURCHILL
LIVINGSTONE

First edition 1989
    Reprinted 1990
    Reprinted 1993 (twice)
Second edition 2005

ISBN 0443071004

British Library Cataloguing in Publication Data
A catalogue record for this book is available from the British Library

Library of Congress Cataloging in Publication Data
A catalog record for this book is available from the Library of Congress

Note
Medical knowledge is constantly changing. Standard safety precautions must be followed, but as new research and clinical experience broaden our knowledge, changes in treatment and drug therapy may become necessary or appropriate. Readers are advised to check the most current product information provided by the manufacturer of each drug to be administered to verify the recommended dose, the method and duration of administration, and contraindications. It is the responsibility of the practitioner, relying on experience and knowledge of the patient, to determine dosages and the best treatment for each individual patient. Neither the publisher nor the authors assumes any liability for any injury and/or damage to persons or property arising from this publication.

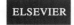 your source for books, journals and multimedia in the health sciences
www.elsevierhealth.com

The publisher's policy is to use paper manufactured from sustainable forests

Printed in China

PREFACE

Many current medical textbooks concentrate on disease entities with an anatomical or physiological orientation. In practice, patients present with symptoms, and doctors must develop a method for assessing such symptoms to approach diagnosis and management based on physiological principles. In paediatrics particularly, symptoms provide a major clue to the underlying disease. This book is designed to provide doctors involved in childcare with a logical approach to interpreting symptoms, rather than a formal review of disease entities. The second edition has been extensively rewritten with many more chapters and includes the most recent information about the investigation of symptomatic paediatric medical conditions.

Each section, chosen for its importance in clinical paediatrics, presents the important physiological principles underlying symptoms and discusses those areas which are often confused by both undergraduate and postgraduate students. Clinical features are then analysed to formulate an appropriate differential diagnosis, and, finally, important investigations are suggested to help establish a final diagnosis.

A true clinical scenario, with relevant questions, is presented at the end of each chapter, and the process of diagnosis for each scenario is detailed. These problems will be useful to examination candidates and others who are reading to improve their understanding of each topic. The chapters and scenarios could also usefully form the basis for a tutorial during a hospital teaching session.

D.J.F.
D.I.
J.S.

CONTRIBUTORS

Adrian Brooke MRCP FRCPCH MD
Consultant Community Paediatrician, Leicestershire and Rutland Specialist Community Child Health Services Leicester, UK
Developmental delay, hearing problems, behavioural problems

Charles R Buchanan BSc (Hons) MRCP FRCPCH
Consultant Paediatric Endocrinologist and Senior Lecturer, Variety Club Children's Hospital, King's College Hospital, London, UK
Ambiguous genitalia, short and tall stature, precocious puberty

Elaine Carter MA FRCP MRCPCH
Consultant Paediatrician, Leicester Royal Infirmary, Leicester, UK
Constipation, noisy breathing, accidental and non-accidental injuries, vomiting

Chris Cowell MBBS FRACP
Clinical Associate Professor
Institute of Endocrinology and Diabetes, The Children's Hospital at Westmead, Westmead, Australia
Failure to thrive

David Field MBBS DCH FRCPCH FRCP DM
Professor of Neonatal Medicine, Department of Health Science, University of Leicester, Leicester, UK
Neonatal convulsions, the ill-looking newborn

Peter Houtman MBBS MRCP BSc MRCPCH
Consultant Paediatrician, Leicester Royal Infirmary, Leicester, UK
Painful joints, urinary tract infection, haematuria, wetting

David Isaacs MD FRCPCH FRACP
Clinical Professor in Paediatric Infectious Diseases, The Children's Hospital at Westmead and University of Sydney, Sydney, Australia
Rash and fever, recurrent infections, persistent or recurrent fever, acute fever

Andrew Kornberg MBBS FRACP
Neurologist, Royal Children's Hospital, Parkville, Australia
Fits and faints, headache in children

Meryta May MBBS
Fellow in Paediatric Infectious Diseases, The Children's Hospital at Westmead, Westmead, Australia
Rash and fever, recurrent infections, persistent or recurrent fever, acute fever

Tina Sajjanhar MRCP FRCPCH DCH DRCOG
Consultant in Paediatric Accident and Emergency Medicine, Children's Hospital Lewisham, London, UK
The crying baby, unexpected/unexplained death and ALTE, the ill-looking child, abdominal pain in children

Elizabeth Sleight MRCP FRCPCH
Consultant Neonatologist, Children's Hospital Lewisham, London, UK
Feeding problems in infancy, sleep disorders, neonatal jaundice, the small for gestational age baby, the floppy baby

The late Richard Stevens FRCP FRCPath FRCPCH
Formerly Consultant Haematologist, Royal Manchester Children's Hospital, Manchester, UK
Bruising and bleeding, anaemia

John Stroobant FRCP FRCPCH
Consultant Paediatrician, Honorary Senior Lecturer, Children's Hospital Lewisham, London, UK
Cyanosis, apnoea, heart murmurs

Kate Wheeler MRCP FRCPCH
Consultant Paediatric Oncologist, John Radcliffe Hospital, Oxford, UK
Cough, lumps, diarrhoea

Fabian Yap MBBS MRCP MMED
Consultant, Endocrinology Service, Department of Paediatrics, KK Children's Hospital, Singapore
Failure to thrive

CONTENTS

APNOEA
John Stroobant

Apnoea, a pause in respiration, can occur at all ages from infancy to adulthood. The causes of apnoea are age dependent and may be *central*, caused by absent neurological drive from the respiratory centre, *obstructive*, where there is temporary blockage of the airway, or *mixed*, a combination of central and obstructive. It is important to recognize that apnoea is a symptom and therefore a search for an underlying cause must be made when it has been recognized. The three commonest apnoea syndromes are apnoea of prematurity, obstructive sleep apnoea and apparent life-threatening events in infancy (ALTEs), although there are also other causes (see Table 1.1). This chapter will deal with the first two of these (see Ch. 37 for ALTEs).

There is no universally agreed definition of apnoea; however, most clinicians recognize that significant apnoea has occurred if the pause in respiration is longer than 20 seconds. In neonates there is considerable variation in breathing pattern and even in normal infants regular rhythmic respiration will be interrupted by periodic breathing, identified as respiratory pauses of 3–10 seconds between phases of regular respiration. There may be regular patterns of this cycle. In obstructive apnoea – an abnormal breathing pattern – there are episodes of breathing movements without airflow which may be followed by absence of respiratory effort and cessation of breathing movements.

Neonatal apnoea

Pathophysiology

Apnoea is commonest in the neonatal period; although it occurs in both preterm and mature neonates, central apnoea is more prevalent in the former. Factors to explain this include:

- Altered responsiveness of respiratory centre to physiological stimuli:

Table 1.1   Causes of apnoea

Age	Central	Obstructive	Mixed
Neonates	Sepsis Meningitis Seizures Intracranial haemorrhage Kernicterus Hypoxia Hypoglycaemia Electrolyte imbalance Hypothermia and hyperthermia Drugs Anaemia Asphyxia Werdnig–Hoffmann Myopathies	Gastro-oesophageal reflux Tracheomalacia Vocal cord paralysis	Respiratory distress syndrome Congenital anomalies Diaphragmatic fatigue Pneumonia Patent ductus arteriosus Seizures
Infancy	Sepsis Seizures Drugs CNS tumours Subdural haemorrhage Central hypoventilation (Ondine's curse) Arrhythmias Metabolic disorders Werdnig–Hoffman Myopathies	Gastro-oesophageal reflux Discoordinate swallowing Tracheomalacia Vascular rings Pierre Robin syndrome	Respiratory syncytial virus infection Seizures Pertussis Upper airway obstruction
Older children	Ondine's curse Arrhythmias Metabolic disorder Myopathies	Gastro-oesophageal reflux Vocal cord paralysis Tracheomalacia Vascular rings	Respiratory infection Upper airway obstruction

a) Decreased responsiveness to high carbon dioxide or hypoxia.
b) Paradoxical response to hypoxia, which may increase depression of the respiratory centre.

- Increased depression of the centre from adverse factors including hypoxia, anaemia, sepsis, dugs, metabolic disturbance, arrhythmias and acidosis.
- Upper airway vulnerability to obstruction; size, less structurally robust.
- Increased upper airway protective reflex.
- Physiological oscillatory breathing patterns in preterm infants.
- Tendency to diaphragmatic fatigue.
- Increased tendency to gastro-oesophageal reflux and discoordinate swallowing.

Differential diagnosis

As apnoea in neonates may be physiological it is important to assess whether the symptoms are consistent with normal variation or represent a pathological process. Factors which help in this decision are:

- Length of apnoea.
- Signs of sepsis, acidosis etc.
- Associated seizures.
- Upper airway infection, e.g. RSV.
- Signs of gastro-oesophageal reflux (although this may occur without external evidence).
- Congenital anomalies.

- Gestation.
- Associated problems, e.g. congenital heart disease.

Assessment and investigations

Investigations should be undertaken on the basis of the likely pathology. The following list suggests those which might be helpful; the first group should be performed in most cases; the second list should be considered depending on clinical suspicions and results of the initial tests.

- Cardiorespiratory monitoring.
- Full blood count.
- Blood gases.
- Investigations for sepsis.
- Electrolytes.
- Cranial ultrasound scan.
- Chest X-ray.

- EEG: standard and a continuous recording.
- pH probe.
- Upper gastrointestinal contrast study.
- Echocardiography.

Sleep apnoea

Normal infants, children and adults will have periods of central apnoea during sleep. Normal respiratory pauses will not usually have associated changes in other physiological parameters such as heart rate, O_2 saturation or sleep pattern. Such normal variations in respiratory patterns occur during REM sleep. Periods of obstructive apnoea have also been observed in normal adults but not in children.

Abnormal upper airway obstruction during sleep or obstructive sleep apnoea (OSA) occurs at all ages. Although commonest in the first 4 years of life, episodes of apnoea may continue throughout childhood and persist into adult life. The causes of apnoea, however, are different in older children (Table 1.1), and although some causes are unlikely to result in significant harm other conditions may associated with significant morbidity and mortality. Chronic upper airway obstruction and subsequent sleep apnoea may result in complications such as sudden death, growth failure, poor school performance, pulmonary hypertension and cor pulmonale, and decreased respiratory function during the day.

Pathophysiology

Airway maintenance

Maintenance of a normal airway both when awake and asleep is dependent on several factors operating interdependently:

- Upper airway muscle tone to maintain normal airway caliber, dependent on normal pharyngeal and respiratory muscle activity, intact neuronal reflexes and functioning connections between the muscles, respiratory centre and the reticular activating system.
- Airway protection reflexes which depend on functioning brainstem reflexes, a normal respiratory drive, intact sensory pathways for upper airway sensation and chemoreceptors (for O_2 and CO_2), normal upper airway muscle activity and a mature sleep arousal mechanism; such arousal is less well developed in children and may just increase their respiratory drive rather than change their sleep state (see below).
- Sleep state: rapid eye movement (REM) sleep is more likely to be associated with a significant decrease in airway tone, diminished respiratory drive and a flattened response to hypoxia and hypercarbia.

Such factors will be further influenced by abnormal anatomical features, e.g. Pierre Robin syndrome, cleft palate, large tonsils and adenoids or a small hypopharynx, and age of the child. In infants, brainstem maturity may not have developed to allow an optimal physiological response to external influences. Hypoxia and hypercarbia may dampen brainstem function or airway protective reflexes may operate in an exaggerated manner to occlude the airway or produce prolonged apnoea.

Sleep state

Different sleep states are normally recognized on the basis of characteristic EEG tracing physical activity and frequency of each state throughout a 24-hour period. Patterns of sleep are determined by age. In neonates and young infants three phases are identified: active sleep is similar to REM sleep in older children and adults and has high-frequency waves apparent on the EEG; quiet sleep is identified by low-frequency waves; and an indeterminate stage is also seen. The proportions of each stage change as the infant matures; while in a neonate there are indistinct patterns of sleep during the night, by 3–6 months a more adult type pattern develops with a distinction between sleep during the day and night.

In older children, the adult pattern normally identified has five stages, including REM sleep, quiet sleep and three other stages.

The importance of identifying sleep state in apnoea lies in the described association between REM sleep and increased likelihood of apnoea.

Indications for investigation of sleep-disordered breathing

- Witnessed breathing difficulty.
- Witnessed apnoea.
- Mouth breathing when awake.
- Daytime tiredness.
- Poor school performance or developmental delay.
- Headaches.
- Enuresis.
- Snoring if there are associated respiratory pauses and other signs of upper airway obstruction.

Assessment

Physical examination, seeking evidence of partial or complete upper airway obstruction:

- Nasal obstruction.
- Adenoidal hypertrophy.
- Neuromuscular disease.
- Facial abnormality.
- Abnormalities of oropharynx.
- Significantly enlarged tonsils.
- Palatal abnormalities, e.g. clefts (which may be submucosal).
- Abnormal chest wall.

Investigations

As most sleep apnoea is caused by enlargement of the adenoids with or without tonsillar hypertrophy, if there is clinical evidence of these abnormalities overnight oximetry will provide a simple and informative screening test. If the cause is not thought to be adenotonsillar enlargement, other tests should be considered:

- Oximetry.
- Transcutaneous pO_2 and pCO_2 monitoring.
- End-tidal CO_2 measurement.
- EEG-based sleep staging.
- Assessment of chest and abdominal wall movement.
- Nasal air flow.
- Blood gases.
- Spirometry.
- Echocardiography.

Clinical problem

A normally well 3-month-old baby was brought to the emergency department by his mother having coughed and turned blue an hour after a feed. He had not stopped breathing and was pink again after 5 minutes, when the ambulance arrived.

A chest X-ray taken on arrival in hospital showed a right upper lobe pneumonia. Aspiration pneumonia was diagnosed and the baby was treated with antibiotics and discharged after 4 days. As he had been taking 180 mL/kg per day of bottle milk it was felt that the high volume of feed had provoked his episode; this was reduced to 150 ml/kg per day and an oral compound alginate preparation was also prescribed.

The baby was readmitted 7 days later having had an unprovoked cyanotic episode associated with at least 30 seconds of apnoea. The mother had commenced basic life support and the baby started breathing again within 10 seconds.

Questions

1. What is the differential diagnosis?

2. What investigations are indicated?

3. Would you offer the mother an apnoea monitor to use at home?

Answers

1. The differential diagnosis for these episodes includes:

- Oesophageal reflux and aspiration.
- Reflux and reflex apnoea.
- Seizures, despite the apparent absence of observed abnormal movement; seizures in babies are sometimes subtle and require electrophysiological investigations to confirm.
- Central apnoea.
- Sepsis is unlikely as the baby has not been clinically unwell either before the first episode or in between.
- Intracranial haemorrhage.

2. Investigations which should be performed include:

- Upper gastrointestinal contrast study.
- pH probe.
- Head ultrasound scan.
- 24-hour oximetry and cardiorespiratory monitoring.
- EEG.

Investigations to consider include:

- Metabolic screen.
- 24-hour EEG.
- Echocardiography.
- Blood gases.

3. There is currently no evidence that apnoea alarms decrease the risk of further apnoea occurring; the underlying abnormality needs determining and appropriate management strategy should be developed.

THE CRYING BABY

Tina Sajjanhar

Babies cry as a means of communicating with their carers. Babies may cry for a number of reasons including hunger, discomfort, pain, illness, heat, cold, a dirty nappy or even boredom and unhappiness. Parents may learn to recognize the type of cry their baby makes and react appropriately. Parents may become very anxious when simple measures have not calmed their baby down. Where there is prolonged crying or the character of the cry changes, parents may seek medical attention. The challenge for the clinician is to decide if the cry is pathological and if not, to reassure the parents. This can only be done after a careful history and examination, and investigations if warranted. Younger babies present more of a problem, as symptoms may be vague and non-specific. Young babies who cry a lot may also be at risk of child abuse due to increasing frustration on the part of the parents.

Differential diagnosis of the crying baby

Infection
- Sepsis.
- Meningitis.
- Urinary tract infection.
- Osteomyelitis.
- Septic arthritis.
- Otitis media.
- Upper respiratory tract infection (URTI).
- Paronychia.

Surgical
- Intussusception.
- Obstruction, e.g. malrotation, volvulus.
- Obstructed hernia.

Gastrointestinal
- Colic.
- Cow's milk intolerance.
- Gastro-oesophageal reflux disease (GORD) with oesophagitis.

- Constipation.
- Oral thrush.

General discomfort
- Hunger.
- Dirty nappy.
- Nappy rash.
- Rashes, e.g. eczema.
- Heat/cold.
- Attention seeking.

Miscellaneous
- Hair tourniquet.
- Fracture (consider child abuse).
- Teething.
- (Parental anxiety).
- Post immunization.

History

The history should include the following:

History	Significance of history
▪ Age	
▪ Length of symptoms	Short duration more likely to be infective
▪ Prodromal symptoms	Infective causes
▪ Type of cry	Irritable cry, worse on handling may indicate meningitis
▪ Pattern of crying	Hunger, discomfort
▪ Localizing pain	Fracture, osteomyelitis, septic arthritis
▪ Feeding pattern, e.g. reduced feeding	Infection
▪ Type of feed, e.g. cow's milk formula, breast fed	Cow's milk protein intolerance
▪ Vomiting, e.g. bilious/milk	GI obstruction, GORD, cow's milk protein intolerance
▪ Drawing up of legs	Colic
▪ Nature of stools, e.g. bloody, hard	Intussusception, constipation

History	Significance of history
▪ Condition between feeds, e.g. sleepy/lethargic	Infection
▪ Episodes of pallor	Intussusception
▪ Red cheeks	Teething
▪ Presence of fever	Infection
▪ Rashes	Infection, eczema
▪ Smelly urine	UTI
▪ Weight loss/failure to thrive	GORD

Additional features should include:

▪ Perinatal history, e.g. prematurity, admission to SCBU	GORD, NAI
▪ History of any previous illness or medical condition	
▪ Development	
▪ Immunization history	Meningitis, post-pertussis reaction
▪ Current medication	
▪ Allergies	
▪ Family history, e.g. first child	May increase parental anxiety
▪ Social history	NAI

Examination

The baby should be undressed and examined fully. For example, it is vital to observe the baby as this may provide a clue to any limitation of movement of any limbs which may otherwise not be evident. The following are important:

- Vital observations: pulse, temperature, respiratory rate.
- Look at the mouth for oral thrush/erupting teeth.
- Fontanelle: bulging in meningitis/depressed in dehydration secondary to poor feeding.
- Neck stiffness: often difficult to elicit in infants, and absence does not exclude meningitis.
- Presence of coryzal signs: babies with nasal congestion may find it difficult to feed.

- Presence of chest signs, e.g. recession.
- General routine cardiovascular examination.
- Abdominal exam for distension, tenderness, organomegaly, hernia: may indicate surgical cause.
- Examination of ears and throat.
- Joints for swelling, reduced movement.
- Limbs for any long bone pain which may indicate fracture.
- Skin for rashes, unusual bruising/marks.
- Hair tourniquet needs to be sought specifically.

Investigation

- This depends on details from history and examination of child.
- Diagnosis may already be obvious and investigation tailored accordingly.

The following may be useful:

Septic screen including full blood count, C-reactive protein, blood culture, urine (suprapubic aspirate/catheter), lumbar puncture	To exclude infective cause
X-ray: chest/limbs/abdomen	To exclude pneumonia, fractures; look at gas pattern in surgical cases
Abdominal ultrasound	Surgical causes
Bone scan	Osteomyelitis
Upper GI contrast study	GORD, malrotation
pH study	GORD
Skeletal survey	NAI

Non-organic causes of crying

A thorough history and examination and appropriate investigations may not reveal a pathological cause for crying, and parents may be advised accordingly.

Hunger

- Babies develop a pattern of feeding, but require increasing volumes of feed as they progress.

- Babies vary in the frequency with which they demand feed – a breast-fed baby will often feed every 2–3 hours, while a bottle-fed baby may require feeding every 3–4 hours. Some babies will wake at night for feeds.
- Parents learn to recognize cries for hunger with time, but any change in pattern of the cry may be concerning.
- Crying will often settle after the baby has fed an adequate amount and will remain alert, happy and well between feeds.

Teething

- Teething often starts around 6 months of age with eruption of the lower incisors, but may be variable.
- First molars erupt at 8 months of age, and by 12 months of age all eight primary incisors are usually present.
- Teething may lead to increased salivation, discomfort and crying.
- Examination may reveal alveolar mucosal erythema.
- Symptoms are maximal a few days before the teeth show.
- The baby may refuse food.
- Often symptoms such as high fever, diarrhoea, fits and vomiting are incorrectly attributed to teething.
- Presence of a facial or perineal rash and a slight fever and loose stools are often present but this may be coincidental.
- Analgesics may be helpful, such as topical gels and oral paracetamol.
- Diagnosis may be made in a child of appropriate age who is otherwise well, and other diagnoses have been excluded.

Colic

- Colic is an ill-defined problem of infancy.
- It is common: up to 1 in 10 infants.
- It peaks at 2–3 months of age but may be present from birth.
- It occurs in both breast-fed and bottle-fed babies.
- The baby may cry inconsolably for many hours, pull up its legs and appear to have abdominal pain.
- Attacks may occur at any time but seem to be commoner in the evening.
- There is no clear pathophysiology.

- It resolves spontaneously by 6 months of age.
- Inconsolable crying may need to be differentiated from other causes, particularly cow's milk protein intolerance or reflux oesophagitis.
- There is no proven benefit from the use of anticolic agents.
- The diagnosis may be made in a baby with no other symptoms such as vomiting, normal bowel habit and where the infant is thriving.

Nappy rash

- This may be due to ammoniacal dermatitis or thrush.
- It can be very irritating for the child.
- It is easily identified on examination.
- Advice and appropriate treatment may be required.

General discomfort

- This may be due to overheating.
- There may be a simple cause such as a dirty nappy.
- Babies may cry because they are bored or demanding attention.
- Crying babies can be a source of great anxiety to the parent, which in turn leads to stress in the child and a vicious circle may be set up.
- A good social history may be useful.
- Support can be offered through the health visitor.

Organic causes of crying

Oral candida infection

- This is common in babies.
- The buccal mucosa has a white appearance.
- It is often mistaken for milk.
- Plaques will not come off easily, even using a tongue depressor.
- It causes discomfort.
- The child may not be able to feed properly.
- Always look for and treat perineal thrush concurrently.
- Diagnosis is made on examination.

Constipation

- There is difficulty or delay in the passage of stools.

- Parents will often attribute crying to constipation, especially if associated with evidence of straining.
- Bowel habits of babies are variable, from opening bowels with every feed to once every few days.
- Bottle-fed babies may have a more regular bowel habit than breast-fed babies.
- In significant constipation, crying may follow development of an anal fissure, which may be apparent on examination.
- Stools may be pellet-like, but may be normal.
- Consider an organic cause if the baby is constipated from birth, if there is severe constipation within the first year of life or if there is failure to thrive.
- Organic causes include:
  - Hirschsprung's disease.
  - Hypothyroidism.
  - Anal stricture.
  - Partial intestinal obstruction.
- Diagnosis is suggested by history; examination may be unremarkable; trial of treatment may be necessary.

Cow's milk protein intolerance

- Damage to small intestinal mucosa by cow's milk leads to villous atrophy.
- Soluble proteins of cow's milk are most important (lactalbumin/lactoglobulins).
- Immunologically mediated reaction (IgA).
- Symptoms include:
  - Colic and crying.
  - Constipation.
  - Diarrhoea.
  - Atopic disease (eczema/asthma).
  - Acute colitis.
  - Occult GI blood loss.
- Remission on withdrawal of milk proves diagnosis.
- Whole protein is absorbed by mother and excreted into breast milk.
- Mother has to be on full cow's milk-free diet if breast-feeding baby.
- Predigested formula, e.g. Pregestemil, may be used.
- There is 10% cross-sensitivity with soya milk.
- Goat's milk may be used but there is still the potential for cross-reactivity.
- Diagnosis is suggested by the presence of crying with or without the above associated symptoms, but is proven on changing the type of feed.

Gastro-oesophageal reflux disease (GORD) with oesophagitis

- Oesophagitis occurs in up to 83% of infants with clinically significant reflux.
- Diagnosis is suspected when crying is associated with irritability and disinterest in feeding.
- There may be associated symptoms of reflux such as severe vomiting, failure to thrive, or respiratory symptoms such as cough, wheeze, apnoea, hoarseness, stridor and aspiration pneumonia, although the absence of these symptoms does not exclude the diagnosis.
- A pH study may be helpful in making the diagnosis.

Infection

- Diagnosis may be apparent if the child is ill.
- In early stages the child may present only with crying.
- Look for other symptoms and signs, for example:
  - Irritability.
  - Poor feeding.
  - Vomiting.
  - Fever – note that absence of fever in young babies does not exclude sepsis.
- Specific infections may be sought or full septic screen performed in very young babies, i.e. under 3 months of age.
- Look for localized infection such as paronychia.

Hair tourniquet

- A strand of hair becomes wrapped around the base of a digit.
- It is not associated with NAI.
- Crying is due to pain.
- It may be deeply embedded and require surgical removal under general anaesthetic.
- It may not be apparent unless a thorough examination is carried out.

Surgical causes

- Crying may be due to abdominal pain related to a surgical condition.
- Look for other specific features including:
  - Bilious vomiting.
  - Abdominal distension.
  - Bloody diarrhoea.
- Look also for non-specific features of irritability, poor feeding.
- Causes include malrotation or volvulus.
- A thorough examination will reveal the presence of an obstructed hernia as a cause for obstruction.

Intussusception

- This condition is where the distal ileum (the intussusceptum) telescopes into the adjoining distal bowel (the intussuscipiens), resulting in intestinal obstruction.
- The peak incidence is at 4–7 months of age.
- It affects 70% of infants between 3 and 12 months of age.
- There is a male preponderance.
- 90% are idiopathic.
- One possible explanation is that an enlarged Peyer's patch in the distal ileum becomes oedematous, possibly due to viral infection, and becomes the apex of the intussusception.
- A viral prodrome may therefore precede intussusception.
- Once intussusception is present, crying occurs as a result of pain (85%), typically colicky, lasting 2–3 minutes, causing the infant to appear pale and draw up the knees.
- Spasms occur at 15- to 20-minute intervals, but after 12 hours may be more continuous.
- Diagnosis may be suspected owing to the presence of other symptoms.
  - Vomiting occurs early then is more persistent once obstruction is established.
  - Passage of a few loose stools occurs early but these are typically of small volume and short duration and due to evacuation of distal bowel.
  - 50% of patients may pass redcurrant jelly stools (blood and mucus) due to congestion of the intussusceptum, but this may occur late.
  - The child is lethargic and unwell even between episodes.
  - An abdominal mass may be present, typically in the right upper quadrant, but it may not be palpable in the presence of abdominal distension.
- The diagnosis should be suspected in a child where persistent severe colic lasts for more than 1–2 hours, especially if other symptoms such as vomiting are present and diarrhoea is absent.

- Diagnosis may be made by abdominal X-ray, which may be normal, show non-specific abnormality or bowel obstruction, or on ultrasound examination.
- Treatment includes treating the presence of any shock, stabilizing the child, giving antibiotics and performing an air enema. If this is unsuccessful the child may need to progress to operative reduction.

Orthopaedic causes

- Orthopaedic infections may present with only crying and may only be identified on careful examination.
- Look for:
  - Swollen joint.
  - Painful joint.
  - Decreased movement of joint or limb.
  - Fever.
  - Local inflammatory signs.
- Osteomyelitis affects the metaphyses of the long bones and is usually due to haematogenous spread.

- The commonest organisms are *Staphylococcus pyogenes*, *Streptococcus pyogenes* and *Haemophilus influenzae*.
- A high index of suspicion needs to be maintained as external signs may not be present in the early stages of infection except for pain and limitation in movement of a limb.
- A plain X-ray excludes a fracture as the cause of pain although is unhelpful in the diagnosis of osteomyelitis in the early stages.
- A bone scan detects early changes and aids diagnosis.
- Septic arthritis is usually due to *Staphylococcus aureus*.
- The joint is swollen and painful to move.
- Fever may not be present in septic arthritis but is often present with osteomyelitis.
- In a crying infant the presence of a painful joint with or without fever should raise the suspicion of septic arthritis or osteomyelitis.
- If an X-ray reveals the presence of a fracture, a careful history for trauma should be taken and the possibility of NAI should be considered.

Clinical problem

A 2-month-old baby is brought to the A&E department at 0200 hours by his mother, with the complaint of crying incessantly. He has had crying episodes since he has been home, but they appear to have grown worse over the last week or so. He has now been crying for 2 hours continuously and his mother is extremely anxious. The crying has always been worse at night and during the evening. His mother has tried giving him colic drops, with no success.

He has not had any vomiting although he has always posseted a small amount after feeds. He is currently taking 3–4 ounces 3- to 4-hourly, and feeds well. He had his last feed 3 hours ago. He has a normal bowel motion and is passing urine.

He is the first child of a 19-year-old single mother. He was born at 34 weeks' gestation, by normal delivery. He was on the 50th centile for weight at birth, but was admitted to the special care baby unit for 1 week due to mild respiratory distress. He required oxygen only for 2 days, and was discharged once feeds were established by 10 days of age. He is currently on the 25th centile for weight. The parent-held record that his mother has shows she has made several visits to the health clinic with similar complaints about his crying, and has been given advice on how to manage him.

On examination the following are noted:

- He appears pink and well perfused.
- He is afebrile, alert and crying intermittently.
- The anterior fontanelle is soft when the baby is not crying.
- He is well cared for and is well hydrated.
- It is difficult to assess the chest.
- The abdomen is slightly distended and soft.
- There is no rash, or marks on the skin.

Questions

1. What is the most likely diagnosis?
   a) Gastro-oesophageal reflux.
   b) Urinary tract infection.
   c) Intussusception.
   d) Infantile colic.
   e) Parental anxiety.

2. What is the next step in the management of this child?
   a) A full septic screen should be performed.
   b) The child should be admitted for observation.
   c) The child should be sent home with an appointment for the baby clinic.
   d) The child should be investigated to exclude an intussusception.
   e) The child should be sent home and referred to the health visitor the next day.

Answers

1. e)

2. b)

This child does not have convincing evidence of organic disease in the history and examination. However, there are many risk factors for social isolation and poor coping mechanisms, including:

- Young mother with no partner.
- Preterm delivery with separation from the mother, which may lead to bonding problems.
- Demanding baby, especially at night, leading to maternal exhaustion.

The cycle needs to be broken, and in these circumstances it may be appropriate to admit the child to hospital and confirm there is no pathology. This would give the opportunity to observe the mother–child interaction, and involve other health professionals such as health visitor and GP to provide more support.

CHAPTER 3

THE ILL-LOOKING NEWBORN
David Field

Introduction

This book contains chapters on both the 'ill-looking baby' and the 'ill-looking child'. The purpose of having these two quite separate accounts is to emphasize the differences both in terms of pathogenesis and also presentation of these two situations. Clearly problems of pregnancy, labour and delivery can all impact on the baby and as a result can affect the baby's well-being in the period immediately after birth, and sometimes for somewhat longer. Many congenital abnormalities will also typically present in the early postnatal period. This chapter focuses therefore on the baby who looks ill either immediately after birth or in the days that immediately follow.

The range of problems to which an individual baby can be exposed is briefly outlined below:

- *Infection.* A range of infections can be acquired during pregnancy and have serious consequences for the baby. Some, such as rubella and toxoplasmosis, can cause severe problems in the baby but, in general, do not result in severe acute problems after birth. Other congenitally acquired infections, e.g. varicella infection very late in pregnancy, can make the child very ill at delivery. However, probably the most important microbial cause of severe disease in the newborn is peripartum-acquired bacterial disease, of which group B streptococcus is the most well known. There is much controversy regarding the exact mechanism and timing involved in the acquisition of such infections during labour and or delivery.
- *Hypoxic ischaemic disease.* During the highly complex biological process of labour and delivery a huge number of physiological changes occur in the baby and mother. As a result there is great potential for some aspect of the process to 'go wrong'. Many of these variations have no significant effect on the baby as there is clearly a range of adaptive processes built into the physiology of the fetus and newborn to allow them to cope with such stresses,

should they arise. It is when labour and delivery become sufficiently abnormal, for whatever reason, to exceed the adaptive capability of feto-maternal physiology that there is a risk to fetal well-being. Although a whole variety of mechanisms can be involved in development of a critical impairment of the feto-maternal exchange (e.g. placental infarction, abruption, cord prolapse) it is the resultant fetal hypoxia that has the most rapid and major effect on the fetus. The brain is the most vulnerable organ, but where the hypoxic insult is sustained renal, liver and cardiac damage may all occur. It is important to understand that sudden and catastrophic blood loss from the fetus (e.g. from a snapped cord secondary to a velamentous insertion) will result in an almost identical insult but with the additional problem of a very low circulating blood volume.

■ *Prematurity.* It is important to remember that prematurity will place the baby at risk of a range of problems, particularly, in those of 32 weeks' gestation or less, respiratory distress.

■ *Congenital abnormalities.* A large number of congenital abnormalities will present either just after birth or in the first few days of life. Although increasing numbers of women in the Western world undergo fetal anomaly scanning, virtually all subtle defects and a proportion of major anomalies will go undetected (e.g. it is not unusual for right-sided diaphragmatic hernias to be missed by such scans). Clearly, congenital abnormalities can potentially cause a variety of serious problems and a significant proportion of these will either manifest at birth or in the first few days of life. 'Congenital abnormality' must always be considered in the differential diagnosis when assessing the sick newborn. In this context 'congenital abnormality' should also include inborn errors of metabolism.

■ *Trauma.* Although birth trauma can result in severe acute illness in the newborn, this is very rare in the developed world. (A small number of babies will suffer non-accidental injury in the period after discharge home. This latter group may present with a variety of serious symptoms and hence it is important that the diagnosis is considered where appropriate).

■ *Maternal disease.* A range of problems in the mother can have consequences for the baby (e.g. maternal diabetes leading to hypoglycaemia, maternal SLE causing heart block in the baby). Worldwide, the commonest problem of this type is HIV

infection, although it is unusual for this to manifest in the newborn period.

■ *Other pregnancy complications.* Other pregnancy-related problems that can result in severe problems for the baby include:

– *Hypertension* (all causes). This is common and can have a variety of effects on the baby. Most important is the association of reduced placental function, hence increasing the risk of hypoxic ischaemic problems described above. Where hypertension has been sustained for much of the pregnancy, deterioration of placental function may have occurred over a more sustained period, leading to growth retardation (see Ch. 6).

– *Blood group incompatibilities.* Although these typically result in problems of jaundice and are not life threatening, if severe haemolysis occurs the baby may go into heart failure (hydrops fetalis).

– *Premature rupture of the membranes.* Early membrane rupture (>24 hours before delivery) increases the risk of infection in the baby, but where it occurs very early in the pregnancy (between 18 and 24 weeks' gestation) uterine compression can cause secondary pulmonary hypoplasia.

Presentations

The term 'ill-looking baby' is non-specific. The following table lists a range of presentations that could be described in this way and indicates the main differential diagnosis for each symptom.

Presenting symptom	Differential diagnosis
Respiratory distress	Surfactant deficient respiratory distress syndrome (RDS) Pulmonary maladaptation (transient tachypnoea of the newborn) Pneumonia Congenital anomaly (e.g. tracheo-oesophageal fistula, congenital diaphragmatic hernia, cystic adenomatous malformation of the lung)

Presenting symptom	Differential diagnosis
Respiratory distress (cont'd)	Metabolic acidosis (all causes including some inborn errors of metabolism)
	Cardiac failure (commonest early-onset causes: transposition of the great vessels and hypoplastic left heart syndrome)
	Abnormal central respiratory control (rare)
Cyanosis	Cyanotic congenital heart disease
	Significant lung disease, e.g. RDS, pneumonia
	Inadequate respiration, e.g. following sedation, and or an encephalopathy
Pallor	Severe acute or chronic blood loss or haemolysis
	Sepsis: impaired circulation
	Poor cardiac function (all causes)
	Structural abnormalities affecting the left side of the heart
Abnormal tone, posture and/or responsiveness	Hypoxic ischaemic encephalopathy
	Metabolic impairment of CNS function, e.g. hypoglycaemia
	CNS infection
	CNS trauma
	Congenital abnormalities of the CNS
	Drug withdrawal syndrome
Fits	Hypoxic ischaemic encephalopathy
	Metabolic impairment of CNS function, e.g. hypoglycaemia
	CNS infection
	CNS trauma
	Congenital abnormalities of the CNS
	Drug withdrawal syndrome
Apnoea	Prematurity
	CNS dysfunction (all causes, including metabolic derangement)

Presenting symptom	Differential diagnosis
Apnoea (cont'd)	Sepsis
	Pertussis, RSV infection
	Congenital abnormalities of the respiratory system and upper GI tract, e.g. tracheo-oesophageal fistula

History

Given the comments above, it should be clear that when a baby presents unwell either at birth or soon after it is important to discover as much as possible about past obstetric history, pregnancy and delivery. Much of this information should be available in the mother's notes and it is important to discover what is already known before trying to get further information by speaking to the parents. However, from one or both sources, it is important to be clear about the following:

1. The outcome of any previous pregnancies. Previous pregnancy losses should be discussed to see if there is any indication that the outcome occurred as the result of a congenital abnormality. This discussion is probably best combined by asking about the subsequent health of any live-born children and whether there is any history of familial disease in the extended family.
2. Maternal health. Points covered should include general issues such as whether the mother smoked or drank alcohol during the pregnancy, as well as more specific questions about any diseases from which the mother suffers. Drug abuse can clearly have major implications for the baby, although mothers will not always volunteer this information even when the baby is clearly unwell.
3. The course of this child's pregnancy. There is a huge number of things that may occur during pregnancy and which may be of relevance to the baby. Focus on all areas perceived by the mother or her carers as being in any way abnormal, but in addition the following are particularly important:
   a) Scans (both for dating and fetal anomaly). Ask whether these occurred and what the results were.
   b) Investigate whether any abnormalities were noted on the serological screening tests.

c) Any concerns about maternal weight gain and fetal growth.

d) Any maternal hypertension noted throughout pregnancy and any accompanying symptoms such as proteinuria.

e) Whether the onset of labour was spontaneous or induced and, if induced, what was the indication. Ask specifically when membrane rupture occurred.

f) The best estimate of the baby's gestation.

g) The course of the labour in terms of duration and any complications noted (it is sensible to ask how the labour was monitored as, if a 'low-tech' approach were adopted, potential abnormalities may have been missed).

h) How the delivery occurred and any problems that were encountered.

i) Any abnormalities noted on inspection of the placenta.

4. Where the 'ill-looking baby' does not present immediately after birth, ask specifically about any problems or abnormalities noted at birth and any action taken.

In those babies who present later and not at delivery, explore carefully the baby's behaviour up to the point that it was realized the baby was ill:

- Has the baby passed meconium and, if so, when? Has the baby passed urine?
- Was the baby *really* entirely well after delivery or was the problem present then (and not felt to be important) and simply allowed to progress?
- Were any abnormal signs noted prior to the baby being clearly unwell, e.g. breathlessness or temperature?
- Had the baby's behaviour previously been completely normal? Feeding records are often helpful in this regard.
- Did any acute event occur that appeared to result in the baby becoming unwell? If so, what were the circumstances, e.g. a choking episode during or immediately following a feed?
- Have any new symptoms emerged since the baby became unwell, e.g. bile-stained vomiting, apnoea?

Examination

Clearly the focus of any initial examination is to establish whether the baby requires resuscitation; however, describing this is outside the scope of this book and hence the remainder of the section will assume that the baby is unwell but stable.

Assess the vital signs:

- *Skin colour.* Look for evidence of anaemia or polycythaemia. Peripheral cyanosis, if present, is not of diagnostic significance but central cyanosis is indicative of serious cardiorespiratory compromise.
- *Perfusion.* Measure the capillary refill time. This will be increased if the circulation (e.g. as a result of blood loss or severe infection) or cardiac function (e.g. as a result of congenital heart disease or hypoxic insult) is impaired.
- *Respiration.* Tachypnoea may result from lung disease and or metabolic acidosis. The presence of respiratory distress implies that the child has a problem of lung function, but this can have a range of causes, e.g. surfactant deficiency, heart failure, pneumonia.
- *Pulse.* Tachycardia is a non-specific response to a variety of underlying conditions and hence is largely unhelpful. A very high heart rate (>200 per minute) is suggestive of a tachyarrhythmia but an ECG may well be necessary before a diagnosis can be made. Bradycardia is an ominous, but once again non-specific, sign generally indicating the need for resuscitation. Less acute causes of bradycardia include drug therapy (e.g. high-dose steroids) or heart block.
- *Blood pressure.* Regular blood pressure measurements are essential in the management of the acutely ill baby but are rarely diagnostic. Readings are normally taken by a non-invasive automated technique which, if not used very carefully, can easily generate erroneous readings. This problem is particularly relevant when 'four-limb blood pressure' measurements are performed. This technique can be helpful in detecting some types of coarctation of the aorta when blood pressure in the legs is consistently less than that in the arms.
- *Temperature.* Babies with a significant infection may well develop a fever but they are less consistent in this regard than older children and adults. Infection may result in hypothermia but this is once again a rather non-specific response in ill children who, in addition, often lose heat rapidly as they undergo various investigations such as venepuncture and lumbar puncture. Always note the site where temperature is being monitored, since peripheral (skin) temperature will be reduced by a variety of factors that impair the circulation. In fact

it is common to assess the adequacy of the circulation by monitoring the difference between a baby's core (rectal, tympanic) temperature and that of the skin of the peripheries (the difference should be no more than 1–1.5°C).

Perform a general inspection, looking specifically for:

- Any evidence of dysmorphism (the child's appearance may be diagnostic, or simply flag the increased likelihood of an underlying congenital abnormality).
- Rashes may be seen in a number of infections and can be characteristic. Petechial rashes are more non-specific, resulting, very often, from deranged clotting.
- Look specifically at *the entire baby* for any abnormal signs such as a distended abdomen, excessive bruising or swelling over the skull.

Complete a general examination, paying particularly attention to:

- Auscultation of the heart.
- Any abnormal respiratory noises.
- The mouth and upper airway to exclude minor congenital abnormalities. Similarly inspect the anus and the genitalia carefully.

Investigations

The title of this chapter is too non-specific to permit a didactic approach to investigation. However, the following are often helpful in managing such children and reaching a provisional diagnosis.

Investigation	Role
Blood gas	Helpful acutely in assessing the adequacy of the child's respiration Provides an objective measure of the severity of any earlier hypoxic ischaemic insult May be suggestive of underlying metabolic disease
Septic screen	A rather loose term covering a range of bacteriological investigations such as blood culture and lumbar puncture – essential in investigating the potentially septic child. Sometimes the term is used to include also full blood count (see below) and measurement of one or more acute-phase reactants, e.g. CRP (see below)
Full blood count	Provides invaluable information about the child's potential problems, including acute blood loss, sepsis (note that in the case of infection in the newborn the white blood count may be high or very low) and clotting problems
Acute phase reactants, e.g. CRP	Used widely as early indicators of infection, but results can be misleading and should be interpreted with caution
Electrolytes	Essential in managing the child and very helpful in pointing to a number of aetiological diagnoses such as underlying renal disease
Chest X-ray	Mandatory where cardiorespiratory signs are present
Abdominal X-ray	Mandatory where abdominal signs such as distension are present
Ultrasound of the heart	Essential where congenital heart disease is suspected
Ultrasound of the head	Particularly helpful in the sick preterm baby, but will not detect peripheral lesions in the term baby, where MRI is the investigation of choice

Clinical problem

A child is brought to the neonatal unit at 48 hours of age, having been noted to have marked tachypnoea. The child, a first baby, was born by normal delivery at 39 weeks and 5 days after an entirely normal pregnancy and delivery. There is no relevant family history.

On examination the child has a respiratory rate of 110 per minute but there is no evidence of difficulty in breathing, such as grunting or recession, and the baby otherwise looks well with no other positive findings.

A blood gas investigation reveals the following: pH 7.02, $PaCO_2$ 2.6 kPa, PaO_2 11.3 kPa, base excess −15.2.

Chest X-ray was normal.

Question

How would you proceed?

Answer

The child has a metabolic acidosis and the tachypnoea is present as a compensatory mechanism (by lowering $PaCO_2$). There is nothing to suggest primary lung disease. The acidosis could have arisen from a variety of mechanisms, including cardiac disease, renal failure, infection and a primary metabolic disorder. The child's well-being makes infection (severe enough to cause this degree of acidosis) unlikely but clearly the possibility of infection must be positively excluded by a septic screen and, in the interim, the child treated with antibiotics. Assessment of renal function, four-limb blood pressure, cardiac ECHO and a full metabolic screen are all reasonable next steps. Poisoning, a potential cause of this picture, seems less important to exclude at this stage. However, inadvertent poisoning (i.e. miscalculating a drug dose) is a common mistake in neonates on any form of medication.

Subsequent metabolic investigations over many weeks failed to identify a precise diagnosis. A lactic acidosis persisted and the child died before 1 year of age.

CHAPTER 4

NEONATAL CONVULSIONS
David Field

Introduction

Convulsions are defined as the manifestations of paroxysmal discharges of abnormal electrical activity in some part of the brain. The terms *fit*, *convulsion* and *seizure* are used interchangeably. Although, of course, they can occur at any age, they are most common in the newborn and especially the preterm infant. This increased risk in the newborn appears to be the result of the brain being in a state of relative excitability compared to older children and adults. As a result, a range of insults can produce convulsions, the convulsion itself being a somewhat non-specific response. Estimating the incidence of convulsions in the newborn is fraught with difficulty since some are difficult to recognize, especially in preterm infants. Identification using combined video and EEG recording represents the gold standard in this regard. There is an active debate about the extent to which uncontrolled convulsions might result in damage to the brain and/or further convulsions.

In general, four different types of convulsion can be recognized:

- *Subtle*. These are the most difficult to identify with certainty as they may involve persistence of otherwise normal activity, e.g. prolonged sucking. Other types of abnormal movement that can occur include 'bicycling', chewing and abnormal eye movements. However, these convulsions can manifest themselves simply as apnoea and or bradycardia alone.
- *Tonic*. Extensor posturing of the limbs and trunk are characteristic of this type of convulsion.
- *Clonic*. Typical clonic jerks are noted but they may be localized or involve several limbs and the face.
- *Myoclonic*. Single myoclonic jerks are 'normal' in the newborn but if they are multifocal and persistent myoclonic jerks are usually the result of electroconvulsive activity.

Aetiology

Causes of convulsions in the newborn include:

- Brain injury (including haemorrhage, infarction and hypoxic ischaemia).
- Infection (meningitis and congenital infections).
- Drug withdrawal.
- Metabolic derangement, e.g. hypoglycaemia, hypocalcaemia and hypomagnesaemia.
- Congenital abnormalities, e.g. abnormal neuronal migration.
- Inborn errors of metabolism, e.g. urea cycle defects.
- Kernicterus.
- Hypertension.
- Fifth-day fits.
- Pyridoxine-dependent convulsions.

Differential diagnosis

Two conditions regularly cause diagnostic confusion:

- Irritability.
- Jitteriness.

Irritability is a rather non-specific term for an infant who, if disturbed even mildly, cries excessively and is difficult to settle. The cause can be obvious, e.g. marked bruising to the head as a result of a difficult delivery, but on other occasions no cause is apparent. The cry may be high pitched but this is a variable feature. Apart from acting as a non-specific symptom which needs assessment in its own right, it has no long-term significance. However, irritability can be caused by a number of conditions which, as they evolve, may produce convulsions. Such conditions include hypoxic ischaemic encephalopathy, meningitis, drug withdrawal and inborn errors of metabolism.

Jitteriness is common in normal newborns. No cause is apparent in most babies and it has no lasting consequence. It presents as a sustained fine tremor following a stimulus such as a sudden noise. The tremor is faster than that noted during a clonic convulsion and stops if an affected limb is held. It does not affect the face and the physiological changes, seen typically during convulsions (e.g. a rise in blood pressure), do not occur.

History

The first goal of the history in a baby presenting with a possible convulsion is to assess the likelihood that a convulsion, as opposed to some other episode, has indeed occurred. A clear description of the attack by an experienced observer can be sufficient, particularly in the case of clonic convulsions. Here the relatively slow (one to four times per second) rhythmic jerking, which cannot not be stopped by holding the affected part of the body, can usually be recognized as being different to jitteriness. Similarly, tonic convulsions can usually be recognized when they arise in a child about whom there is pre-existing concern perhaps because of a prior diagnosis of hypoxic ischaemia or infection. However, in relation to both tonic and subtle convulsions where the child has previously been well, descriptions of the child's behaviour and/or the movements seen are rarely sufficient to be clear that a convulsion has occurred. In this situation other changes noted at the time of the attack such as eye deviation or changes in blood pressure, in a child being continuously monitored, can be very helpful. Multifocal myoclonic jerks are difficult to separate from jittering on the basis of description alone.

The age of the child at the onset of convulsions is important in relation to the underlying aetiology. Convulsions resulting from a hypoxic ischaemic event in utero virtually always start in the first 48 hours of life. Similarly, convulsions resulting from focal infarction of the brain typically occur in the first few days after birth. While this is also true of most infants who suffer fits as a consequence of maternal drug addiction, onset can be delayed until the second or third week of life.

In taking the history of any possible convulsion as well as assessing the 'attack', it is also important to make a judgement about the child's risk of having suffered a convulsion. This is helpful both in putting the 'attack' into context and, if on balance it seems likely that the child has suffered a fit, looking for a cause.

In relation to all problems of the newborn, details of the pregnancy and delivery are vital in trying to identify a particular diagnosis. This is especially true in relation to convulsions in the newborn period.

Clues from the antenatal period:

- Gestation of the baby at delivery? (Both the risk of convulsions occurring and the range of likely aetiologies vary with gestational age.)

- History of familial fits?
- History of thrombophilia in the family?
- History of maternal drug abuse?
- Any abnormal growth detected to suggest the baby could be syndromic or suffering congenital infection?
- Any abnormal antenatal scans noted, suggesting the presence of a cerebral anomaly?
- Is the baby at high risk of perinatal infection, e.g. known maternal carriage of group B *Streptococcus*.

Clues from the labour and delivery:

- Evidence of intrapartum hypoxic ischaemic insult:
  - Abnormal cardiotocogram (CTG).
  - Antepartum haemorrhage.
  - Passage of thick meconium.
  - Delay in second stage.
  - Abnormal fetal blood sample.
- Evidence of intrapartum infection:
  - Fever in labour.
  - Spontaneous preterm onset of labour.
  - Offensive liquor.
  - Prolonged rupture of the membranes.

Clues available immediately following delivery:

- Abnormal cord pH (<7.0 is suggestive of significant intrapartum asphyxia).
- Depressed baby (Apgar ≤ 4) needing resuscitation (can have multiple causes but is compatible with intrapartum asphyxia and infection).
- Appearance of baby including birth weight (e.g. severe growth retardation – risk of hypoglycaemia – baby may have been noted to have features suggestive of an inherited disorder/syndrome).

In terms of the baby's later course further useful information can be gained:

- Had the baby been previously well prior to the convulsion?
- If the baby had not been well, what were the antecedents? (This question could reveal a range of scenarios from the preterm baby on the ventilator who has been on very high ventilator pressures for 12 hours and then starts fitting – compatible with a cerebral haemorrhage – to the term baby who had been feeding poorly for 12 hours and had been noted to have a temperature in the 6 hours prior to the fit – suggesting infection.)

Examination

Again two issues have to be addressed:

1. Is there evidence to suggest that the baby is fitting or is likely to have suffered a fit?
2. If yes, is there information available from the baby regarding the likely aetiology?

The examination must be general and take in all of the major systems:

- *General*
  a) What is the baby's general condition? (This is an important contextual issue in that the baby may appear entirely normal or require full ventilation because of central depression.)
  b) Is the baby normally alert and responsive? (The presence of a cerebral insult could result in irritability or general depression with lack of response.)
  c) Are there any obvious dysmorphic features or injuries, especially injuries to the head?
  d) Any signs of systemic upset, e.g. high or low temperature (both compatible with infection), raised respiratory rate?
  e) Is the baby's state of perfusion normal? It may be impaired as a consequence of septicaemia or major cerebral bleed.
- *Neurological.* A full neurological examination is required. Clearly, the extent of the examination will be governed by the baby's overall condition and gestation. However, it should be possible to determine whether there is evidence of abnormal neurology or not. This might manifest in a variety of ways, including abnormalities of posture, tone, primitive reflexes, tendon reflexes, eye movements, breathing pattern and, in the face of massive cerebral damage, loss of sphincter tone.
- It is also important to note any abnormal movements that occur during the examination. Where this happens to occur in a baby whose vital signs are electronically monitored, useful information can be gained by noting whether the abnormal movements are associated with changes in heart rate and blood pressure (typical of a convulsion).
- *Other systems.* The examination should be completed in order that a full picture of the baby's condition is obtained. Again particular attention should be paid to evidence of infection (e.g. sticky umbilical stump) and congenital abnormalities/syndromal diagnosis.

Investigations

Diagnosis	Features/investigations
1. Hypoxic ischaemic encephalopathy	Commonest cause of fits in mature babies. Diagnosis usually rests on the history, which typically reveals clear evidence of an intrapartum insult, although this may not be so in the face of a more chronic insult. Some biochemical upset may occur as a secondary feature, e.g. hypoglycaemia and hypocalcaemia. Ultrasound scans may be essentially normal or be non-specifically bright as a result of cerebral oedema. MRI scans of the head may be helpful in revealing cortical damage or enhanced brightness of the basal ganglia – commonly seen following hypoxic ischaemia
2. Intracranial haemorrhage	This is the commonest cause of fits in the preterm baby and is usually seen readily on cranial ultrasound
3. Localized cerebral infarction	This too may occur in preterm babies but again is readily seen on ultrasound. In term babies peripheral cortical lesions may occur in the territory of the middle cerebral artery in otherwise well babies. These are usually diagnosed on MRI scan being too peripheral to detect on ultrasound
4. Drug withdrawal	This condition is becoming increasingly common. Mothers will often volunteer information about their own drug use. Where this is not the case, diagnosis is made on urine toxicology preferably from mother and baby
5. Infection	Congenital infection of the CNS and acute meningitis can both present with convulsions. With congenital infection other features are almost always present. Meningitis may present with convulsions and no other features and then progress rapidly – untreated perhaps to death – in a few hours. Unless a clear contraindication is present all babies presenting with convulsions should undergo lumbar puncture
6. Metabolic upset, e.g. hypoglycaemia, hypocalcaemia, hypomagnesaemia	A variety of metabolic upsets can cause fits either alone or complicating another condition, e.g. sepsis. Estimations of blood glucose, calcium, magnesium and electrolytes should always be part of the assessment of a child presenting with fits
7. Inborn errors in metabolism	A variety of rare inborn errors of metabolism can cause convulsions in the newborn period and some may present in this way. Blood pH, glucose, pyruvate, lactate, ammonia and amino acids plus urine amino acids and organic acids should be sufficient to indicate if such a diagnosis is possible. More detailed assessment will require consultation with a specialist laboratory
8. 'Other causes'	A number of other rare conditions (e.g. pyridoxine-dependent fits) can present with convulsions in the newborn period. Diagnosis of these conditions is best made in consultation with a paediatric neurologist

The role of EEG

This is a somewhat contentious area, with recent work suggesting that only combined EEG and video monitoring can be relied on to identify convulsions. The results where EEG is used alone are certainly difficult to evaluate. Simplified (averaged EEGs/cerebral function monitors) are commonly used in intensive care units by non-specialists but opinions vary regarding their usefulness.

Reference

Boylan GB, Rennie JM, Pressler RM, et al. Phenobarbitone, neonatal seizures, and video–EEG. Arch Dis Child, Fetal Neonatal Ed 2002; 86:F165–F170

Clinical problem

Baby J presented at 24 hours of age with what appeared to be right-sided clonic fits affecting both her arm and leg.

She was a first baby born to healthy parents who were both in their twenties. The pregnancy, including dating and diagnostic scans, had been quite uneventful until 38 weeks when the mother's blood pressure became raised. A decision was made to induce the labour and this took place the following day. Mother was fully dilated after 11 hours. The CTG was felt to be non-reassuring at that point and the mother was exhausted. The obstetric registrar therefore decided to proceed to a forceps delivery, which was achieved with some minor difficulty. The baby's Apgar score was 7 at 1 minute and 9 at 5 minutes. Cord pH (two separate vessels) was 7.28 and 7.32. Birth weight was 3.8 kg.

She went to the postnatal ward and was generally felt to be satisfactory, although her feeding had been slow, until the onset of fitting. On admission to the neonatal unit she was having repeated right-sided clonic convulsions lasting 1–2 minutes. She was generally lethargic and not very responsive. Investigations were as follows:

- Urea and electrolytes: normal.
- Calcium, magnesium and glucose all within the normal range.
- CRP < 5.
- Full blood count: normal.
- Cranial ultrasound scan: normal.

Following a loading dose of phenobarbital she suffered a series of apnoeas and required ventilation. Because her fits continued she was started on phenytoin 6 hours later and no further fits occurred.

Questions

1. What other investigations are required?

2. What is the most likely diagnosis?

Answers

This is a well-grown baby who seems to have had an uneventful pregnancy and delivery. Investigations are all reassuring but two key tests appear not to have been done:

1. *Lumbar puncture.* The story is clearly compatible with meningitis and in the absence of contraindications a lumbar puncture must be performed.

2. *MRI scan.* In a term baby such as this, assessment using ultrasound alone is not adequate.

In fact the lumbar puncture was normal but the MRI revealed a small area of infarction in the left parietal area. The baby made a good recovery. A thrombophilia screen was normal. It remained unclear whether the forceps was significant in producing the damage to the parietal cortex.

CHAPTER 5

NEONATAL JAUNDICE
Elizabeth Sleight

Introduction

What is jaundice?

Jaundice is the yellow appearance in skin and conjunctivae caused by an increase in circulating bilirubin. It is important to define its cause and treat if necessary; sustained high levels of bilirubin may have serious consequences, in particular, kernicterus.

Bilirubin is produced exclusively from the breakdown of haemoglobin or haem within the reticuloendothelial system. Haem can be produced from the breakdown of cytochrome P450; otherwise it is produced from either senescent red blood cells (RBCs), extravasated RBCs or from RBCs being prematurely destroyed.

Hyperbilirubinaemia in the newborn period can therefore occur because of:

- Increased bilirubin production, e.g. in a haemolytic state, reabsorption of blood from an intraventricular haemorrhage or gastrointestinal (GI) bleeding.
- Impaired hepatic uptake, e.g. sepsis where decreased binding to albumin occurs or there are low levels of ligandin due to immaturity.
- Impaired hepatic excretion, e.g. low activity of glucuronyl transferase, e.g. Gilbert's disease, or physical blockage, e.g. biliary atresia or a choledochal cyst.
- Increased enteric reabsorption, e.g. upper GI obstruction/atresia.

Alternatively, hyperbilirubinaemia can be considered to be:

- Physiological in nature.

This is thought to be due to a low level of ligandin, low activity of glucuronyl transferase (see below) and increased level of bilirubin production because of increased fetal RBC breakdown (see Fig. 5.1).

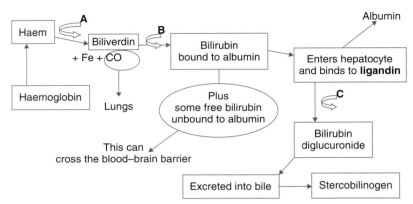

Fig 5.1 Bilirubin metabolism. **A** = haem oxygenase, **B** = biliverdin reductase, **Ligandin** concentrations are low at birth and can also be increased by the administration of phenobarbital, **C** = bilirubin uridine diphosphate glucuronyl transferase

What is kernicterus?

Kernicterus is a devastating complication of unconjugated hyperbilirubinaemia.

Once serum proteins have been saturated by bilirubin, the excess crosses the blood–brain barrier and can cause irretrievable brain damage, classically causing sensorineural deafness and damage to the basal ganglia, which leads to choreoathetoid cerebral palsy.

Some years ago there was a theory that babies without any high-risk factors would not develop kernicterus, and this led to a 'kinder' approach to assessment, with fewer babies undergoing estimation of their serum bilirubin. There were frightening case reports of kernicterus in apparently healthy term babies with no risk factors.

It is therefore important to remember that any baby can develop hyperbilirubinaemia to such an extent that they could develop kernicterus, but in general the following are thought to be risk factors.

Risk factors for developing kernicterus

- Gestational age younger than 37 weeks and birth weight less than 2500 g.
- Haemolysis due to maternal isoimmunization (mother Rhesus negative or group O), G6PD deficiency, hereditary spherocytosis or other cause.
- Jaundice at less than 24 hours of age.
- Signs of sepsis.
- The need for resuscitation at birth.

Factors from and investigations that would help distinguish causation

1. Haemolytic disease is more likely in the following circumstances:
   - Onset in the first 24–48 hours.
   - Pallor.
   - Hepatosplenomegaly.
   - Phototherapy merely controlling, rather than causing fall in serum bilirubin.
   - Mother's blood group Rhesus negative or blood group O.
   - There may also be a history of a sibling needing phototherapy or a blood transfusion in the newborn period. Haemolytic causes lead to an unconjugated hyperbilirubinaemia that might need treatment with exchange transfusion and may lead to continued anaemia due to continued RBC breakdown.

2. Timing:
   a) Onset first noted in the first 24 hours (Fig. 5.2):
   - Sepsis (review risk factors for congenital bacterial sepsis, such as maternal carriage of group B streptococcus, maternal fever in labour, prolonged rupture of membranes, fetal distress).
   - Haemolysis (immune or non-immune).
   - Crigler–Najjar syndrome: a rare disorder where low levels of bilirubin uridine diphosphate glucuronyl transferase lead to rapidly rising unconjugated hyperbilirubinaemia. The serum bilirubin may be over 700 µmol/L. Treatment is initially with exchange transfusion and then with lifelong phototherapy or liver transplantation.

b) Started second/third day of life (Fig. 5.3):
- More likely to be 'physiological' in nature.
- Breast milk jaundice is *not* the same as breast-feeding jaundice. The second is the more commonly seen condition where babies are establishing breast-feeding and physiological jaundice is compounded by poor calorie intake/relative dehydration.

c) Started in first week of life, but persisting over 14 days of age (Fig. 5.4):
- *Must exclude* obstructive causes – see conjugated hyperbilirubinaemia.
- Breast milk jaundice – only if unconjugated. This is thought to be a combination of an as yet undiscovered factor that increases entero-hepatic recirculation of bilirubin and an inhibitor of glucuronyl transferase. The timing is typically of a jaundice which becomes more noticeable towards the end of the first week and becomes more pronounced in the second week.
- Hypothyroidism – only if unconjugated. Consider in babies with Down's syndrome.
- Panhypopituitarism – may be conjugated or unconjugated.
- Urinary tract infection.

3. Ethnicity:
- Glucose 6-phosphate dehydrogenase deficiency is more common in people from tropical Africa, the Middle East, tropical and subtropical Asia, some areas of the Mediterranean and Papua New Guinea. It is X-linked, but homozygous women can be affected. It causes an unconjugated hyperbilirubinaemia that might need treatment with exchange transfusion. If this is found to be the cause, it is important to advise the family about which drugs to avoid and and to consider favism.

4. Positive family history:
- Rhesus incompatibility – sensitization increases with subsequent pregnancies.
- Hereditary spherocytosis – did the mother or father have splenectomy, cholecystectomy or was on regular folic acid supplementation? Most cases are caused by an RBC membrane defect caused by spectrin deficiency, which leads to the

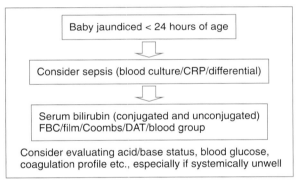

Fig 5.2   Jaundice with onset in first 24 hours.

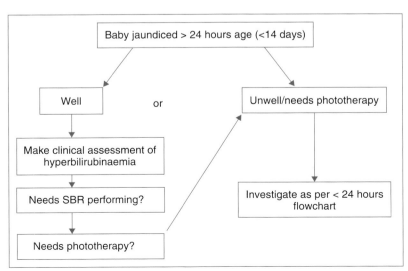

Fig 5.3   Jaundice with onset during second and third days of life.

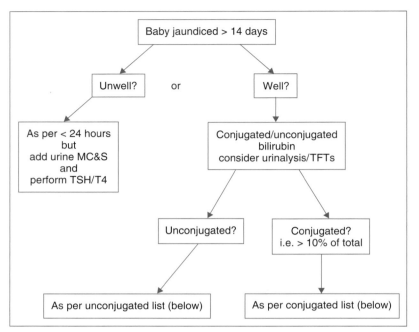

Fig 5.4   Jaundice persisting after 14 days.

formation of spherical RBCs. These are scavenged more rapidly from the circulation, leading to chronic haemolysis. The homozygous state is lethal. Incidence is 1 in 5000 northern Europeans. The condition causes an unconjugated hyperbilirubinaemia that might need treatment with exchange transfusion.

- Alpha-1-antitrypsin deficiency – early-onset emphysema (especially in non-smokers) or cirrhosis? This is caused by deficiency in antiprotease, which should normally be released from hepatocytes. Its lack leads to an excess of proteases, which causes alveolar/hepatic damage. It is uncommon in non-Caucasian races. There are 24 variants of the alpha-1-antiprotease molecule and the most common allele is PiM. People homozygous for this (PiMM) produce normal levels of antiprotease. People homozygous for PiZZ produce deficient levels and may develop illness and this is thought to affect up to 1 in 3000 white people. The condition causes a conjugated hyperbilirubinaemia.
- Gilbert's disease – family history of intermittent jaundice. The condition causes an unconjugated hyperbilirubinaemia. Inheritance may be auto-

somal dominant or recessive. The gene is located on chromosome 2. It occurs predominantly in men, but all races are affected and incidence in the USA is quoted as between 3% and 7%.

- Consanguinity – risk for Crigler–Najjar syndrome and other metabolic conditions.

5. Sepsis/galactosaemia:
- Vomiting.
- Lethargy/poor feeding.
- Apnoea.
- Temperature instability.
- Tachypnoea.
- Acidosis.
- Coagulopathy – a normal coagulation profile makes galactosaemia very unlikely.

The condition causes an unconjugated hyperbilirubinaemia. Galactosaemia is caused either by galactokinase deficiency, uridine diphosphate galactose 4-epimerase deficiency or galactose 1-phosphate uridyl transferase (GalPUT) deficiency. The gene is located at 9p13. It is thought to have an incidence of 1 in 40 000 people and can be screened for on newborn screening programmes. Otherwise it presents with vomiting, lethargy, hepatosplenomegaly and cataracts.

6. Cholestatic jaundice:
- Pale stools – point to something the family can see to identify 'putty' colour. A modern colour to describe this would be 'linen' or 'off-white'.
- Dark urine – 'does the urine look like tea *before* you add milk?'
- Persistence over 14 days of age.
  The condition causes a conjugated hyperbilirubinaemia (Fig. 5.5).

General serum liver function tests

Gamma-GT and alkaline phosphatase may be raised but the level does not help distinguish the cause of cholestasis. Raised transaminases may be more suggestive of an idiopathic hepatitis.

Extra-hepatic biliary atresia (EHBA)

- This may be a difficult diagnosis to make. The condition may be associated with situs inversus and polysplenia/asplenia. It rarely occurs in the preterm infant, and there is currently no single causative agent.
- The USS needs to be performed after a 3- to 4-hour fast; if a baby has just fed, the gallbladder might be normally contracted and thus not seen. Do not rely on the result of a USS in isolation.
- A hepatobiliary scintiscan, e.g. DISIDA nuclear scan, is helpful if normal; it confirms bile duct patency, but if abnormal does not confirm EHBA.
- A percutaneous liver biopsy may need to be repeated, as there may be an evolving histopathological pattern of cholestasis with ductular proliferation, inflammation and sometimes fibrosis.

CONJUGATED HYPERBILIRUBINAEMIA

General principles

Exclude UTI and hypothyroidism
Arrange abdominal USS after 3–4 hour 'fast'
Start on phenobarbital 5 mg/day
Arrange DISIDA scan 2–3 days later
If no gallbladder seen/delayed excretion on isotope scan, contact specialist paediatric liver unit

---

Fig 5.5   Causes of conjugated hyperbilirubinaemia.

- The diagnosis can sometimes only be made by an intraoperative cholangiogram or exploration of the porta hepatis.

Choledochal cyst

- Perform liver USS initially – an ERCP/cholangiogram may be needed.

Alpha-1-antitrypsin deficiency

- Measure serum alpha-1-antitrypsin level *and* phenotype.
- LFTs are likely to be affected.
- If a liver biopsy is performed there may be cholestasis, but PAS-positive granules, which are not digested by diastase, will also be seen.

Panhypopituitarism

- Low serum cortisol and TSH are very suggestive; growth hormone evaluation may need to be repeated, especially after the first year.

Cystic fibrosis

- Immunoreactive trypsin and stool elastase analysis are indirect indications.
- The gold standard remains the sweat test. On a sweat sample weighing more than 100 mg, a sweat sodium level of 60 mmol/L is diagnostic.
- Genotyping: there are over 900 known mutations of the cystic fibrosis transmembrane conductance regulator gene. Delta508 is the commonest mutation found in northern Europeans.

Idiopathic neonatal hepatitis

- Diagnosis of exclusion! Transaminases may be more elevated in this condition than in other causes of cholestasis.

Alagille's syndrome

Bile duct hypoplasia is associated with cardiac lesions (peripheral pulmonary stenosis is the classical association), elfin-like facies, skeletal abnormalities (classically butterfly vertebrae seen on chest X-ray) and posterior embryotoxin or other abnormalities will be seen on a full ophthalmic examination. The incidence is thought to be ~1 in 100 000 and is an autosomal dominant condition caused by a variable deletion of the JAG 1 gene on the short arm of chromosome 20.

Viral causes

Toxoplasma, rubella, cytomegalovirus and herpes simplex can all cause a neonatal hepatitis, as can enteroviruses, Ebstein–Barr and varicella. Rarely cytomegalovirus, rubella and hepatitis B infections can also cause bile duct hypoplasia leading to cholestasis.

Other metabolic disease

Most authorities would suggest analysing amino and organic acids to exclude conditions such as tyrosinaemia. Hypoglycaemia should prompt you to exclude glycogen storage disease, galactosaemia and fructosaemia. A raised ammonia level should lead to a urea cycle disorder being excluded. A high ferritin may be caused by idiopathic neonatal haemochromatosis, but if associated with hypotonia; other features of Zellweger's syndrome should be sought.

Unconjugated hyperbilirubinaemia

Alloimmune haemolysis

- The condition is caused by Rhesus (D, C and E), AB or Kell, Duffy, Kidd antibodies.
- Positive direct Coombs test and direct antigen test (DAT) – DAT may be negative in ABO incompatibility.
- Spherocytes may also be seen in ABO incompatibility.
- Anaemia/neutropenia/thrombocytopenia may also be features.
- Hypoglycaemia may occur due to islet cell hyperplasia leading to hyperinsulinaemia.

Galactosaemia

- Urine-reducing substances may be positive.
- A coagulopathy is often noted. Hyperbilirubinaemia is frequently unconjugated but may become conjugated.
- Confirmatory tests may need to be repeated if the baby has been transfused acutely; otherwise ask the reference laboratory to analyse GalPUT levels in RBCs.

Glucose 6-phosphate deficiency

A full blood count with reticulocyte count should be performed; the actual level of glucose 6-phosphate dehydrogenase activity should be measured, rather than the level of protein, as a high reticulocyte count will interfere with the assay.

Hereditary spherocytosis

- Combination of spherocytes seen on a blood film, along with a brisk reticulocytosis and unconjugated hyperbilirubinaemia.
- The most specific test is the incubated osmotic fragility test, where the RBCs are incubated for at least 24 hours at 37°C. The spherocytes will undergo lysis.

Crigler–Najjar syndrome

- Markedly high unconjugated hyperbilirubinaemia in the presence of normal liver function tests.
- Bilirubin uridine diphosphate glucuronyl transferase levels can be measured. Type II CNS is distinguished by higher levels of enzyme activity and, classically, a response to phenobarbital.

Summary and learning points (see Fig. 5.6)

Remember – jaundice is a symptom, not a diagnosis

Consider the *timing*

- First 24 hours

- Or between 24 hours and 14 days

- Or after 14 days

the type of hyperbilirubinaemia

- Conjugated or unconjugated

and

- Is the patient in a high-risk group?

Consider the consequences of misdiagnosis – could the patient

- develop kernicterus or

- have you missed the early signs of sepsis or another significant underlying diagnosis or

- have you missed the opportunity to make a timely diagnosis of extra-hepatic biliary atresia in the late presenting or conjugated group?

If the bilirubin rises at greater than 12 μmol/L per hour despite phototherapy, an exchange transfusion is highly likely to be needed

Fig 5.6   Summary and learning points.

Clinical problem

Edward was born by normal vaginal delivery at term and received no active resuscitation.

He is the third child of unrelated Caucasian parents and he was successfully breast-fed. His mother sought advice in the second week of life because of ongoing jaundice. She was reassured. At 5 weeks of age he presented to hospital with a 1-day history of bruising on his back, bleeding from his gums, pallor and poor feeding.

On examination, he appears pale, jaundiced and shocked.

Questions

1. What are your initial investigations?

2. What specific direct questions should you ask, and what information should be sought from other sources?

Your initial investigations reveal a haemoglobin of 5 g/dL, a prolonged APPT and a total bilirubin of 150 µmol/L with a conjugated fraction of 50. You give i.m. vitamin K and order cryoprecipitate and fresh frozen plasma. His initial blood sugar was normal.

Despite being given several boluses of crystalloid and FFP and administering broad-spectrum intravenous antibiotics, Edward becomes more unstable and is intubated and ventilated.

A chest X-ray confirms adequate endotracheal tube placement but a large mediastinal mass is seen. Blood gases are normal. A CT of his chest is performed.

A large intrathymic haemorrhage is seen, and coincidentally, no gallbladder is seen.

3. What is the encompassing diagnosis?

4. What further investigations need to be considered once Edward is stable to confirm this diagnosis?

Answers

1. a) Sepsis screen (*not* an LP); include blood culture/urine culture/CRP or equivalent FBC and film.
b) Coagulation screen.
c) Liver function tests including conjugated/unconjugated bilirubin.
d) Blood sugar.

2. a) Received vitamin K and by what route?
b) Did mother have group B streptococcus during her pregnancy?
c) Family history of haemophilia/bruising problems?
d) Are siblings on at-risk register? Is the family known to social services? Does the family have a social worker?

3. a) Extrahepatic biliary atresia leading to a vitamin K-dependent coagulopathy, causing the intrathymic bleed.

4. a) DISIDA scan.
b) Abdominal/biliary USS.
c) Liver biopsy.

CHAPTER 6

THE SMALL FOR GESTATIONAL AGE BABY

Elizabeth Sleight

Definitions

- Being born small for gestational age (SGA) is said to have occurred when a baby's birth weight lies below the 10th centile irrespective of completed gestation. Some textbooks use the 3rd centile as the defining centile.
- Intrauterine growth retardation (IUGR) is said to have occurred when the rate of fetal growth is less than normal for the genetic potential of a specific fetus.

This would therefore imply that a dynamic process is occurring in which a baby is being monitored in utero by serial ultrasound measurements and its growth parameters are seen to change over time.

In the past, the term was applied to babies who were born and were then found to have a weight which was not appropriate to – i.e. not in proportion to – the baby's length/head circumference centiles. Another way of thinking about this is to ask the question: 'Is this low-birth-weight baby asymmetrical or symmetrical?'

Another term that is used in this context is *intrauterine growth restriction*. There is evidence that babies who have symmetrical growth restriction may have suffered an insult earlier in pregnancy (e.g. chromosomal disorder, congenital infection) and the prognosis for catch-up growth in childhood is poorer than an asymmetrically affected baby who may have been 'starved' of nutrients in the third trimester only.

- A baby is said to have been born preterm if delivered at less than 37 completed weeks after the first day of the mother's last menstrual period.
- Low birth weight (LBW): the birth weight is less than 2.5 kg.
- Very low birth weight (VLBW): the birth weight is less than 1.5 kg.
- Extremely low birth weight (ELBW): the birth weight is less than 1.0 kg.

Thus a 980 g baby born at 25 weeks will be designated ELBW but not SGA, whereas a 2800 g baby born at term will be SGA (9th centile) but will not have suffered IUGR if the baby's length is also on the 9th centile.

General factors influencing birth weight (whether SGA or AGA)

The most obvious determinant is gestational age at delivery. The next most important variables are:

- Maternal race (increased rate of LBW in African/Caribbean/Indian mothers).
- Maternal height.
- Obesity.
- Pregnancy weight gain.
- Age (birth weight lower in both young and older mothers).
- Parity (first baby often lighter).
- Fetal sex (male babies are heavier than female babies).

Maternal nutrition is an obvious factor; women exposed to long periods of malnutrition or undernutrition during the Second World War in Europe and Russia delivered babies who weighed 300–500 g less than expected.

Specific factors which may lead to low birth weight

- Cigarette smoking (also influences prematurity rates) and narcotic/substance misuse.
- Increased alcohol intake (see below).
- Chronic hypertension.
- Pregnancy-induced hypertension.
- Infection: viral, e.g. rubella, toxoplasmosis, CMV (see below).
- Chromosomal abnormality/malformation.
- Maternal illness during pregnancy, e.g. SLE, congenital heart disease.
- Placental abnormalities.

Estimation of fetal weight and antenatal management

Palpation/measurement of fundal height has long been used as a proxy for fetal size but is recognized to be inaccurate.

Obstetric ultrasonographers use many different measurements to arrive at an estimated weight; current available algorithms can use combinations of the fetal biparietal diameter, abdominal circumference, femoral length and head circumference measurements. Studies show that fetal biometric data is more sensitive and specific at detecting abnormalities when employed in pregnancies at under 37 weeks' gestation rather than near term. However, most authors still quote an accuracy of ±10%.

Other measurements that are thought to reflect fetal well-being include estimations of blood flow in uterine, placental and fetal blood vessels.

Signs of chronic fetal distress associated with the greatest risk of imminent demise include reversed diastolic flow in fetal arteries plus increased umbilical venous pulsation and reversed flow in the fetal abdominal aorta.

Consequences of being SGA irrespective of gestation

Neonatal

- Mother more likely to develop pregnancy-induced hypertension or suffer an abruption.
- More likely to be delivered by emergency caesarean section because of abnormalities of fetal heart rate.
- Higher death rates; the figure of 88% survival at 27–28 weeks can be further broken down to 68% survival if <5th centile for birth weight and 90% survival if >25th centile for birth weight.
- Increased rate of need for admission to a neonatal intensive care unit, which may be due to:
  - *Asphyxia.* Acute or chronic hypoxia is more likely, presumably because these babies are receiving suboptimal nutrition from the placenta and hence have poor carbohydrate reserves on which to call at times of intrauterine stress.
  - *Meconium aspiration.* See above.
  - *Hypothermia.* SGA babies may be more likely than AGA babies to become cold. One obvious cause is a thinner layer of fat to insulate the baby but also they have less brown fat to actually produce heat once cold and an impaired ability to generate glucose from fat.
  - *Polycythaemia/hyperviscosity.* A central venous haematocrit of >0.65 is thought to occur in ~40% of near term SGA babies. The mechanism

is thought to be relative fetal hypoxia secondary to poor placental function leading to increased production of erythropoietin. The debate about whether polycythaemia = hyperviscosity (and hence requirement for treatment) will not be addressed here.

– *Symptomatic hypoglycaemia.* The SGA infant is at risk of hypoglycaemia in the first 48–72 hours for many reasons. Lower glycogen stores and impaired gluconeogenesis may be compounded by asphyxia, polycythaemia and hypothermia. These babies also have an impaired response to hypoglycaemia; adrenaline does not increase as dramatically as expected. Most neonatal units would suggest close monitoring of LBW babies in the first 24–48 hours, including glucose monitoring. One must not forget, however, that SGA babies can become hypoglycaemic for other reasons and sepsis must always be considered; if hypoglycaemia is profound or refractory, other causes must be sought.

– *Persistent pulmonary hypertension.*

– *Increased rate of significant intraventricular haemorrhage.* One reason for this might be the lower platelet count and raised prothrombin and partial thromboplastin times that frequently occur in SGA babies.

– The incidence of *necrotizing enterocolitis* (NEC) is said by some authorities to be increased in IUGR babies, but the link with prematurity per se is greater. Some authors have described increased NEC rates in preterm babies who had abnormal intrauterine Doppler studies. However, other studies do not support this, although it would seem logical that a baby whose gut may have received a suboptimal level of nutrition during development may be at higher risk of a later ischaemic insult, especially if compounded by hyperviscosity.

■ Incidence of surfactant deficiency/respiratory distress syndrome is thought to be decreased in near-term SGA babies; reports vary when describing the incidence in the preterm SGA baby. Many reports describe the need for more prolonged ventilation if SGA and preterm, but this may be compounded by these babies having a lower muscle mass and therefore needing ventilatory support for reasons other than surfactant deficiency per se. SGA preterm babies are also more likely to be delivered by caesarean section and their mothers are less likely to be labouring; further independent risks for surfactant deficiency disease should be performed.

Post-neonatal

The concept of fetal programming and the 'Barker hypothesis' have resulted from epidemiological studies. It would appear that obesity, insulin resistance, diabetes and cardiovascular disease may be more common in adults who had evidence of IUGR.

Appearance of an IUGR baby at term

In general, these babies have a very characteristic appearance. Their faces appear 'old' and wizened. They appear to have a disproportionately large head/long body and they look as if they need to 'grow into their skin'. Often the usual vernix is lacking and their skin is cracked and flaky due to increased exposure to amniotic fluid.

The CANS score (clinical assessment of nutritional status) describes nine signs, each scoring 1–4, with 4 representing 'normal' and 1 the most abnormal which nicely describes the state of nutrition of a term baby.

	4	*1*
■ Hair	Good amount, silky	Thin with depigmented stripe
■ Cheeks	Plump	Narrow, flat face
■ Chin/neck	Double chin, can't see neck	Thin chin, loose folds evident
■ Arms	No free folds of skin to lift from triceps area	Loose folds readily grasped between finger and thumb
■ Back	Difficult to lift free skin from interscapular area	Easily lifted
■ Buttocks	Full gluteal fat pads	Skin of buttocks and posterior thigh loose

	4	1
■ Legs	No free folds of skin to lift	Loose folds readily grasped between finger and thumb
■ Chest	No ribs visible	Prominent ribs with loss of intercostal muscles
■ Abdominal wall	Full, no loose skin	Scaphoid with loose wrinkled skin folds

Possible investigations to consider in a non-IUGR, SGA baby

If there is nothing obvious in the antenatal history which explains why an apparently otherwise healthy baby is small, when should one investigate, or ask more detailed questions of the parents?

This list of indications is not exhaustive:

- Consider investigation if the baby requires admission to the neonatal unit for treatment of symptoms.
- Consider investigation the greater the growth discrepancy.
- Chromosomal/congenital abnormality more likely if:
  - Symmetrically small baby with 'normal'-sized parents.
  - Family history of consanguinity.
  - Dysmorphic features noted.
  - Congenital abnormality found.
- Congenital infection more likely if:
  - Mother not vaccinated against rubella.
  - Flu-like illness in early pregnancy.
  - Hepatosplenomegaly.
  - Low platelet count.

Fetal alcohol syndrome

Ethanol and acetaldehyde alter fetal development by disrupting cellular differentiation and growth. Fetal alcohol syndrome (FAS) is said to affect up to 2 per 1000 births in the USA and is thought to affect 4% of heavily drinking mothers. Its effects are in the following areas: dysmorphology, intrauterine *and* postnatal growth retardation and CNS damage, leading to cognitive and behavioural difficulties.

- *Craniofacial abnormalities.* Midface hypoplasia, long philtrum, retrognathia, thin upper lip, short palpebral fissures and cleft lip/palate are features.
- *CNS abnormalities.* Microcephaly, hypotonia and irritability in infancy, with cognitive and developmental delays in childhood. Poor coordination, language impairment, echolalia and cerebral palsy are also seen.
- *Other organ-specific damage.* Congenital cardiac defects, hydronephrosis, inguinal and abdominal hernias, gastroschisis, biliary atresia and skeletal and ocular defects are well documented.
- *Miscellaneous.* Hypoplastic nails, infantile hirsutism and neoplastic change.

Congenital cytomegalovirus infection

If primary infection occurs during pregnancy, approximately 40% of fetuses will be infected and most will show signs/symptoms at birth. If reactivation of the mother's disease occurs, only ~1% will be affected. This is characterized by IUGR, hepatosplenomegaly, thrombocytopenia, petechiae, microcephaly and chorioretinitis. It is estimated that up to 90% of affected babies will go on to develop long-term sequelae. Diagnosis is by culture of CMV from any bodily fluid or tissue – usually urine obtained before 3 weeks of age. CMV IgM assays are unreliable. Cranial CT may show ventriculomegaly, cerebral atrophy and intracerebral calcification. Cranial USS may also show calcification of the lenticulostriate arteries and germinal matrix. Hearing impairment is the most significant association and screening must be repeated, as the deafness is progressive.

Clinical problem

You are called to the delivery suite to attend the birth of a baby of uncertain gestation. The mother is 15 years of age and she had not booked for antenatal care. Her blood pressure is raised and she has 3+ for protein in her urine. There are late decelerations on the cardiotocograph.

The baby is delivered and is vigorous, with no need for active resuscitation.

His birth weight is 2100 g with a length of 50 cm. You make an assessment that the baby is an IUGR near-term baby. You make a plan that the baby should stay with its mother but you have a transitional care ward to which they can be admitted.

Questions

1. What instructions should you give the midwives looking after the baby?

2. Describe five symptoms that may be caused by hypoglycaemia in a term baby.

3. The baby is admitted to the neonatal unit at just 48 hours of age with a blood sugar of 1.9 mmol/L and a core temperature of 35.9°C, despite receiving 2-hourly nasogastric tube feeds at 90 mL/kg.
Outline your next five immediate actions:

4. Despite performing a dilutional exchange transfusion when it was discovered that the baby's venous haematocrit was 70% and using 12% dextrose, the baby's blood sugar is between 1.2 and 1.8 mmol/L.

If it is receiving 12% dextrose at 120 mL/kg per day, (a) what is its glucose utilization rate and (b) is this normal?

Answers

1. Ensure baby is warm; if necessary care for in a pre-warmed incubator or on a heated mattress.

2. a) Tremors or jitteriness.
   b) Convulsions.
   c) Apnoea.
   d) Respiratory distress.
   e) Poor feeding/apathy.
   f) Hypotonia.
   g) Abnormal cry.
   h) Cyanosis.
   i) Hypothermia.

3. a) Place in a thermoneutral environment (incubator/under radiant heater).
   b) Address ABC by monitoring heart rate, respiratory rate and oxygen saturation.
   c) Obtain venous access.
   d) Take blood culture/serum glucose.
   e) Administer 2 mL/kg of 10% dextrose and then a continuous infusion of 10% dextrose at 120 mL/kg per day.
   f) Start i.v. antibiotics to cover the usual pathogens (group B streptococcus etc.).
   g) Ensure baby is not polycythaemic.

4. a) 12% glucose contains 12 g of glucose per 100 mL.
   The baby is receiving 120 ml × 2.1 kg
   = 252 mL/day of fluid
   = 12 × 2.52 g of glucose per day
   = 30.24 g/day.
   The glucose utilization rate = glucose in mg/kg per minute.
   Thus, glucose per day × 1000 divided by weight, divided by 24, divided by 60
   = 30.24 × 1000 divided by 2.1 divided by 24 divided by 60 = 10 mg/kg per minute.

b) *No, this is not normal.* Anything over 8 mg/kg per minute is abnormal. Hyperinsulinaemia as a cause for the hypoglycaemia should be considered if the utilization rate is particularly high.

5. What investigations should now be sent?

5. a) Laboratory glucose.
  b) Serum cortisol.
  c) Plasma insulin (on ice).
  d) Lactate/beta-hydroxybutyrate/free fatty acids.
  e) Acyl carnitine.
  f) Urine for intermediate metabolites.

6. The cortisol comes back as 50 nmol/L, leading to a provisional diagnosis of hypoadrenalism. What are the causes of this?

6. Congenital adrenal hypoplasia is rare. Although the frequency has been estimated in Japan at 1 in every 12 500 births, clinical experience indicates that this disease is not as common as congenital adrenal hyperplasia due to 21-hydroxylase deficiency (incidence is approximately 1 per 10 000–15 000 births worldwide).

Congenital adrenal hypoplasia is a lethal disease unless promptly recognized and appropriately treated. With proper medical treatment patients do well, unless they also are affected with Duchenne muscular dystrophy.

Glycerol kinase deficiency, if present, does not result in morbidity but will result in hyperglyceridemia. This is due to a factitiously elevated serum triglyceride concentration.

FAILURE TO THRIVE

Chris Cowell

Introduction

Children with failure to thrive (FTT) usually present to primary care paediatricians or general practitioners. The term *failure to thrive* is not a diagnostic label but a descriptive term for infants and young children failing to gain weight appropriately, the cause of which is not immediately known. Therefore, children with FTT may pose a diagnostic challenge as the differential diagnoses encompass all of paediatrics. It is important to recognize FTT promptly, as it can potentially lead to physical and intellectual delayed development. Furthermore, it may be associated with child abuse.

The central cause of FTT is inadequate nutrition, either because insufficient calories are consumed or delivered, or more than normal calories are required. When adequate calories are supplied, most children with FTT will demonstrate normal catch-up growth, whether or not organic disease is present.

Traditional medical practice has focused on the exclusion of organic disease. However, sufficient attention should be accorded to non-organic contributors of FTT, not only because most children have a non-organic basis for their FTT, but also because non-organic issues may still be present in those with underlying medical illness. Indeed, there is growing recognition of the role of infant and toddler mental health in the pathogenesis of FTT. This is reflected in the recent development of specific criteria in the *Diagnostic and Statistical Manual of Mental Disorders* (DSM-IV-TR) that may be used in diagnosing children with feeding disorders.

The 'food chain'

The provision of adequate calories primarily requires the availability of food – food that is of sufficient nutritional quantity and quality, administered by a parent or caregiver proficient in the technique of feeding a child who is receptive to oral nourishment, and whose intestine is capable of absorption of these

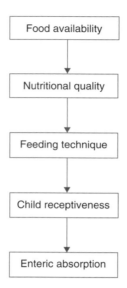

Food availability

↓

Nutritional quality

↓

Feeding technique

↓

Child receptiveness

↓

Enteric absorption

nutrients. Each element of this 'food chain' must be assessed in a child with FTT even in those with organic disease but especially in those without.

Definition

The key point is to recognize that *weight* is the primary parameter affected in children with FTT. Indicators that a child may be failing to thrive are:

- An attained weight <3rd percentile.
- Downward crossing of weight ≥2 major percentiles on the National Center for Health Statistics (NCHS) growth chart, where the space between two major percentile lines is equivalent to 0.67 SD scores.
- Documented sustained weight loss.

Secondary growth consequences of being chronically underweight include compromised *height* gain (known as stunting) and suboptimal increase in *head circumference*, particularly if the FTT is severe or prolonged.

An accurate definition of FTT must acknowledge the limitations of each criterion and exclude normal variants of weight growth.

1. By definition, 3% of the normal population will be below the 3rd percentile for weight. It is important to appreciate that within this group are normal children who belong to a statistical cohort

at greater risk of having FTT. A *constitutionally light child* who weighs <3rd percentile but gains weight at an appropriate rate does not have FTT (Fig. 7.1).

2. Since an infant's birth weight is a function of maternal, placental and genetic factors, the relative position on the percentile chart at birth may not be maintained after the first months of life. The weight of these otherwise healthy children may exhibit 'catch-down growth' and cross percentile lines until their constitutional weight is achieved. This phenomenon is exaggerated in children who are constitutionally light or those exclusively breast-fed in the first 12 months (Fig 7.2).

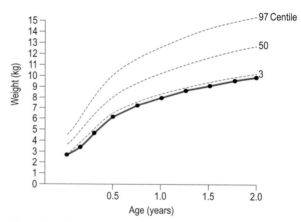

Fig 7.1   The constitutionally light child.

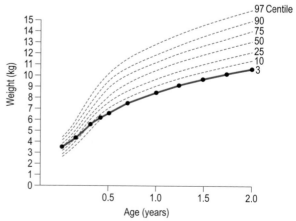

Fig 7.2   Infant demonstrating catch-down growth.

3. A far greater proportion of the body weight of a child under 2 years old, compared with that of an adult, is comprised of extracellular water. For this reason, young children are predisposed to *transient weight loss* during acute illnesses, particularly when oral intake is reduced. Such children should not be considered as having FTT.

4. The effect of prolonged breast-feeding on growth is controversial and caution must be taken in labelling an infant who is exclusively breast-fed as having FTT. This is because no growth charts for *breast-fed infants* are available and a normal growth pattern of a breast-fed baby may seem to be lower on the growth channel of currently available growth charts, which were established by studies on infants who were mostly formula-fed.

Classification

Organic FTT (OFTT) is attributable to major systemic or chronic disease. Although the specific diagnoses are myriad, careful assessment in the history for disease symptoms usually identifies the affected system. However, occult conditions must be considered and excluded accordingly.

Non-organic FTT (NOFTT) is traditionally attributable to environmental and psychosocial factors, and includes feeding disorders of infancy and childhood. The DSM-IV criteria for the diagnosis of *feeding disorder of infancy* include:

1. Feeding disturbance manifested by persistent failure to eat adequately with significant failure to gain weight or significant weight loss over at least 1 month.
2. Manifestations that are not due to associated gastrointestinal or other medical conditions.
3. Manifestations that are not better accounted for by another mental disorder or lack of food.
4. Onset before 6 years of age.

Mixed-cause FTT implies a combination of OFTT and NOFTT, and occurs in up to 35% of children with FTT. More than 50% of children with OFTT have NOFTT compounding their organic disease. Conversely, the presence of an adverse social environment should not discourage the clinician from investigating for underlying disease, if indicated in the history and physical examination.

Sequential assessment of failure to thrive

Element	Evaluate
Food availability	Social environment
Nutritional quality	Nutrition
Feeding technique	Care giver's application of feeding techniques
Child receptiveness	Child's behaviour & oral motor function
Enteric absorption	Gastrointestinal function
Medical disease	History of significant medical disease
Occult disease	For undiagnosed medical disease

The social environment

Failure to thrive in any child should take into account the child's *macro-environment*; that is, the country, state or community in which he or she resides. The incidence of FTT is significantly higher in poorer compared to more affluent communities. Additionally, it is important to consider the immediate *domestic environment*, including the family social economic status and state of the parental relationship.

Many risk factors can be identified by a clinician trained in the collection of information pertaining to the parents (education, psycho-emotional dysfunction, habit disorders), family (arguments, separation, income) and their surroundings (disorganized homes, children raised by daycare providers) that may potentiate the development of FTT. Likewise, careful neurobehavioural assessment of the child within the home environment, including observation of parent–child interaction, can identify characteristics that contribute to the FTT.

Nutritional assessment

Nutritional evaluation should include collecting dietary data observed from a 24-hour recall or, more preferably, a food diary for 3–7 days. It should include the frequency of feeding as well as the composition of food and fluids provided to the child. Sufficient calories for weight and height but not age implies an inadequate intake for catch-up growth to occur. If an inappropriate diet is suspected, formal evaluation by a dietician or nutritionist is indicated.

Feeding assessment

There is increasing recognition of the importance of eating problems in young children. Proper assessment must include observation of parental feeding techniques, child behaviour and receptiveness during feeding, oral motor function of the child, as well as parent–child interaction during the feeding process. This is often neglected in a busy general practice, as it is a time-consuming process.

Appropriate referral to the speech therapist may provide the opportunity to observe the entire feeding process and identify childhood disorders of oral motor function and feeding behaviour. Formal multidisciplinary evaluation and management of feeding disorders of infancy should involve gastroenterology, behavioural psychology, nutrition and occupational therapy.

Assessment of underlying disease

The existence of any chronic disease that places a burden on the family's social economic dynamics or influences the child's feeding and intestinal absorption abilities and metabolic requirements can result in FTT. The majority of underlying medical or surgical disease causing FTT involves existing illnesses

that can be identified from detailed history taking (Table 7.1).

Chronic neurological disease, such as cerebral palsy, mental disability and neurodegenerative disorders, may be associated with *inadequate feeding* and consequently a higher incidence of FTT. Chronic suppurative lung disease, hyperdynamic congenital heart disease and malignancies are associated with *increased metabolic demand* and will result in FTT if higher calories than normal are not provided to the suffering child. Chronic liver disease such as the obstructive jaundice syndrome of infancy, inflammatory bowel disease, chronic exocrine pancreatic insufficiency such as cystic fibrosis and the short gut syndrome following necrotizing enterocolitis result in *suboptimal quantity or malabsorption of nutrients*, resulting in FTT.

Any serious disease can cause growth failure but FTT usually implies that the cause is not immediately apparent. It must be appreciated that some conditions are occult, requiring careful physical examination and laboratory investigation for diagnosis.

Assessment for occult disease

In an asymptomatic child without pre-existing illness, the search for an underlying disease entails careful physical examination and a high index of suspicion. Except for gastro-oesophageal reflux disease, occult conditions causing failure to thrive are usually related

Table 7.1   Chronic conditions causing failure to thrive

Category	System	Diagnoses
Inadequate feeding	Neurological	Cerebral palsy, mental disability, neurodegenerative disorder
	Malignancy	Anorexia associated with malignancy and/or its treatment
Increased metabolic demand	Cardiovascular	Congenital heart disease with left-to-right shunting, heart failure, chronic cyanosis
	Respiratory	Chronic suppurative or non-suppurative lung disease
	Malignancy	Leukaemia, lymphoma or solid neoplasms
Malabsorption	Intestinal	Inflammatory bowel disease, chronic exocrine pancreatic insufficiency, coeliac disease
	Hepatic	Obstructive jaundice syndromes, chronic liver disease

Table 7.2 Occult conditions causing failure to thrive

Category	Diagnosis	Identification
Increased metabolic demand	Mild–moderate acyanotic congenital heart disease with L-to-R shunt	Cardiac murmur
	Occult hyperthyroidism	Thyroid function testing
	Occult malignancy	Hepatosplenomegaly, lymphadenopathy
Malabsorption	Coeliac disease	Antibody testing
	Parasitic infestations	Stools for ova, cysts and parasites
Renal tubule disease	Diabetes insipidus (including central DI)	Electrolytes, water deprivation testing
	Renal tubular acidosis	Serum electrolytes, urine Dipstix and electrolytes
Chronic infection	Tuberculosis	Mantoux test, chest radiograph, electrolyte sedimentation rate
	Acquired immune deficiency syndrome (AIDS)	HIV serology

to increased metabolic demand, intestinal malabsorption or an undiagnosed tubulopathy (Table 7.2).

Asymptomatic congenital heart disease with left-to-right shunting, such as moderate-size ventricular or atrial septal defects, undiagnosed hyperthyroidism, undiagnosed malignancy and the obstructive sleep apnoea syndrome, lead to increased metabolic demands and FTT. Intestinal infestation with parasites such as *Giardia lamblia* and coeliac disease, in its early stages, is associated with intestinal malabsorption and FTT. The difficulty of diagnosing diabetes insipidus in neonates and infants often results in a delay in its diagnosis, which requires a high index of suspicion. Tubular loss of hydrogen, phosphate, glucose and/or amino acids occurs in renal tubular acidosis and the Fanconi syndrome, and is strongly associated with FTT. In any child with anorexia cachexia an undiagnosed malignancy or a chronic infection such as tuberculosis or HIV should be strongly suspected.

Although occult conditions causing FTT are uncommon, the identification of an underlying cause usually results in an improved weight gain following treatment of the underlying disorder.

Management of FTT

The management of FTT involves a thorough evaluation process, such that four key considerations are addressed, namely:

1. What is the severity of malnourishment?
2. Is there evidence of child abuse?
3. Are there severe parent–child interaction issues?
4. Has underlying organic disease been optimally managed?

Further management then proceeds according to the algorithm (Fig. 7.3).

Nutritional rehabilitation

The inability to achieve an adequate caloric intake is the focal point of FTT. Therefore, nutritional management is the cornerstone of therapy. The goals of nutritional rehabilitation are:

1. The achievement of ideal weight for height and correction of nutrition deficits.
2. Allowance of catch-up growth with preservation of normal body composition.
3. Parental education on the nutritional requirements and feeding of the child.

Nutritional rehabilitation involves the use of modified infant formulas, carbohydrate supplementation using glucose polymers, medium-chain triglycerides and multivitamin preparations that include iron and zinc. Approximately 25–30% more energy is required for catch-up growth than in a normal child, with doubling of the amount of protein needed. Ensuring high

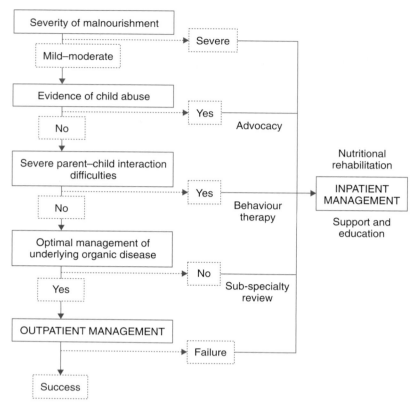

Fig 7.3   Management of failure to thrive.

Psychosocial support and education

Besides nutritional rehabilitation, psychosocial support and education are equally important in the management of FTT, where the primary care physician has a critical role. He or she must be an advocate for the child without becoming an adversary of the parents, so that trust can be attained and sustained. Trust is important in solving social and emotional problems that may have contributed to FTT, and facilitates long-term success of intervention. Where indicated, involvement of the social worker or behavioural psychologist may be necessary. Provision of education on the cause of FTT follows the attainment of trust

protein content (≥15%) preserves normal body composition and avoids excessive adiposity during catch-up growth.

and can be delivered in the primary healthcare setting. Psychosocial support and education are important, particularly in FTT predominantly attributable to family and psychosocial maladaptation.

Behavioural therapy

Behavioural therapy may be required in the management of feeding disorders of infancy. This usually requires inpatient management involving the developmental paediatrician, nutritionist, psychologist and gastroenterologist. Initial separation of the child from the parent during feeding has been recommended, while the parent undergoes specific education on child feeding and nutrition. The parent is then gradually introduced into the feeding process under guidance.

Advocacy

Everyone involved in the care of a child with FTT has a role as an advocate for his or her well-being. Identification of high-risk situations for child abuse, intended or otherwise, should be identifiable if all team members play their respective roles responsibly. Regular follow-up and management coordination is usually required. Therefore, care provided by the primary care physician forms an important basis of the management structure.

Clinical problem

A 6-month-old girl is admitted to hospital with failure to thrive. Five days ago she had two loose stools and had begun vomiting. She has not had her bowels open since, but continued vomiting once a day despite administration of an oral glucose–electrolyte solution. There is no history of steatorrhoea and no other symptoms to suggest chronic illness.

She is the only child of unrelated parents. Her father is a long-distance truck driver, home only at weekends, and her mother, aged 21, is at home. The baby was born at term weighing 3200 g and bottle-fed from birth. Solids were introduced at 4 months. Clinic charts showed that she was growing above the 50th percentile for weight at 5 months, and photos at 5 months showed a fat, bonny baby. Her development is age appropriate.

Questions

1. What is your differential diagnosis for the cause of this baby's failure to thrive?

2. What investigations would you do?

On examination she is thin with muscle wasting of the buttocks and thighs, and has a protuberant abdomen. She smiles readily and relates well to her mother. Her length and head circumference are on the 50th percentile, but her weight is on the 3rd percentile. Her abdomen is distended but soft and non-tender. She has mild, generalized hypotonia, but her head control is good and she has no ptosis. The remainder of the examination is normal. She sucks vigorously from a bottle.

She is admitted to hospital with her mother, who stays with her constantly. Over the next week she feeds well, but continues to vomit once a day. Her urine output is normal and her bowels open once a day, with stools of normal consistency, not smelly and with no blood or mucus. At the end of a week she has lost a further 400 g in weight.

Discussion

This baby has marked weight loss and hypotonia developing over a month, despite a good appetite. The problem does not appear to be inadequate caloric intake, because she lost weight in hospital despite an apparently adequate diet.

Could she have a major systemic disease? Diabetes mellitus is rare in infancy, but can occur, and a blood sugar and urinalysis were performed and were normal. Metabolic disease may present this way, so urine was sent for amino and organic acids, which were also normal. Renal tubular acidosis was excluded by normal serum electrolytes and urinalysis. The patient was passing large quantities of urine of low specific gravity, which might have been due to excessive fluid intake. A diagnosis of diabetes insipidus (DI) was entertained, despite the normal serum electrolytes, and a water deprivation test was performed. A first test, stopped according to protocol, after 5% loss of body weight, showed minimal concentration of urine. A second test was stopped after 6 hours of anuria, when the patient had lost almost 7% body weight. The last urine showed minimal concentration, but the degree of anuria was felt to exclude DI.

Malabsorption is possible without steatorrhoea. The most likely causes were cow's milk protein intolerance and coeliac disease. Anti-endomysial

IgA antibodies were absent, and a small bowel biopsy showed normal mucosa, with no enteropathy. Stool microscopy and culture showed no pathogens. Abnormal bowel pathology was further investigated radiologically, but a barium meal and follow-through was normal.

A central cause was considered, in view of the hypotonia, and in particular the diencephalic syndrome, a condition of weight loss often with good appetite and alertness, due to a cerebral tumour. A brain scan was normal.

After 3 weeks weight loss was continuing, and some staff expressed concern about the mother's intense relationship with her baby. She never left the baby, always fed her, and on one occasion said the staff were trying to overfeed her and would make her vomit. She then disappeared into the bathroom and returned 'triumphantly' with a bowl of vomit. There is a described association between absentee husbands, particularly long-distance truck drivers, and Munchausen by proxy syndrome. The staff felt unsure if the mother was really giving all feeds and/or inducing vomiting. The mother refused to see a social worker or psychiatrist. Eventually it was decided to explain the staff's concerns to the mother, and tell her that a nurse would have to be with the baby at all times. It was intended that if the mother refused, a Court Order would be sought. The mother was hurt and angry, and threatened to discharge the baby. When it was explained that the alternatives were the nurse or a Court Order, the mother reluctantly agreed to stay. Over the next week the baby fed well, there was no vomiting, but her weight loss continued at the same inexorable rate.

An endocrinologist felt that DI had not been adequately excluded. A third water deprivation test showed total inability to concentrate urine even after 10% weight loss, and a marked rise in plasma osmolality. The baby was started on intranasal vasopressin, and thrived. Regular cranial imaging will be performed, because of the risk of a microscopic hypothalamic tumour being the underlying cause of the DI.

CHAPTER 8

AMBIGUOUS GENITALIA
Charles R Buchanan

Abnormalities of genital development leading to ambiguous genitalia can best be understood in the context of the physiology of normal genital development.

Normal genital development

The mammalian fetus has an inherent tendency to develop into a female. If the gonads of fetal rabbits are destroyed early in fetal life, the rabbits develop female genitalia regardless of their karyotype.

The primitive human gonad starts to develop between the fourth and sixth weeks of fetal life, deriving from cells of endodermal origin that migrate from the yolk sac to the genital ridge. The gonad is initially bipotential and becomes a testis or an ovary depending upon karyotype and normal function of several genes that determine normal testicular development.

The initial early determinant of the male phenotype (see Fig. 8.1) is the Y chromosome. A gene on the short arm of the Y chromosome is necessary to initiate testicular differentiation from the seventh week of fetal life. This gene has been called the 'SRY' gene, as it was initially recognized as the sex-determining region of the Y chromosome. Other genes essential to testis development have since been identified on the autosomes. By the 8th week of fetal life the testes are beginning to secrete hormones. The testes produce two types of hormone: testosterone, a steroid synthesized in the Leydig cells, and anti-Müllerian hormone (AMH), a glycoprotein. AMH is produced by the Sertoli cells and, by local diffusion, inhibits the development of the adjacent Müllerian ducts, which would otherwise develop into the internal female structures of fallopian tubes and uterus. Thus functional testes are necessary for inhibition of Müllerian duct development.

The Leydig cells, in response to stimulation by human chorionic gonadotrophin (HCG) from the placenta, produce testosterone. Testosterone acts

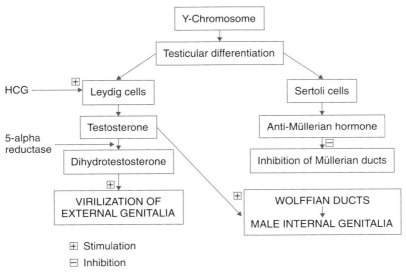

Fig 8.1 Male genital development.

locally to stimulate the development of the Wolffian ducts to form male internal genitalia (seminal vesicles, vas deferens and epididymis). Testosterone itself is a relatively weak stimulus for virilization of the external genitalia, but is converted intracellularly to the more potent derivative dihydrotestosterone (DHT) by the microsomal enzyme 5-alpha-reductase. Virilization of the external genitalia requires binding of DHT to a specific cytoplasmic receptor. There is a critical period of maximum sensitivity of fetal tissues to the action of hormones, between the 8th and 14th weeks of gestation, and exposure of a male or female fetus during this period to inappropriate or exogenous androgens may cause virilization of the external genitalia.

Male genital development, therefore, depends on the presence of the testis-determining genes on the Y chromosome and autosomes, testicular hormone production and normal responsiveness of the androgen-dependent tissues.

Normal female genital development is a spontaneous process that is independent of hormonal influences, and will arise by default if there is complete failure of the above mechanisms for masculinization. With a female karyotype (XX), and the absence of the testis-determining genes on the Y chromosome, the primitive gonads develop into ovaries. The Müllerian ducts do not involute (as AMH is not produced) but develop into the female internal genitalia: oviducts, fallopian tubes, uterus and upper vagina. The lower third of the vagina forms from the urogenital sinus.

The external female genitalia develop spontaneously in the absence of the virilizing effects of testosterone/DHT. Since Müllerian duct development depends upon the absence of a functioning testis, subjects with ovarian dysgenesis (e.g. Turner's syndrome, in whom karyotype is X0 or XvariantX) will have otherwise normal female internal structures and also have normal female external genitalia. With some complex karyotypes, notably with some residual or mosaic Y chromosome material, individuals may develop a mixture of male and female internal structures and/or external appearances, the latter presenting as genital ambiguity.

Ambiguous genitalia

Children born with ambiguous genitalia may be subdivided into three groups: the virilized female, the undervirilized male and the child with abnormal gonadal differentiation (Fig. 8.2). Clinically, the former group have no palpable gonads, the undervirilized males will usually have two gonads of equal size located in the scrotum, groin or labial folds, and the third group may have asymmetrical gonads or only a single palpable gonad. This distinction is useful clinically, but is not an absolute guide to aetiology, which can only be determined by endocrine investigations and karyotype, and sometimes requires full assessment of the internal pelvic structures.

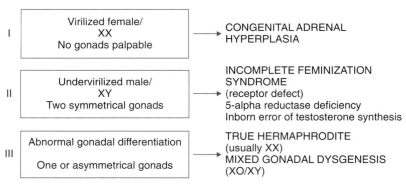

Fig 8.2   Categories of ambiguous genitalia.

When a child is born with ambiguous genitalia it is best to tell the parents that the baby's sex is uncertain and that naming of the child should be deferred. This is preferable to the child 'changing sex' after several days or weeks.

The virilized female

The karyotype is 46XX. In the absence of a Y chromosome the internal genitalia are female, but there is virilization of the external genitalia owing to abnormal production of fetal or maternal androgens, or rarely an exogenous androgen source. The degree of virilization can vary from mild to marked clitoral enlargement and/or labial fusion, with the appearance of male external genitalia without testes.

The most important cause of the virilized female is congenital adrenal hyperplasia (CAH). This condition is the result of a recessively inherited deficiency of an enzyme in the pathway of cortisol synthesis, which leads to overproduction of intermediate steroids and increased testosterone production. Inadequate cortisol production stimulates adrenocorticotrophic hormone (ACTH) production, which increases the inefficient adrenocortical steroidogenesis. The commonest enzyme defect in CAH is 21-hydroxylase deficiency, which is responsible for over 90% of cases. In 21-hydroxylase deficiency, the principal cortisol precursor is 17-hydroxy (17-OH)-progesterone, which is usually markedly elevated in the circulation. 17-OH progesterone is converted within the adrenal to androstenedione and thence to testosterone, which virilizes the external genitalia. In most patients, production of the mineralocorticoid aldosterone is also impaired, resulting in a salt-losing state, which can present with life-threatening dehydra-

tion and collapse in the neonatal period. In the rarer 11-hydroxylase deficiency, there is an inappropriate excess of deoxycorticosterone in addition to testosterone; the former is a potent mineralocorticoid, salt-losing does not occur and 10–15% of these subjects will develop hypertension in later childhood.

Rarer causes of the virilized female are a maternal androgen-secreting tumour (usually an adrenal adenoma) and exogenous maternal androgen exposure, for instance as in the case of progestin, which was at one time given for threatened abortion.

The undervirilized male

The genital anomaly in the undervirilized male can vary from severe hypospadias to apparently female external genitalia. The prognosis for normal male pubertal development is variably poor and, when the definitive diagnosis has been reached, the possibility of rearing the child as a girl may need to be considered, although this involves complex ethical and psychological problems. The parents must understand that such a child would be infertile. Full disclosure of the nature of the underlying medical disorder and future implications for the child as an adult need to be considered in the context of management by a specialist multidisciplinary team embracing the knowledge and skills of the paediatric endocrinologist, genitourinary surgeon and psychologist.

In the undervirilized male, the gonads are usually palpable in the groins/labia or scrotal sac and are symmetrical. The karyotype is 46XY, and testicular differentiation and suppression of Müllerian structures by AMH have usually occurred. The major causes of undervirilization are:

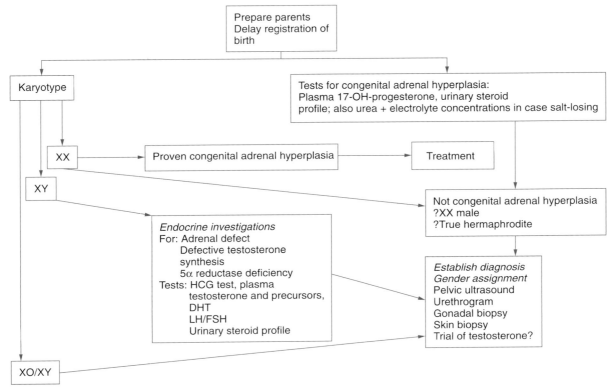

Fig 8.3 Management of baby born with ambiguous genitalia.

1. Abnormal testicular function:
   a) Inborn errors of testosterone biosynthesis.
   b) Leydig cell hypoplasia.
2. Abnormal peripheral androgen activity:
   a) 5-alpha-reductase deficiency.
   b) Androgen insensitivity: a receptor defect resulting in complete (testicular feminization) or incomplete phenotypes.

Undervirilization occurs as a result of defects in three main steps in the pathway. The first mechanism is testosterone biosynthesis, which may be impaired because of an inborn error (e.g. 17-beta-hydroxysteroid deficiency). Secondly, conversion of testosterone to DHT depends upon the enzyme 5-alpha-reductase; thus deficiency of this enzyme results in ambiguous external genitalia, but normal male internal genitalia (which are testosterone dependent). Thirdly, there may be complete or incomplete insensitivity of the peripheral tissues to androgens, probably resulting from a defect in the cytoplasmic receptor to which testosterone and DHT bind. Complete androgen insensitivity syndrome (CAIS, previously known as testicular feminization syndrome) results in female external genitalia. This is the commonest identifiable cause of the undervirilized male, and may be inherited as an X-linked recessive trait since the cause is a mutation or deletion of the androgen receptor, which is carried on the X chromosome. These children are usually reared as girls and undiagnosed until adolescence, when they fail to establish menses and are realized also to have failed to develop pubic and axillary hair. Breast development can occur normally at puberty, as a result of aromatization of testicular-derived testosterone to oestradiol. The internal genitalia are rudimentary: AMH causes Müllerian duct regression but the Wolffian ducts do not develop as the tissues lack androgen sensitivity. Incomplete forms of the androgen insensitivity syndrome (AIS) result from mutations in the androgen receptor gene that permit reduced androgen responsiveness and embrace a spectrum of incomplete virilization from perineal hypospadias to almost female external genitalia. There can be remarkable degrees of phenotypic variation within a family despite siblings carrying the same abnormality of the androgen receptor. A trial period of topical treatment with DHT or large parenteral doses of testosterone can sometimes help the decisions necessary to plan gender of rearing and surgery.

Abnormal gonadal differentiation

The two most important causes of the rare condition of abnormal gonadal differentiation, in which one gonad is usually palpable, are true hermaphroditism and mixed gonadal dysgenesis.

True hermaphrodites have both mature testicular tissue, with seminiferous tubules and Leydig cells, and ovarian tissue with follicles. They are usually 46XX, although subjects with a 46XY karyotype and some with sex chromosome mosaicism have been described. At puberty features of virilization and feminization both occur.

Mixed gonadal dysgenesis usually results from 46XX/45XO or 46XY/45XO mosaicism. Patients have a streak ovary (as in Turner's syndrome) and a testis (which may be dysgenetic or fully functional) and often have phenotypic features of Turner's syndrome.

Rarer causes of abnormal gonadal differentiation include 46XX males and children with micropenis and rudimentary testes. Some of these cases result from defective genes that not only regulate testis/sex steroid production but are also involved in development of the adrenal gland and glucocorticoid/mineralocorticoid synthesis. These infants, like those with CAH, are at risk of hypoglycaemia and serious salt-losing illness in early life or under stress.

Investigations

When a baby is born with ambiguous genitalia the parents should be warned to delay registration of the birth. Initial investigations in clinical practice would be a karyotype and tests to identify CAH, which will be responsible for about 50% of cases. A scheme for further investigations is suggested in Figure 8.3.

Clinical problem

A baby was noticed at birth to have ambiguous genitalia. The baby was the first child of unrelated European parents. The father was a 26-year-old engineer and the mother a 24-year-old teacher. The pregnancy had been uneventful and the mother had been well and had not received any medication throughout pregnancy. She went into labour spontaneously at 39 weeks' gestation and after a 12-hour labour delivered a live infant who cried at birth and did not require resuscitation.

The mother gave no history of previous illnesses and there was no family history of ambiguous genitalia nor of adrenal problems and, to the parents' knowledge, no one in the family was on steroid replacement therapy.

At 2 hours of age the infant was sleeping peacefully, having sucked well for 5 minutes at the breast. There were no dysmorphic facial features and the body habitus was normal. There was no abnormal pigmentation and the baby was pink in air. The rectal temperature was 36.9°C. The heart sounds were normal, the heart rate was 130 beats per minute and the blood pressure, measured by Doppler technique, was 60/35 mmHg. Respirations were 45 per minute and the chest shape and movement was normal. The abdomen was soft, the liver was palpable 1 cm below the costal margin but no other masses were felt.

The baby had a small phallus with perineal hypospadias, the labia were fused and two symmetrical gonads, about 1 mL in volume, were palpable in the labioscrotal folds.

Questions

1. What are the two most likely diagnoses?

2. What investigations would you perform?

Discussion

If no gonads had been palpable, as occurs in most cases of ambiguous genitalia, the most likely diagnosis would have been a girl with congenital adrenal hyperplasia. The presence of two equal gonads means the patient is most likely to be a boy with karyotype 46XY and with either insensitivity to testosterone or impaired biosynthesis of testosterone. Insensitivity to testosterone occurs because of a defect in tissue testosterone receptors: when the defect is complete the patient is phenotypically female but partial defects cause ambiguous genitalia usually with two palpable gonads. This is the commonest cause of an undervirilized male. In androgen receptor defects, the testes are of normal size. If testosterone synthesis is impaired by an enzyme defect, male internal genitalia fail to develop through a lack of testosterone, and external genitalia because of a lack of DHT.

Rarely the karyotype is found to be 46XX despite the presence of palpable gonads; these patients are either hermaphrodites with bilateral ovotestes or 46XX males with complex genetic disorders. A gonadal biopsy and extensive genetic studies may be required to distinguish these conditions.

The patient's karyotype must be determined in all cases of ambiguous genitalia. In clinical practice, electrolytes and blood glucose must be checked and adrenal steroid synthesis (e.g. plasma renin activity, aldosterone and Synacthen test for cortisol production) should be evaluated while awaiting the chromosome cultures. The plasma testosterone and DHT response to HCG stimulation should be documented to exclude a defect in testosterone biosynthesis or 5-alpha-reductase deficiency. A pelvic ultrasound and subsequent urethro/sinogram and laparoscopy can define the anatomy of the pelvic structures. Gonadal biopsy may be indicated if the karyotype is 46XX or complex mosaic.

Summary

This patient had a 46XY karyotype and normal testicular androgen production, and a diagnosis of incomplete testicular feminization syndrome due to a receptor defect was made. After long discussions with the family, the patient was reared as a girl and underwent genitoplasty. Oestrogen therapy to produce breast development will be given at the age of puberty.

PRECOCIOUS PUBERTY
Charles R Buchanan

The normal age of onset of puberty is between 8 and 13 years for girls and between 9 and 14 years for boys. Pubertal changes starting before or after these ages should be considered abnormal and investigated appropriately. There is, however, considerable variation in the normal age of onset and most cases of apparently delayed puberty in both sexes are due to constitutional delay in growth and puberty.

Normal puberty

The complex interactions of the hypothalamic–pituitary–gonadal (H-P-G) axis in the initiation of puberty in humans are only partially understood. The hypothalamus secretes gonadotrophin-releasing hormone (GnRH or LHRH), which stimulates secretion of both gonadotrophins (luteinizing hormone (LH) and follicle-stimulating hormone (FSH)) from the anterior pituitary. These in turn stimulate sex hormone secretion by the gonads.

Before puberty, circulating levels of gonadotrophins are low, with H-P-G activity quiescent for most of the time from early infancy. As puberty progresses, the pattern of pituitary hormone secretion evolves from one in which the FSH response to GnRH predominates, to a situation in which LH is the principal hormone. Interestingly, in pubertal girls with anorexia nervosa, there is usually a prepubertal pattern of pituitary hormone production, with low or near-absent LH and FSH levels.

At puberty, the hypothalamus releases GnRH in pulses for a few minutes every 2–3 hours. This occurs predominantly during the night from the onset of puberty and eventually extends throughout 24 hours in later puberty when menses are established with the monthly cycle of H-P-G feedback interactions. Pulsatile GnRH secretion is necessary for gonadotrophin production by the pituitary, as continuous GnRH secretion actually inhibits the release of gonadotrophins. This phenomenon can be applied in clinical practice using GnRH analogues with enhanced potency and delayed clearance to suppress precocious puberty.

FSH promotes development of the seminiferous tubules in boys, and consequent testicular enlargement, which is the first easily recognized clinical sign of male pubertal development (attainment of testis volume of 4 mL). LH secretion stimulates the Leydig cells to produce testosterone, which is responsible for development of the male secondary sexual characteristics. In girls, FSH stimulates oestrogen production by the ovarian follicles. There is a remarkable change, as puberty progresses, from negative to positive feedback of oestrogen on the production of pre-ovulatory LH and, to a lesser extent FSH, which permits the LH surge that precedes ovulation.

In both sexes, secretion of the adrenal androgens (androstenedione and dehydroepiandrosterone (DHEA)) increases markedly within a few months of onset of puberty (and occasionally before puberty). This is known as adrenarche. The initiating mechanism is unknown but adrenarche is not caused by a rise in adrenocorticotrophic hormone (ACTH) levels. In both sexes the adrenal androgens contribute to the development of sexual hair, a change to adult type body odour, greasy skin and acne.

with premature sexual maturation. True precocious puberty is said to occur when the normal pubertal process starts before 8 years in girls and 9 years in boys, through activation of the H-P-G axis. This is best known as 'central' or 'gonadotrophin-dependent' precocious puberty.

In contrast, pseudo-precocious puberty results from sex steroid production independent of the H-P-G axis. It is usually distinguishable clinically from true precocious puberty because pubertal changes are not concordant with the normal pattern of pubertal development. For instance, extensive breast development might occur in the absence of development of pubic or axillary hair as a consequence of autonomous ovarian oestrogen production.

A third category is incomplete precocious puberty or dissociated puberty, in which pubertal changes are again incomplete and the significance for these children becomes cosmetic rather than medical after an underlying medical abnormality has been excluded (these include thelarche, adrenarche and, rarely, isolated menarche).

The commonest causes of true and pseudo-precocious puberty in boys and girls are shown in Figure 9.1.

Sexual precocity

The terminology of sexual precocity can be confusing. The classification presented here is perhaps the easiest for understanding the clinical presentation of children

True precocious puberty

In boys, the main clinical feature differentiating true precocious puberty from pseudo-precocious puberty is testicular size. True precocious puberty is diagnosed

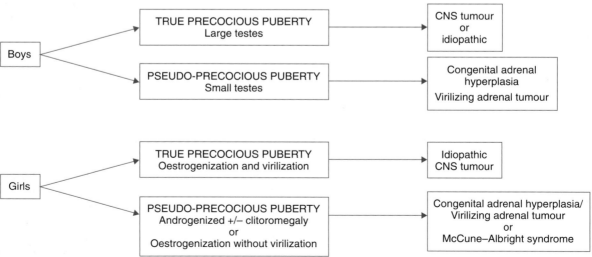

Fig 9.1   Commonest causes of true and pseudo-precocious puberty.

if the testes are 4 ml or greater in volume in addition to features inappropriate for age of androgen production, which are common to both true and pseudo-precocious puberty (i.e. rapid growth with advanced bone age, pubic and axillary hair development and enlargement of the penis). Confusion may arise when a tumour causes testicular enlargement, but this is usually unilateral. Rarely, however, bilateral testis enlargement may occur in cases of pseudo-precocious puberty. Examples are virilizing congenital adrenal hyperplasia (CAH), when there may be aberrant adrenal-rest tissue in the testes which enlarges in response to ACTH, or if a tumour such as a hepatoblastoma is secreting human chorionic gonadotrophin (HCG), which stimulates the testicle Leydig cells to enlarge. The milder variants of CAH which escape diagnosis in infancy can also be associated with true precocious puberty as a consequence of the brain and hypothalamus having been exposed to inappropriately raised sex steroid levels over many years.

In girls with true precocious puberty there are signs of effects of oestrogen and androgens. Oestrogen causes breast development, changes in the vaginal mucosa and eventually menstruation if allowed to progress untreated. Androgens cause pubic and axillary hair development, greasy skin, acne and a change to adult-type body odour. Clitoromegaly will only develop as a consequence of inappropriate androgen excess as may occur in pseudo-precocious puberty. Rare adrenal or ovarian tumours can secrete both oestrogen and androgens, and functional adrenal tumours may also secrete cortisol and present with features of Cushing's syndrome.

Causes of true precocious puberty

There are important sex differences in the aetiology of true precocious puberty. In boys, about half the cases have CNS tumours and about half are idiopathic. In girls, however, 75–95% of cases are idiopathic, often with a family history of constitutional early pubertal development. Imaging of the brain, preferably by magnetic resonance imaging (MRI) of the brain, is nevertheless indicated in all cases of true precocious puberty in either sex. Some causes of true precocious puberty are as follows:

1. Idiopathic.
2. CNS lesions (e.g. previous trauma, infection, radiotherapy or tumours).
3. Neurofibromatosis.
4. McCune–Albright syndrome (mainly girls).
5. Hypothyroidism (severe, untreated).

Idiopathic true precocious puberty may be sporadic or familial and a family history should always be sought. Almost any space-occupying CNS lesion or congenital abnormality may be associated with sexual precocity. Congenital lesions include porencephalic or arachnoid cysts, hydrocephalus and midline defects such as agenesis of the corpus callosum and septo-optic dysplasia. CNS trauma (including cranial radiotherapy given as leukaemia prophylaxis) and infections (particularly encephalitis or meningitis associated with residual tissue damage, such as tuberculosis) are well recognized as predisposing factors. CNS tumours are usually localized in the hypothalamus (notably benign hypothalamic hamartoma), pineal gland, median eminence (in particular a germinoma) or they may exert pressure on the floor of the third ventricle. Many of these are malignant tumours and may secrete tumour markers (alpha-fetoprotein, HCG and placental alkaline phosphatase). True precocious puberty may occur in neurofibromatosis as a result of intracranial neurofibromata but also in the absence of an identifiable lesion.

McCune–Albright syndrome results from autonomous activation of endocrine secretory pathways as the result of an activating mutation in the intracellular hormone signalling events which generate cyclic AMP. In its typical form this results in precocious puberty, thyrotoxicosis, characteristic patches of café-au-lait skin pigmentation and the lytic bony lesions of polyostotic fibrous dysplasia. The sexual precocity usually results from autonomous oestrogen secretion from the ovaries (i.e. pseudo-precocious puberty) but can sometimes occur by pituitary secretion of gonadotrophins, predominantly FSH (i.e. true precocious puberty).

True precocious puberty may occur following perinatal CNS insults such as severe hypoxia, and in severe untreated hypothyroidism.

Laboratory differentiation

Differentiation between true and pseudo-precocious puberty depends primarily on the GnRH (LHRH) test. In true precocious puberty there is a pubertal FSH and LH response to administered GnRH, as opposed to a lack of (suppressed) FSH and LH response in subjects with gonadal or adrenal sex steroid secretion which is not regulated by GnRH of pituitary origin. Measurement of the plasma level of the cortisol precursor 17-OH-progesterone, or a urinary steroid profile, is essential to exclude virilizing CAH in all boys and in girls with features of androgenization and a clinical picture of discordant puberty (e.g. a history of pubic hair development before breast development). Adrenal androgen levels in blood (DHEA sulphate, androstenedione) and testosterone or estradiol levels, unless markedly elevated, do not usually help distinguish true from pseudo-precocious puberty.

Pseudo-precocious puberty

Pseudo-precocious puberty may be clinically diagnosed in boys with sexual precocity and prepubertal testicular size (volume less than 4 mL as measured by the Prader orchidometer), and in girls with evidence of androgenization. For girls with oestrogenization (breast development or vaginal blood loss) it is usually only after a GnRH test or pelvic ultrasound (to look for ovarian cyst development or a bulky uterus) that a distinction between true and pseudo-precocious puberty can be made.

In boys, the commonest cause of pseudo-precocious puberty is congenital adrenal hyperplasia, and the next most common is a virilizing adrenal tumour. Testicular tumours are even rarer, and are usually malignant embryonic/germ cell tumours, as are tumours of non-endocrine tissues, such as hepatoblastoma, that produce gonadotrophin-like substances (e.g. HCG).

The two most common causes of androgenization in girls are congenital adrenal hyperplasia and a virilizing tumour of adrenal or ovarian origin. Clitoromegaly is a very important sign of abnormal androgenization. Ovarian tumours causing oestrogenization are usually of granulosa cell origin and are also rare. More common are functional follicular cysts, which may have been active over a period of time then involute spontaneously. Exogenous administration of oestrogens or androgens (orally or transdermally) may cause similar signs.

Some causes of pseudo-precocious puberty are as follows:

1. Congenital adrenal hyperplasia.
2. Adrenal tumours.
3. Ovarian or testicular tumours.
4. Tumours of non-endocrine organs (liver, dysgerminoma) producing gonadotrophic hormones.
5. Exogenous.

Dissociated or incomplete precocious puberty

These conditions are considered separately from true and pseudo-precocious puberty because of the different prognosis. Three categories will be considered: premature thelarche, premature adrenarche (or pubarche) and premature menarche.

Premature thelarche

Isolated early breast development in girls below 8 years of age, usually bilateral, is called premature thelarche. Growth rate is not usually accelerated. The usual age of presentation is during the second year of life. Breast enlargement may resolve completely within 2 years or may persist as a mild degree of normal breast development. It is probably caused by a brief or intermittent increase in H-P-G axis activity with relatively low and transient ovarian oestrogen production. It may be cyclical in nature with regression of breast volume before subsequent recurrence to a limited degree that does not progress to full breast development. In the absence of such cyclical events or when it is not yet clear that the degree of breast development is no longer progressive, this cannot be distinguished on clinical grounds from precocious puberty.

Premature adrenarche

The early development of pubic hair (below the age of 9 years in either sex) without other secondary sexual characteristics (pubarche) is common, particularly in girls. It is usually accompanied by observation by the parents of an increase in the child's body odour (adult type), usually predating the appearance of body hair, and sometimes with the additional sign of axillary hair; rarely this may appear before pubic hair. If, as is usual, the biochemical evidence supports physiological (albeit early) adrenal androgen secretion the term premature adrenarche is preferred.

Adrenarche is distinguished from pseudo-precocious puberty by the absence of inappropriate excess androgenization. Thus, in premature adrenarche, there is only slight increase in growth rate and bone age and there is no clitoromegaly. Occasionally mild acne and increased greasiness of the skin are noted. The mechanism for these changes is unknown other than the understanding that the adrenal cortex undergoes a degree of hypertrophy in mid-childhood which is accompanied by increased synthesis of the adrenal androgens. Children with structural CNS abnormalities (hydrocephalus in particular) more frequently show early adrenarche, suggesting that a CNS factor may partly regulate the onset of adrenarche. Children with a history of prenatal growth restriction are also more likely to undergo early adrenarche, suggesting that prenatal 'stress' events may alter the intrinsic programme of the timing of maturational events in the adrenal gland.

The signs of adrenal androgen activity are usually not recognized independently of pubertal endocrine events when puberty starts before adrenarche, as is the usual circumstance. Other features of puberty generally occur at the normal age, although some children with early adrenarche will also enter true precocious puberty as a feature of constitutionally advanced development of that child ('an early developer'). The possibility of a virilizing tumour (adrenal or ovarian) and mild, virilizing CAH should be excluded. A minority of girls with premature adrenarche seem to be at risk of developing hyperandrogenism and related metabolic and endocrine abnormalities of polycystic ovary syndrome as teenagers/young adults, but a common specific mechanism to link these disorders has not yet been identified.

Premature menarche

Isolated early menses or vaginal spotting may occur and the cause is unknown, although the mechanism of cyclical menses is presumably mediated through the H-P-G axis. These girls might have a more sensitive oestrogen response in uterine compared with breast tissue, mediated through tissue specific expression of variant oestrogen receptors. Patients with McCune–Albright syndrome may present with premature menarche, and a careful physical and endocrine evaluation is necessary for other features of this disorder.

Investigations

A scheme for possible investigations in true and pseudo-precocious puberty is shown in Figure 9.2. Bilateral testicular enlargement may in extremely rare circumstances be caused by bilateral tumour but, in general, the clinical differentiation between true and pseudo-precocious puberty may be used and appropriate investigations performed.

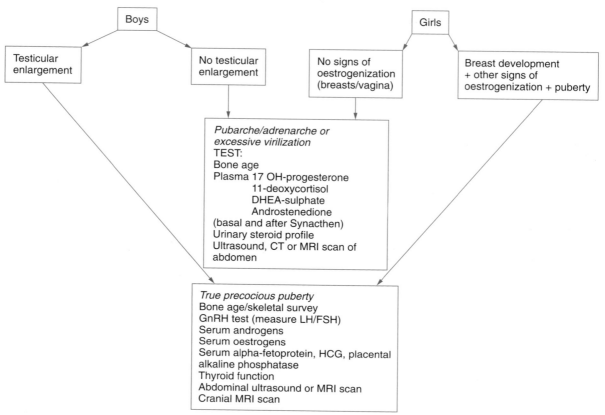

Fig 9.2 Investigation of premature development of secondary sexual characteristics.

Clinical problem

A 6-year-old boy was referred because of premature sexual maturation. His parents said that they had noticed his penis getting bigger over the previous 6 months, that he was having frequent erections and that he had started to develop pubic hair.

He was born by vaginal delivery at term, weighing 3.7 kg. He was bottle-fed from birth and there were no neonatal problems. His development was normal and he had been fully immunized. He started at nursery school at 3 years of age and was then of average height. However, he thereafter grew at an excessive growth rate, was always needing new shoes, and by 6 years of age was one of the tallest in his class. He loved school, was popular with teachers, had several friends and could read and write well for his age. Neither his parents nor his teachers had noticed any change in his behaviour.

His health had been generally good apart from several episodes of acute otitis media in infancy. He complained of occasional headaches. There was no history of visual problems, polyuria or polydipsia. The family had a locked medicine cabinet, which contained only aspirins and vitamins.

His father was an accountant, 1.73 m (5 ft 8 in) tall, and his mother a part-time secretary, 1.65 m (5 ft 5 in) tall. He had a 3-year-old sister who was on the 50th centile for height and weight. There had been one stillbirth 4 years previously. There was no family history of early sexual development.

On examination, he was a tall, muscular boy with facial acne and pubic and axillary hair (Tanner stage 2). He had a single circular café-au-lait patch 5 cm in diameter on his left arm. His height was above the 97th percentile and weight on the 90th percentile for age. His penis was enlarged (Tanner stage 4) and testes were 2 ml in volume, of equal consistency. Examination was otherwise normal.

Questions

1. What is the most likely cause of his sexual precocity?
2. What investigations would you perform?

Discussion

This 6-year-old boy presents with a 6-month history of rapid growth and penile enlargement, and physical examination reveals acne and pubic and axillary hair. These findings are consistent with either activation of the H-P-G axis (true precocious puberty) or exogenous androgens (pseudo-precocious puberty). If this were true precocious puberty, however, one would expect testicular enlargement at or greater than 4 mL by this stage of sexual development. The patient's testes are only of prepubertal size (at 2 mL). Thus, on clinical grounds, this patient has pseudo-precocious puberty.

The presence of a single café-au-lait patch is insufficient to support a diagnosis of McCune–Albright syndrome which, in a boy, would usually present with testicular enlargement, whether true or pseudo-precocious puberty. (In girls with McCune–Albright syndrome and pseudo-precocious puberty their bulky ovaries are revealed by pelvic ultrasound). In neurofibromatosis there would be true precocious puberty (gonadotrophin dependent), which would cause testicular enlargement.

This clinical picture would be consistent with administration of exogenous androgens, although there is no history to support that in this child. Nevertheless, as in all cases of non-accidental ingestion or exposure, a full history may not be immediately forthcoming. Oestrogen ingestion from the contraceptive pill is commoner than exposure to a pharmaceutical androgen preparation.

The most likely cause of this boy's pseudo-precocious puberty is either congenital adrenal hyperplasia or a virilizing adrenal tumour. The most useful single initial investigation would be a urinary steroid profile, which would identify a characteristic pattern of steroid metabolites for either of these disorders. An elevated plasma/serum 17-OH-progesterone level would identify CAH (21-hydroxylase deficiency). In practice one would also look for raised adrenal androgen levels by measuring plasma DHEA sulphate and androstenedione, together with testosterone, and confirm that the patient had pseudo-precocious puberty by showing suppressed LH and FSH levels after administration of GnRH (LHRH). Imaging of the adrenal glands (ultrasound, MRI or computed tomographic scan), and testes if necessary, would localize a virilizing tumour.

Summary

The patient had congenital adrenal hyperplasia and was started on hydrocortisone treatment. He would need to be further investigated to determine the need for mineralocorticoid replacement. The family were counselled that there was a 25% risk to future offspring, and were advised to increase the patient's hydrocortisone therapy during intercurrent illnesses.

SHORT AND TALL STATURE

Charles R Buchanan

Growth is highly complex and this is reflected in the fact that abnormalities in several different bodily systems may result in impairment of normal growth.

Physiology of growth

The regulation of growth is dependent on several factors, and these are summarized in Figure 10.1.

Nutritional influences

The intake, digestion, absorption and metabolism of adequate calories are the primary requirements for normal growth potential to be fulfilled. Children who are obese are often tall for their age and family background. Increased calorie intake is probably responsible for a degree of advanced rate of physical development through interaction between insulin and the growth hormone–insulin-like growth factor (IGF) signalling pathways. Conversely, children with inadequate calorie intake may show impairment in weight gain and later in height. Malabsorption, as for example in coeliac disease, will eventually impair growth if caloric deprivation is severe, although in many cases additional factors such as the inflammatory mediating cytokines (e.g. interleukins, tumour necrosis factor) very likely play a role as in other chronic inflammatory disorders (e.g. inflammatory bowel disease, chronic juvenile arthritis). Malnutrition may be revealed by anaemia, and inflammation may be revealed by elevation of the platelet count (thrombocytosis), sedimentation rate (ESR) or C-reactive protein (CRP). Growth may be transiently impaired during active disease with subsequent 'catch-up' recovery, or may be permanently impaired with stunting of final height. Once food is absorbed it has to be appropriately metabolized and metabolic defects, as for example in the glycogen storage disorders, also lead to short stature, commonly with delayed puberty, if untreated.

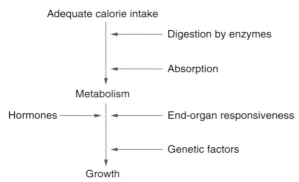

Fig 10.1 Regulatory factors in growth.

Genetic influences

Genetic factors are important determinants of final height. Children with short parents are likely to be short, while many children with major chromosomal abnormalities, such as trisomy 21 (Down's syndrome), Turner's syndrome or Prader–Willi syndrome, are all much shorter than their 'normal' genetic potential – presumably through defective regulation of genes specific to the growth process.

The end-organs must be able to respond to genetic influences to attain normal growth; children with deficient cartilage growth potential, as for example in the chondrodystrophies (e.g. achondroplasia, hypochondroplasia, epiphyseal dysplasia), will not grow normally. Presently there are about 250 clinically defined chondrodystrophy disorders, with an overall incidence of approximately 1 in 2500 births. Children with multiple fractures due to severe osteogenesis imperfecta (fragile bones resulting from genetically abnormal collagen structure) will also be short.

Hormonal influences

Postnatal growth is largely regulated by hormonal control. Normal statural growth throughout childhood and adolescence is dependent in particular on growth hormone and thyroxine, with the additional requirement of sex steroids to accelerate growth at puberty. Abnormal secretion of these hormones, whether increased or decreased, leads to abnormal growth. Growth hormone stimulates chondrogenesis, probably acting both directly on chondrocytes in bone epiphyses and also via the IGFs (originally known as somatomedins): peptide growth factors produced within the growth plate epiphyses under the control of growth hormone and other locally active growth regulators.

Thyroid hormones, in contrast, act mainly on osteogenesis. Thyroxine deficiency (hypothyroidism) delays the rate of maturation and cell proliferation in the long bone epiphyses, leading to a reduction in growth rate. In contrast, the rarer childhood condition of thyroxine excess (thyrotoxicosis) causes accelerated growth, but usually only for a relatively brief period before other obvious signs and symptoms reveal the disorder.

Gonadal steroids are unimportant in normal prepubertal growth. However, the pubertal increase in sex hormone secretion drives the pubertal growth spurt. Testosterone (and possibly oestrogen) stimulates proliferation of growth cartilage cells synergistically with the two- to three-fold increase in pituitary growth hormone secretion. In both sexes oestrogen (derived in males by aromatization from testosterone) is responsible for epiphyseal fusion.

Normal bone development requires normal calcium and phosphate homeostasis, which in turn depends primarily upon parathyroid hormone, vitamin D and normal function of gut, kidneys and bone to achieve the balance of an ever-changing milieu.

The physiological role of adrenocortical hormones in regulating growth is unclear, although the rise in adrenal androgens with adrenarche may contribute to a small 'mid-childhood' growth spurt in some children. Glucocorticoid deficiency does not prevent normal growth. However, glucocorticoid excess from steroid therapy or Cushing's syndrome causes growth impairment by inhibiting cell replication through suppression of effects on DNA synthesis in growing cells. An excess of androgenic adrenocortical hormones (in particular excess testosterone), such as occurs in congenital adrenal hyperplasia, causes accelerated bone development. Statural growth is initially accelerated, and fusion of the epiphyses may occur early if inadequately treated so that final height may be severely reduced.

Emotional factors

Emotional factors are important in normal growth. Children with an adequate calorie intake but in a disadvantaged social situation may not grow normally until the social situation is altered, when catch-up growth should occur. Such 'psychosocial deprivation' can be associated with growth hormone deficiency which is reversible through changes in lifestyle, home placement and other aspects of care.

State of health

Normal health is necessary for normal growth, and many chronic inflammatory conditions of childhood will result in growth impairment that can only partially be explained by poor calorie intake. In chronic heart failure, for example, both reduced calorie intake and increased work of breathing have been shown to be important in impairing growth. In severe asthma, short stature may respond dramatically to improved treatment of the asthma, even if systemic steroids need to be prescribed. In children with cystic fibrosis malnutrition, chronic infection and diabetes may contribute to the delayed or permanently stunted growth observed, particularly in teenagers when puberty may be late.

Assessment of stature

Measurement

Accurate measurements are necessary to assess and monitor stature. Stadiometers capable of accurate and precise measurement to within 1–2 mm are available, and weight and head circumference should be measured as accurately as possible. Height velocity (statural growth rate) may be calculated from two accurate measures of height. Height velocity standards (and charts) are available to compare year-on-year growth rates with normal ranges/reference values for age and sex. Extra care must be taken to interpret growth rates over intervals other than a full year, and in the context of pubertal status rather than just the age of a child. Height velocity is more useful than a single measurement of height in assessing normality, since it represents current growth rate rather than the summed effect of growth rates since birth. It is particularly useful to assess the response to treatment of children with growth impairment.

A useful diagnostic measure of body proportions is the comparison of standing and sitting heights (a special stadiometer is available to measure the latter). The upper:lower segment ratio is increased in children with short-limbed growth disorders (many chondrodystrophies) and decreased in disorders with tall stature, such as those with Marfan's or Klinefelter's syndromes.

Bone age

Skeletal maturation can be determined by radiological assessment of 'bone age'. The progressive development of epiphyseal ossification centres in the hand and wrist is compared with standard 'normal' radiographs for different ages.

Short stature

Short stature is a somewhat arbitrary definition of relative extreme smallness from the population range. A convenient definition is height below the 3rd centile for age as this approximates to −2 standard deviations (SD) below mean for population (more accurately the 2.5th centile is 2 SDs below the mean for age). Other convenient thresholds according to the desired application may be 5th, 2nd or 0.4th, according to one's country of residence. Any threshold may have a purpose for application of health management programmes according to specificity or sensitivity of diagnostic value and local resources. Children below such a threshold will include those with 'constitutional' short stature (delayed normal growth), in whom bone age is delayed and where normal adult height in relation to family background will be achieved late; or 'familial' short stature, in which bone age is consistent with chronological age, where the parents are short (parental height target below average for the population) and the child's final height will be short. Thus, constitutional and genetic short statures are the commonest causes of short stature. The further a child lies more than 3 SDs below the mean for height, the more likely a pathological cause for the short stature will be present.

Causes of short stature

Some of the more important causes of short stature are listed in Table 10.1, using the same classification as in Figure 10.1, which considers the factors regulating growth. An eighth category has been added in which the final stature, if untreated, is short but where children often present with accelerated growth. The more important causes of short stature, in terms of frequency and the likelihood of children with these conditions presenting undiagnosed at growth clinics, are shown.

Management of a child with short stature

The history and examination of a child presenting with short stature are directed towards recognizing whether

Table 10.1 Some important causes of short stature

1. *Inadequate calorie intake*
   Intrauterine growth restriction (IUGR) without
     'catch-up'
   Malnutrition
   Chronic heart failure
   Chronic infections

2. *Deficient digestion*
   Cystic fibrosis
   Shwachmann's syndrome (congenital pancreatic
     exocrine deficiency with syndromic short
     stature)

3. *Deficient absorption*
   Coeliac disease
   Crohn's disease
   Chronic obstructive liver disease

4. *Chronic disorders*
   Chronic lung diseases (e.g. asthma, bronchiectasis)
   Chronic heart failure
   Chronic renal failure/renal tubular acidosis
   Nephrogenic diabetes insipidus
   Glycogen storage diseases
   Vitamin deficiency (e.g. rickets)
   Emotional (psychosocial) deprivation

5. *Neuroendocrine disorders*
   Hypopituitarism
   Hypothyroidism

6. *End-organ hyporesponsiveness*
   Achondroplasia
   Chondrodystrophies
   Growth hormone insensitivity

7. *Genetic factors*
   Constitutional short stature
   Familial short stature
   Turner's syndrome
   Noonan's syndrome
   Down's syndrome
   Other chromosomal abnormalities (e.g.
     Prader–Willi syndrome)

8. *Reduced final height after premature sexual
   maturation*
   True precocious puberty (with underlying CNS
     abnormality)
   Pseudo-precocious puberty (tumours secreting
     excess androgen or oestrogen)
   Congenital adrenal hyperplasia (with or
     without pseudo-precocious puberty)

the child looks normal or abnormal, whether short stature is of recent onset or long-standing and whether it is likely to be familial. Standing and sitting height, weight and head circumference should be measured and a radiograph of the hand and wrist obtained to estimate bone age. Heights of the parents should be measured and plotted on centile charts, and parental target height range calculated and marked on the chart. Familial short stature is likely if the child's height centile is within the parental target range, the bone age is normal for chronological age and the rest of the history and examination are normal. Routine investigations to screen for causes of short stature are still usually performed to avoid failure to recognize the commonest causes of poor growth. The child should be reviewed after a period of at least 6 months to measure the height velocity: if this is normal then further tests are not usually necessary unless there are additional phenotypic/clinical features to arouse concern. For example, an overweight child with a smallish penis might have growth hormone deficiency. Constitutional delay as a cause of short stature is likely if the child looks normal, height centile is low for parental target range but bone age is delayed sufficient to yield a final height prediction within parental target range, and height velocity over 6–12 months is normal.

Children who look abnormal may have a recognizable syndrome or may have bodily disproportion. The commonest diagnosed pathological cause of short stature in girls is Turner's syndrome. Girls with the full clinical phenotype have webbed neck, cubitus valgus, a broad chest with wide-spaced nipples and dysplastic finger and/or toe nails (hyperconvex with a narrow base). A history of marked oedema of the hands and feet in the neonatal period should be sought. The femoral pulses should be checked and blood pressure measured because of the association with coarctation of the aorta and essential hypertension. Girls with 45XO/46XX mosaicism or an XvariantX karyotype may look normal or have subtle phenotypic abnormalities (many pigmented naevi, pseudoptosis). Girls with Turner's syndrome reach a final height approximately 20 cm below their genetic potential had they been normal. Up to 40% remain above the 3rd centile for height in early childhood with progressive slowing of growth until 95% are below the 3rd centile by 12–13 years old, emphasized in many during the latter 2 years through lack of the pubertal growth spurt.

Children with increased upper:lower segment ratios and short limbs may have a chondrodystrophy and appropriate radiological investigations (long bones, spine and lateral skull) may yield a definitive diagnosis. Achondroplasia is always readily recognizable but more subtle disorders which may escape clinical definition fall into this category.

Most children with chronic disease as a cause for short stature will look normal and be of normal proportions. Short and fat suggests an endocrine disorder. Short and thin should suggest chronic inflammation or malnutrition. In coeliac disease there may be a history of diarrhoea rather than steatorrhoea, abdominal pain and malaise. When small bowel biopsies were performed on all children with no recognized cause for short stature up to 10% were found to have coeliac disease without any gastrointestinal symptoms. Children with coeliac disease may have an iron or vitamin B_{12} deficiency, but not always. Routine availability of serological detection with antigliadin, antiendomysial and/or tissue transglutaminase antibodies has enabled screening before biopsy to detect these children. Children with acquired hypothyroidism may give a clear history of lethargy, cold intolerance, weight gain and constipation, and in advanced disease they may be anaemic with a classic lemon-yellow appearance (hypercarotenaemia). In both coeliac disease and hypothyroidism there may be a history of normal growth with or without other symptoms for years followed by arrested growth, as suggested for example by the child's height changing relative to his or her peers in school. Hence the inclusion of coeliac serology screen and thyroid function tests as routine assessment for 'poor growth'.

Some children with congenital growth hormone deficiency have a history of a difficult birth (e.g. breech, or birth asphyxia). Obesity is common and skinfold thickness is increased. Boys often have small genitalia (a small penis can be the consequence of growth hormone deficiency with or without coexisting gonadotrophin deficiency). A history of hypoglycaemia in the neonatal period or infancy should be sought since this occurs in growth hormone deficiency with or without ACTH deficiency. About half the children with growth hormone deficiency also have deficiency of other pituitary hormones. Children with growth hormone deficiency resulting from a cranio-pharyngioma or other suprasellar tumour (e.g. germinoma) will usually present with visual field defects or neurological symptoms of raised intracranial pressure. Short children with congenital visual field defects/blindness may have septo-optic dysplasia, and others with hypotelorism and other midline facial defects may have a congenital hypoplasia of the pituitary gland. The onset of growth retardation in growth hormone deficiency is variable, sometimes manifest in infancy and often not until mid-childhood or at puberty.

Routine investigations for short stature/slow growth should be considered as follows:

1. Full blood count (FBC) with ferritin/iron status and ESR/CRP.
2. Serum free thyroxine and TSH.
3. Serum creatinine.
4. Serum calcium, phosphate and alkaline phosphatase.
5. Coeliac disease serology.
6. Urinalysis for pH, protein and sugar.
7. Bone age (X-ray left wrist and hand).
8. Karyotype (all girls, increasingly so in boys).
9. Serum insulin-like growth factor I (unfortunately not specific for growth hormone deficiency, but normal level can exclude growth hormone deficiency).
10. Sweat test (consider for failure to thrive in the younger child).

Growth hormone secretion may be assessed by one of several stimulation tests. Practices vary between countries. Unfortunately, an exact threshold to distinguish sufficient/normal growth hormone status from growth hormone insufficiency/deficiency does not exist. A diagnosis of growth hormone deficiency requires a clinical and endocrine evaluation with CNS imaging and, possibly, analysis of genes regulating pituitary embryogenesis and analysis of the growth hormone gene for rare mutations resulting in reduced growth hormone bioactivity. Two tests using different stimuli may be required, because the response may be variable, unless a recognized intracranial cause for growth hormone deficiency is already established (in the UK, only one test is then required). Insulin-induced hypoglycaemia or 'stress test' is potentially the most dangerous; 0.1 U/kg of soluble insulin is given intravenously, sometimes in conjunction with thyrotrophin-releasing hormone (TRH). Hypoglycaemia stimulates pituitary release of growth hormone and ACTH, while TRH stimulates TSH release, and the pattern of response can be evaluated for evidence of hypothalamo-pituitary dysfunction. Alternative growth hormone stimulation tests employ intramuscular or subcutaneous injection of glucagon, intravenous arginine infusion or oral L-dopa. Screening tests of growth hormone secretion are less useful than these provocation tests, and include a single blood sample after vigorous exercise, several samples during deep sleep and even multiple (e.g. 20-minute) sampling overnight or through 24 hours. The extended sampling tests have replaced provocation tests in some specialized centres outside of the UK. Random growth hormone assay without provocation is not a useful screening test for growth hormone deficiency (although an undetectable growth hormone level will exclude hypersecretion of growth hormone from a pituitary tumour if gigantism is suspected – see below).

Tall stature

Tall stature can be defined as a height above the 97th centile for age. Like short stature, this extreme 3% of the population will include mostly normal children, and referrals to growth clinics of children with tall stature are relatively rare; it is evidently more socially acceptable to parents that their children be too tall rather than too short.

Causes of tall stature

Some causes of tall stature are shown in Table 10.2. In practice, the diagnosis is usually more easily made than in short stature, since many have syndromic features and growth hormone excess is easier to exclude than it is to confirm growth hormone deficiency.

Marfan's syndrome is a clinical diagnosis based on the classical features. Children with homocystinuria share many clinical features with Marfan's syndrome, but urinary amino acid analysis will allow diagnosis of homocystinuria with certainty.

Boys with Klinefelter's syndrome (47XYY) may look normal or may have eunuchoidal body proportions and be tall for parental target range. Karyotype analysis should be considered for all boys presenting with tall stature, particularly in the prepubertal boy or older boy with testis volumes less than 6 mL, and for

Table 10.2 Major causes of tall stature
1. CNS True precocious puberty (possible reduced final stature)
2. Hormonal Thyrotoxicosis Congenital adrenal hyperplasia (possible reduced final stature) Androgen/oestrogen-secreting tumours (possible reduced final stature) Pituitary gigantism
3. Metabolic Homocystinuria
4. Genetic Familial tall stature XYY, XXY Marfan's syndrome Sotos' syndrome Beckwith–Wiedemann syndrome

those with learning difficulties, behavioural problems or a small penis. Hyperthyroidism is relatively rare as a cause for tall stature and eye signs and goitre are usually present.

In Sotos' syndrome (cerebral gigantism) the birth length is usually over the 90th centile and rapid linear growth occurs for the first 4 years followed by a relatively normal rate of growth thereafter, often above the 97th height centile, but modified by parental target range. Patients characteristically have large hands and feet, a large head with prominent forehead, down-slanting eyes, a high arched palate, and usually learning and behavioural difficulties. Bone age is advanced. A candidate gene has recently been identified, defects in which result in this syndrome, and routine testing should hopefully soon be available.

Children with precocious puberty or pseudo-precocious puberty have accelerated growth associated with premature development of secondary sexual characteristics. Their investigation is considered in the chapter on precocious puberty.

Clinical problem

An 8-year-old boy was referred because of short stature. At school entry at the age of 5 years, he had been among the taller boys in his class but was now the shortest. His parents did not think he had grown at all in the past 3 years and he could still fit the shoes and clothes that he wore when he was aged 5 years.

He was born by normal delivery at term, his birth weight was 3.6 kg and he was breast-fed for 6 months with good weight gain. Solids were introduced from 6 months and well tolerated. His growth and weight gain were quite satisfactory until school entry and comparable with that of his brother and sister. He had received all his immunizations, including preschool boosters.

The patient first wheezed at age 1 year; since then he had tended to wheeze with colds. The wheezing episodes were initially well controlled with oral salbutamol but from the age of 4 years he began to have significant night cough and became wheezy after exercise. At the age of 5 years he was started on regular inhaled disodium cromoglicate and had two to three episodes of wheeze per year, which were treated with inhaled salbutamol. He had never required admission to hospital for his asthma. He did not have eczema or hay fever but did occasionally complain that his tummy hurt, although this resolved spontaneously after 1–2 days. His stools tended to be loose at this time and were generally rather less formed than those of his siblings.

The patient had worn glasses since the age of 5 years, having been diagnosed as short-sighted at the preschool medical examination. His eyes were tested once yearly and there had been no change in his vision. He had occasional headaches, about once a month, which resolved within 1–2 hours after being given paracetamol.

He had always been of above average academic ability at school but had recently not been doing quite so well, although the teachers were not unduly concerned with his progress. He was now about average in all subjects.

His mother had asthma and eczema as a child and his father had recently suffered from hay fever in the spring. His father was 5 ft 10 in (178 cm) tall and his mother 5 ft 8 in (173 cm). He had a 6-year-old brother who had grown taller than him in the last year.

Examination revealed a small, thin, rather pale boy who wore glasses. He was not dysmorphic and he had 6/36 vision in both eyes. Fundoscopy was normal and there was no visual field loss. He had a cold with rhinitis and a soft, generalized wheeze on auscultation. There was no chest deformity and chest expansion was good. His peak expiratory flow rate was on the 25th centile for his height. His abdomen was minimally distended but not tender, and there were no palpable masses or organomegaly. The remainder of the examination was normal.

Investigations

■	Haemoglobin	9.1 g/dL
–	White cells count	6.4×10^9/L
–	Neutrophils	45%
–	Lymphocytes	50%
–	Eosinophils	5%
■	Platelets	252×10^9/L
■	Serum iron	4.1 µmol/L (normal range 11–34 µmol/L)
■	Serum ferritin	10 µg/L (normal range 16–300 µg/L)
■	Serum folate	8 nmol/L (normal range 6–21 nmol/L)
■	Serum vitamin B_{12}	520 mmol/L (normal range 150–1000 mmol/L)
■	Urea	4.1 mmol/L
■	Sodium	136 mmol/L
■	Potassium	4.6 mmol/L
■	HCO_3	24 mmol/L

Question

1. What further investigations would you perform?

Discussion

This 8-year-old boy presents with short stature, apparently of fairly recent onset, iron-deficiency anaemia, failure to thrive, asthma and short-sightedness. His normal appearance and normal growth until school entry virtually exclude a congenital cause for his short stature.

Asthma is common with a prevalence of about 10% at this age. His asthma seems to be well controlled and it is unlikely that this is responsible for his growth failure. Lung function tests might be indicated if other investigations were negative but, in view of the anaemia, other diagnoses should be excluded first.

Congenital hypopituitarism may present as late as this although the anaemia would be atypical. His visual fields and fundi are normal and his headaches are not abnormal; however, acquired abnormalities would only be expected if a craniopharyngioma was the cause of hypopituitarism.

The history of abdominal pain is not a very convincing one, but Crohn's disease should be considered – particularly if other more likely diagnoses have been excluded. A high ESR or CRP would add weight to this diagnosis, although if normal would not exclude it. Anaemia, often iron-deficiency anaemia as in this boy, is usual in Crohn's disease; contrast studies of the bowel of indium-labelled white cell and oral technetium-labelled sucralfate scans could identify areas of bowel inflammation. Colonoscopy with multiple biopsies would be performed as the investigation of choice if Crohn's disease was still suspected.

The combination of abdominal pain and discomfort, loose stools, anaemia and failure to thrive is suggestive of chronic malabsorption. Parasite infestation or chronic bacterial infection should be excluded by stool examination and culture. Coeliac disease causes anaemia, which initially is an iron-deficiency anaemia, and only late in the disease does folate deficiency occur. Antiendomysial and antigliadin antibodies should be sought and, if positive, a small bowel biopsy is strongly indicated. Cystic fibrosis should also be excluded in view of the suggestion of malabsorption and respiratory symptoms. Wheeze may be prominent in cystic fibrosis and occasionally patients with cystic fibrosis do not have florid chest symptoms.

Summary

The boy's serum was positive for antiendomysial antibodies. A small bowel biopsy showed subtotal villous atrophy consistent with coeliac disease. Within 1 week of starting a gluten-free diet there was a dramatic improvement in abdominal symptoms and well-being. He has had considerable catch-up growth with his height and weight now on the 75th centile.

CHAPTER 11

FEEDING PROBLEMS IN INFANCY

Elizabeth Sleight

Introduction

The pattern of feeding adopted by healthy infants varies considerably. Most mothers and fathers learn to recognize correctly the various 'cues' given by their baby in relation to feeding and enjoy feeding times. However, this is not always the case. Difficulties can be divided into two main groups:

- Lack of parental understanding regarding normal feeding practice – including normal variations in behaviour and bodily functions.
- Physical problems with the child preventing normal feeding.

In both situations presentation can take a wide variety of forms, including:

1. Failure to thrive.
2. Excessive weight gain.
3. Vomiting.
4. Diarrhoea.
5. Constipation.
6. Constant crying (pain).
7. Choking.
8. Refusing feeds.
9. Difficulty in feeding.

It should be recognized that this list is not exhaustive and that the presentation may be with a combination of symptoms. When seeing a family whose child has presented with an apparent feeding problem it is important to pursue three primary aims:

1. To exclude serious underlying disease as the cause of the feeding difficulties.
2. To identify and advise parents regarding any unhelpful feeding practices.
3. Where appropriate (i.e. the vast majority of cases) to reassure the family that the baby is essentially healthy.

Fundamental to this process are, as always, the history and examination.

History: general

Family history is important not only because it may reveal evidence of familial disease but also because it provides information about the experience of the parents in terms of feeding other children and the amount of support available in the home. This latter point may be very important where the mother is not supported and has a particularly demanding child.

Pregnancy history, including the results of any scans, is particularly important when problems arise in the period immediately after birth. Evidence of a congenital gut abnormality is often available from the antenatal course and scans, e.g. polyhydramnios, may be the result of the baby's inability to swallow liquor in utero.

Where feeding problems have arisen de novo outside the newborn period, always discuss with parents changes that were made around the same time, e.g. constipation after the introduction of solids.

Always ask about the baby's overall health, since it is important to ensure that there are no symptoms that suggest any feeding difficulty is secondary to some other problem, e.g. breathlessness secondary to congenital heart disease, which prevents the baby from sucking vigorously.

Ask in detail about the actual feeding practice. This must be done with particular care. Where the child is bottle-fed ask specifically about how the bottles are made up and calculate the volume taken and compare this to the babies requirement (150 mL/kg per day during the first 4–5 months of life). Babies with any kind of feeding difficulty have often been tried on a variety of milks. This rarely produces any benefit but it is sensible to enquire carefully about any change in symptoms that seemed to result from the use of a different milk. Where babies have been 'put on a cow's milk-free diet' ask carefully about what has actually been done. In the child who has been weaned this may mean the use of soya milk while continuing with other cow's milk products such as yoghurt, i.e. the child is not on a cow's milk-free diet. In breast-fed infants ask about the infant's behaviour as one means of assessing adequacy of the milk supply; for example, ask how often the baby feeds and whether the child seems satisfied at the end of a feed. Stool colour (golden yellow in the healthy well-nourished breast-fed baby) can be helpful as the stools tend to be green and pellet-like if the supply of breast milk is inadequate.

Physical examination: general points in relation to 'feeding problems'

In an infant presenting with feeding difficulties, the examination can be helpful in providing a rapid indication of whether the feeding problems have actually impaired the nutritional state of the child. An accurate weight and head circumference are the most useful measures in young children and these should be plotted on a centile chart and interpreted in conjunction with knowledge of the parents' height and habitus. Evidence of wasting is clearly worrying and is often most clearly seen over the buttocks. More objective measures, such as skinfold thickness, are rarely necessary for clinical practice.

Whenever possible it is sensible to observe a feed. Not only does this allow symptoms to be observed first hand, but it also allows 'technique' to be checked. This is especially important in relation to a mother establishing breast-feeding for the first time. For example, 'fixing' the baby to the breast correctly (with the mouth wide open and the whole areola drawn in) is vital if the baby's sucking is to be effective and the mother is to avoid sore nipples. If necessary, such observation can be done with advice from a nursing or midwifery colleague.

The mouth and face must be examined; in particular:

- Look at the breathing for evidence of airway obstruction; inspect the jaw since a small mandible can lead to airway impairment during feeding.
- Examine the mouth carefully and feel the palate in order to identify any minor clefts.
- Ensure that the baby does not have thrush. This can be difficult to separate from milk curds on inspection alone but the latter are easily wiped away.

A general examination should be completed to exclude evidence of a significant underlying condition.

Dealing with specific problems

Some problems that could be considered as 'feeding problems' have been allocated a whole chapter and will not be covered in detail here. However, a number of situations merit further consideration.

Vomiting

This topic is covered in detail elsewhere. However, persistent vomiting is one of the most common presentations of feeding difficulty. The history alone can point strongly to the diagnosis in many cases. In particular:

- Vomiting in the first few weeks after birth that becomes progressively worse and is accompanied by weight loss is typical of pyloric stenosis.
- Vomiting that varies in timing and volume over many weeks suggests gastro-oesophageal reflux as the cause. Rarely this will lead to other symptoms such as breathing difficulties and/or failure to thrive, but most infants with this problem are otherwise entirely well and thriving.

Poor suck

Problems of not being able to suck long enough and or hard enough are most commonly seen in the newborn rather than later childhood. Common causes include:

- Prematurity (sucking normally develops around 35 weeks of gestation).
- Congenital or acquired neurological impairment: feeding difficulty may be the presenting symptom in an infant with cognitive impairment.
- Primary muscle disease (very rare).
- Significant underlying disease, e.g. chronic lung disease/severe breathlessness.

In general, each of the above is easily recognized because of the previous history and/or associated symptoms.

Choking/apnoea

In the normal newborn some incoordination of sucking and swallowing is common. Occasionally such infants will suffer an apnoea as a result of the airway obstruction. This is almost always self-correcting but can be more persistent as a problem in infants who were originally born prematurely. Where the episodes of choking show no sign of resolution with increasing maturity or they are particularly severe, it is sensible to exclude:

- Gastro-oesophageal reflux.
- 'H-type' tracheo-oesophageal fistula.
- Other structural anomalies such as minor clefts of the palate or larynx.
- Abnormal swallowing. Problems resulting from in coordinated swallowing may be isolated or part of a pre-existing neurological problem. Assessment

requires very careful, specialist investigation using contrast studies of the child swallowing.

It is common for choking attacks to occur during the early stages of weaning, presumably as the child learns to adjust to a more 'lumpy' diet. Unless these are persistent or associated with other symptoms (e.g. tachypnoea suggesting that the child has aspirated food into the lungs) no specific action is required.

Constipation

Constipation as a problem in the period between birth and weaning merits specific consideration as it is common, causes much distress to parents and child and is often relatively difficult to treat. The topic has been given a whole chapter but specific points in relation to very early childhood include the following:

- Establish that constipation is present. Infants, especially if breast-fed, vary enormously in the frequency of their bowel habits. Infrequent (e.g. once a week) bowel actions do not constitute constipation unless the child clearly struggles to pass stool.
- Ask carefully about advice already given to parents and action already taken. Increasing the amount of water offered can help enormously, especially during hot weather. Simple measures such as this should always be tried before the introduction of any kind of laxative.
- Remember that a small percentage of children presenting in this way will have an underlying surgical problem, e.g. anal stenosis or Hirschsprung's disease. Those with particularly severe problems at presentation or who fail to respond to therapy may need a surgical review and/or rectal biopsy.
- Certain 'therapies', for example thickeners for the treatment of gastro-oesophageal reflux, tend to promote hard stools and constipation. Therefore, the relative severity of any coexisting conditions and the effect of any treatments should be always be considered.

Pain and crying

Parents, not surprisingly, find persistent crying in a baby very distressing. A natural response is to try and feed the child and where this fails to improve the situation there is often an assumption that the child has abdominal pain. This belief is reinforced when the child does seem more distressed with the offer of milk or when crying is accompanied by a drawing up of the knees. This is a very difficult situation to assess since, even in a baby who has a long history of persistent crying, a new and serious condition can arise. Therefore such situations cannot be dismissed lightly. Where the presentation is of persistent crying each of the following should be carefully considered:

- Infection: all possible sites. Otitis media, osteomyelitis, septic arthritis, urinary tract infection, oral thrush and meningitis must all be seriously considered and excluded by history, examination and, if necessary, investigation.
- A variety of acute abdominal problems may present in this way, e.g. intususception. Again such a diagnosis should be positively excluded. Oesophagitis, secondary to gastro-oesophageal reflux, is a common cause of recurrent pain.
- Trauma: consider non-accidental injury. This is really only relevant where other evidence (e.g. a torn frenulum) raises the possibility.

Even where the child does have an established history of persistent crying, the above diagnostic possibilities remain important because they may have been missed hitherto and because something new may have developed. However, if such a child is found to be essentially well, a diagnosis of 'colic' is often made. This diagnosis has no real scientific basis and yet is widely accepted. The assumption is that the child suffers from intermittent bowel spasm causing sudden bouts of pain. The fact that there is no specific treatment or proven intervention (although a number are available) provides an additional reason why all possible organic causes of the child's distress must be eliminated before accepting that the child has 'colic'.

Behavioural problems

Abnormal feeding behaviour typically takes the form of being reluctant to feed. Parents of such children often become concerned as they believe that their child is having an inadequate intake and is at risk of dietary insufficiency. Reluctance to feed is most commonly seen in the period following weaning and in fact is common right up until school age. This type of abnor-mal feeding behaviour may begin when, in very early childhood, the parents offer some sort of bribe to encourage the child to eat or drink a little more. Over a period of time the bribe becomes the norm and the child realizes not eating is more rewarding than eating. As a result, every meal may become dependent on the presence of, for example, the cat, the video or some music. Breaking this type of pattern is very difficult since the parents have to confront the very situation that created the problem in the first place. Certainly the children do not simply grow out of this behaviour. From the paediatrician's point of view the first steps in dealing with this situation are to exclude significant organic disease and to make sure that the parents understand the child has nothing physically wrong. This is usually straightforward as the child's growth is unaffected by the pattern of nutrition.

The allergic infant

Many children with 'feeding problems' are considered at some stage to be suffering from an allergy, particularly where there is a family history of atopy. Although true allergies can be the cause of a wide range of feeding-related symptoms they are relatively unusual in this role. Symptoms and signs that point particularly to an underlying allergy include:

- A temporal relationship between exposure to the food and the symptoms and signs appearing.
- Rashes produced by contact with the food.
- The combination of symptoms, e.g. poor weight gain, recurrent rashes and wheezing.

The pattern of symptoms shows great variation and hence a 'characteristic presentation' does not exist. Where there is suspicion that allergy is the cause of the child's problem this is best tested by a therapeutic exclusion of the food. With ubiquitous foods such as milk this needs careful management and ideally the help of a dietician.

Investigations

Although most infants with feeding problems do not require investigation, where appropriate (see text) the following should be considered:

Symptom	Investigation
Vomiting	Ultrasound can be helpful in confirming a diagnosis of pyloric stenosis.
	pH probe is the best method of diagnosing significant gastro-oesophageal reflux
Constipation	Plain abdominal X-ray will demonstrate the extent of constipation and this can be helpful in explaining the child's problems to parents.
	Rectal biopsy is necessary to exclude Hirschsprung's disease
Choking	Video contrast studies of the child while swallowing allows investigation of the swallowing action and in particular whether swallowed food (dye) enters the airway.
	Contrast studies are also helpful in diagnosing 'H-type' tracheo-oesophageal fistula

Clinical problem

A female infant presented to the paediatric outpatient department at the age of 10 months. The mother had recently returned to the area to be nearer her extended family. The father was a soldier and until 4 weeks previously the whole family had lived at an army camp 50 miles away. The child's father was frequently away for long periods and the mother had become increasingly lonely and this had precipitated the family's move.

The girl was an only child and both parents were healthy. She had been born normally at term weighing 4.02 kg and had been discharged home at 12 hours. By 1 week of age the child had become difficult to feed – spitting out milk and crying during some feeds – while other feeds were taken normally. There had been some vomiting but without any clear pattern and her stools had been normal. In addition to these problems, weight gain had progressed slowly between the 3rd and 10th centiles. Numerous visits to the child health clinic and general practitioner had been made but on each occasion examination had been entirely normal and therefore a clinical diagnosis of infantile colic and maternal depression had been made. The mother had been prescribed antidepressants, which she stopped after 6 weeks.

Having moved house, the child's mother reported that things were better than before but the grandmother felt that the child remained a very poor feeder and it was she who had requested this referral. There were no other specific problems.

On examination the child was bright and alert. Height and head circumference were on the 50th centile and weight a little above the 10th. Development was normal for 10 months and there were no other positive findings. She was observed during a feed and was seen to be uninterested in her food, taking very little.

Question

How would you manage this child now?

Discussion

It is always difficult to assess a clinical situation after the peak of the problem. No investigations had previously been performed and it is difficult to know how carefully the diagnoses of colic and depression were made. Following the move, nearer the maternal grandmother, there seems to have been a slight improvement in weight gain. In addition, no physical abnormality was apparent. The child was observed to be a poor feeder but this may have been a reaction to the strange surroundings. Many organic pathologies could have been responsible for her previous difficulties but, in view of her current well-being, extensive investigation does not seem appropriate. Continued follow-up on a regular basis seems indicated in order that the child's progress can be closely monitored. This has two benefits:

- It allows any return of symptoms to be promptly dealt with.
- It affirms to the family that the difficulties are being taken seriously.

In fact at the initial consultation a full blood count was taken and a urine microscopy and culture performed. The latter showed a pure growth of *E. coli*, with many red and white cells in the urine. Subsequent investigation showed the child to have a duplex collecting system on the right and she went on to have recurrent urinary tract infections requiring long-term antibiotic prophylaxis. It seems very likely that this was the basis of her initial problems. This case exemplifies the danger of diagnosing a feeding problem as colic without excluding organic pathology.

CHAPTER 12

DEVELOPMENTAL DELAY

Adrian Brooke

Introduction

Developmental delay occurs when the achievement of the well-recognized schedule of milestones falls behind that of other children of the same chronological age. As with most biological variables, there is a spread in the ages at which children attain developmental milestones and therefore the definition of delay is arbitrary. In a commonly used developmental screening tool (Denver Developmental Screening Test), delay is identified when the milestone remains unachieved by a child at an age when greater than 90% of contemporaries have already done so. While this definition is useful for screening purposes, a large proportion of children with delayed development identified in this way will not have any recognized cause found. Estimates of the prevalence of developmental delay will necessarily be imprecise, but it is thought to occur in 1–2% of the childhood population. The correct identification of delay is heavily reliant upon the skill and knowledge of the clinician, as accurate assessment demands knowledge of the sequence, timing and variability of neurodevelopment in all domains interrogated. Although delay may be temporarily seen during acute illness, or may be influenced by an adverse environment or temperament of the child, these reasons should not be accepted as proof that the child is normal. In such situations, the child should be retested at a later date. Delay in development may also be the first sign of developmental regression, which requires another particular set of differential diagnoses to be considered and investigated.

Developmental delay can be:

- Global (all areas of development affected).
- Specific (for example, expressive speech delay or motor delay).

Outline

When approaching the differential diagnosis of developmental delay, it is important to realize that the clinician is dealing with a symptom complex rather than a diagnosis.

An approach to the initial management is to differentiate global delay from delay in a specific area, specify which area is affected and the degree of delay, and to identify whether there are features to suggest developmental regression.

The most commonly recognized causes of developmental delay are:

- Chromosomal abnormalities, e.g. Down's syndrome and fragile X.
- Intrauterine infections, e.g. CMV, rubella, toxoplasmosis, HIV.
- Perinatal or early childhood disorders, e.g. hypoxic–ischaemic encephalopathy, meningitis, encephalitis, non-accidental injury (shaken baby syndrome): these conditions often lead to cerebral palsy.
- Cerebral malformations, e.g. tuberous sclerosis, Dandy–Walker syndrome.
- Child abuse and neglect.
- Hypothyroidism.
- Metabolic abnormalities, e.g. phenylketonuria, mucopolysaccharidoses.
- Autism (predominantly speech and social delay).

It is important to realize that even in children with severe developmental problems the exact cause will only be apparent in a minority of cases.

Differential diagnosis

Children may be referred with concerns about development that in the event are not substantiated. These are commonly:

- Bottom shufflers referred because of delayed crawling or late walking.
  Bottom shuffling is a developmental variant whereby the infant progresses from sitting to bottom shuffling and then usually directly to standing and walking. Crawling is not usually a feature of these children's development and may cause concern. They will often walk later than children who progress through the crawling stage. There is often a family history of a similar pattern of motor devel-

opment and the child attains all other milestones normally. Bottom shufflers will often 'air sit' (remain in a seated position with the hips flexed when lifted by the paediatrician) on motor examination.

- Children failing one element of a battery of surveillance tests where the result is taken out of context with the child's overall developmental performance.
  Children are sometimes inconsistent during assessments and may not successfully complete one element of a developmental assessment. This can lead to concern unless the child's performance is viewed within the context of their wider development and performance. For example, a child may be referred because of the inability to hop on one foot, when in fact the other indicators of motor development and coordination are age appropriate.
- Children failing one or more elements of surveillance testing where the child is unwell with an intercurrent illness, the circumstances/environment of the testing have not been taken into account or the result is taken out of context with the history of the child's overall developmental performance.
  Children assessed for screening during acute illnesses may fail elements of assessment and should be retested when well rather than referred, particularly if there is no concern with regard to development from the carers. Many toddlers are at times shy, wilful and inattentive and so any concerns need to be reflected via the family's view of the child's functioning.
- Late-talking children from bilingual households.
  Children raised in bilingual households often speak later then monolingual peers and this is a normal phenomenon.

History

The main aim of the history is to clarify the exact nature and extent of the developmental concerns and to put this into the wider context of the child's medical, social and environmental history.

The age of onset of difficulties should be ascertained and the subsequent developmental progress noted. For example, the speech and communication difficulties of children with four-limb cerebral palsy will have a different onset and developmental trajectory from those of a child with an autistic spectrum disorder. The rate of skill attainment may indicate the severity of the problem whereas loss of skills already present may point to a neurodegenerative process.

A history of significant illnesses or symptomatology in the child should be recorded and specific enquiry regarding neurological and behavioural symptoms made. For example, a child with global developmental delay may also be having fits that are unrecognized by the parents and may inform diagnosis and/or contribute to secondary handicap. A child referred with speech delay may in fact show a behavioural phenotype consistent with an autistic spectrum disorder.

Early development including difficulties with establishing feeding and the timing of early milestones should be sought. The child's development across all domains (gross motor, fine motor, hearing, vision, understanding and use of language, social and self-care) should be recorded and brought up to date and the outcome of any previous assessments ascertained. It should be established whether skills previously acquired have been lost, as for example in neurodegenerative diseases (e.g. Batten's disease, mucopolysaccharidoses) or whether skills acquisition has reached a plateau and seemingly stopped; this pattern of developmental arrest may occur in Rett's syndrome. Loss of learnt language and communication skills may be consequent upon an acquired epileptic aphasia (Landau–Kleffner syndrome) and some regression of early language skills is sometimes seen in autistic spectrum disorders.

A family history of any developmental and learning problems should be determined and any consanguinity noted. A history of unexplained miscarriages or previous fetal losses may point to a genetic or metabolic disorder.

Health during pregnancy should be noted and should include maternal health problems, multiple birth, gestation, threatened miscarriage, teratogen exposure (including recreational drugs and alcohol), fetal movements, labour, delivery and any resuscitation. Details of any subsequent admission and progress on a neonatal intensive care unit should be recorded, including details of any investigations performed (e.g. cerebral ultrasound, metabolic tests). Thus for a child presenting with motor delay a history of prematurity necessitating neonatal intensive care and documented abnormalities on cerebral ultrasound identified at that time may well help inform diagnosis.

Examination

Examination of the child with developmental delay has two principal purposes:

- First, to hone the range of diagnostic possibilities that may be raised during the history taking.
- Second, to attempt to define more accurately the nature and extent of a child's developmental problems.

The height and weight of the child should be measured and plotted on the appropriate charts. Further information may be available from the parent-held child health record (red book in the UK). Some conditions that affect development also affect stature, with the most obvious examples being Down's syndrome (short stature), Sotos' syndrome (causing tall stature) and Prader–Willi syndrome (causing obesity). Poor growth is often seen in children with severe developmental problems, for instance the poor somatic growth seen in Rett's syndrome.

The child should be carefully examined for any dysmorphic features. The head circumference should be recorded and plotted. Children with hydrocephalus have macrocephaly, as do those with chronic subdural haematomata, Sotos' syndrome, fragile X and mucopolysaccharidosis. Microcephaly may be present in children with conditions that restrict brain growth such as cri du chat, Angelman's syndrome and congenital infections. Head shape should also be noted; for example, the child with Apert's syndrome with characteristic acrocephaly.

The appearance of the face may be characteristic; for example, the obvious dysmorphism of Down's syndrome, the triangular facies and prominent ears of fragile X, or the narrow forehead, carp-shaped mouth and plethoric facies of an obese child with Prader–Willi syndrome. All features should be described, with particular attention to the size, shape, configuration and location of the pinnae (for example, the low-set ears of Di George's or Noonan's syndrome). Similarly, the eyes merit close attention for diagnostic clues (e.g. angulation of the palpebral fissures in Down's syndrome, increased intercanthal distance – hypertelorism – seen in agenesis of the corpus callosum, cataracts and retinal abnormalities, both of which may occur after congenital infection). The skin should be examined for the presence of neurocutaneous stigmata (e.g. café-au-lait patches in neurofibromatosis, shagreen patches in tuberous sclerosis) and other skin abnormalities (e.g. midline spinal dimple in neural tube defect, eczematous and infected skin in children with HIV encephalopathy, or coarse features in mucopolysaccharidoses). An examination using a Wood's light should be considered to detect depigmented patches characteristic of tuberous sclerosis.

Much of the diagnosis in dysmorphic children with developmental delay is based on pattern recognition, although many delayed children have dysmorphic features that do not fit neatly into particular syndromes. Careful recording of unusual features (including clinical photography where indicated) may allow the clinician to interrogate a dysmorphology database (or book) where necessary.

Careful examination of the cardiovascular system should aim to detect murmurs or other abnormalities (Down's, fetal alcohol syndrome etc). The abdomen should be carefully palpated for signs of organomegaly (mucopolysaccharidoses, galactosaemia, other inborn errors of metabolism etc.) and the genitalia examined (hypogonadism in Prader–Willi or Klinefelter's). The spine should be examined for scoliosis and integrity of the vertebral arches. Neurological examination should aim to detect abnormalities of attitude, tone, posture, reflexes, movement (gross and fine) and gait.

The movement of the child may give specific clues; for instance, the ataxic gait of a child with Angelman's syndrome or wringing hand movements seen in Rett's syndrome. Their behaviour should also be observed; for example, abnormal non-verbal communication in a child with speech delay may indicate the possibility of an autistic spectrum disorder.

Finally developmental examination will need to complement the developmental history obtained and should include some assessment of the child's cognitive development.

Investigations

The range of diagnoses that may cause developmental delay of one type or another means that it is not possible to give a comprehensive commentary on investigation. The following represents an outline approach of some of the more common presentations.

Problem		Investigation	Possible diagnosis
Motor delay		Thyroid function tests	Congenital hypothyroidism
		FBC	
		Ferritin	
		Calcium, phosphate and vitamin D	Rickets
		Creatinine kinase	Neuromuscular disease, e.g. Duchenne muscular dystrophy
		Muscle biopsy	Neuromuscular disease, e.g. Duchenne muscular dystrophy
		EMG	Neuromuscular disease, e.g. Duchenne muscular dystrophy
	With abnormal neurological signs or cranial abnormality	MRI/CT	Previous cerebrovascular insult (CP); CNS malformation
		Serum copper and caeruloplasmin	Wilson's disease
	With ataxia	MRI/CT and alpha-fetoprotein, chromosome irradiation	Ataxia telangiectasia

Problem		Investigation	Possible diagnosis
Speech delay	Moderate to severe	Karyotype	Klinefelter's
		Fragile X	Fragile X syndrome
		VDRL/HIV	Syphilis/HIV encephalopathy
		EEG (sleep deprived)	Landau–Kleffner syndrome
Global delay		As for speech delay *and* motor delay	
		TORCH screen	Congenital infections, e.g. congenital rubella, CMV
		Serum lead levels	Lead poisoning
Plus dysmorphic features	If recognized syndrome suspected	Specific testing may be available	e.g. Prader–Willi, Angelman's, Down's
	No recognizable features	Karyotype	
		Sub-telomeric testing	May be relevant after discussion with cytogenetics team
Recognizable behavioural phenotype		Conner's questionnaire	ADHD
		Use of diagnostic criteria	Autism, ADHD etc.
Regression of skills		Test for metabolic diseases, mitochondrial diseases	May require referral to specialist metabolic or paediatric neurology unit

Clinical problem

A 3½-year-old boy was referred to the child development clinic with concerns about speech and motor delay, having recently arrived from his birthplace in Africa. Concerns emerged at 1 year of age, when he had only progressed to sitting. He did not stand alone until 3 years old and began walking independently at 3½. His first words did not emerge until he was 3, but by 3½ he was speaking three- to four-word sentences and enjoyed singing. He had developed sufficient fine motor skills to turn the pages of a book, use a spoon well, but had not developed a hand preference. There were no concerns about his hearing, vision or his social development.

He had been admitted to hospital at 1 year of age with an unexplained illness and had received a blood transfusion. At 18 months of life he developed an abscess on the neck that required incision, drainage and a course of antibiotics. He was noted at this time to have poor weight gain and loose stools. Over the months prior to being seen in clinic he had developed a rash which had been diagnosed as eczema. In the weeks prior to assessment he had developed some sores on his head that were discharging at the time of the appointment.

The boy was the second child of unrelated parents whose mother had died suddenly after a respiratory illness in Africa which had been felt initially to have been due to tuberculosis. A cousin had a history of mild (and transient) developmental delay.

On examination his height and weight were on the second centile. He was not dysmorphic but had bilateral parotid and submandibular swellings. He had a dry excoriated rash on the extensor surfaces of his forearms and lower legs.

Cardiovascular and respiratory examination was unremarkable. He demonstrated an immature wide-based gait with normal tone.

Questions

1. What investigation(s) is likely to be most useful?

2. What is the most likely diagnosis?

Answers

HIV testing (after suitable counselling) is required. The history of the child's birthplace, transfusion history, the sudden, and not entirely explained, death of the mother, together with the developmental history and findings on examination make HIV encephalopathy the most likely diagnosis. HIV infection was confirmed on serology and direct detection of virus by PCR.

The case exemplifies the need to consider the child's entire medical history even when the focus of the presentation is on the child's development. Here the history provides a whole range of clues to the diagnosis but in other situations any clues may be much more subtle, such as:

- The paucity of movement in utero often noted in children with Prader–Willi syndrome.
- The child with motor delay and signs of cerebral palsy who had a brief admission to the neonatal unit after birth with possible fits which were in fact a manifestation of hypoxic ischaemic encephalopathy but not recognized as such at the time.

CHAPTER 13

THE FLOPPY BABY
Elizabeth Sleight

Introduction

Significant and persistent hypotonia may be a feature of many serious conditions.

Tone is defined as the resistance felt by the examiner when a joint is moved passively. The patient being examined needs to be 'relaxed' or at ease; this may be difficult to achieve with a baby!

An assessment of tone is often described as having been made in a patient's medical notes when what has actually been described is the baby's posture. The assessment of tone and a careful description of posture are both important features of the neurological examination of a newborn baby. It is also important to make repeated reassessments and to document them accurately.

Hypotonia may, or may not be associated with muscle weakness. Muscle weakness may be central or peripheral. The level of general 'activity' or alertness also needs to be accurately assessed.

Remember that a term baby may be described as being 'floppy' by parents or midwives when what they are actually describing is an unresponsive baby. Be alert to the many causes of this, such as sepsis, hypoglycaemia or hypothermia.

Preterm babies possess a different pattern of tone from term babies; their tone is predominantly extensor rather than flexor.

A 28-week gestation baby has little tone in either upper or lower limbs and will remain in the position it is nursed. By 32 weeks gestation tone should have developed in the lower extremities and by term all four limbs should be held in moderate flexion if the child is held in the prone position.

Hypotonia without muscle weakness

- Down's syndrome (see separate box).
- Prader–Willi syndrome (see separate box).
- Rett's syndrome (see Ch. 39).

- Marfan's and Ehlers–Danlos syndromes.
- Benign congenital hypotonia.

Hypotonia with muscle weakness classified by site of major pathology

Central nervous system

- Hypoxic–ischaemic:
  - Global, presenting in the mature baby as hypoxic–ischaemic encephalopathy (HIE).
  - Local, e.g. arterial infarction.
  - Generalized insults to the preterm brain resulting in antenatal periventricular leukomalacia (PVL).
- Major intracerebral bleeding (more likely in preterm).
- Metabolic conditions, e.g. organic acidurias/Zellweger's syndrome.
- Developmental, e.g. lissencephaly.
- Drugs: maternal alcohol, barbiturates, lithium, benzodiazepines, propranolol and magnesium sulphate used in labour.
- Trauma, e.g. extradural haemorrhage.

Peripheral nervous system

- Cervical spinal cord injury at birth.
- Anterior horn cell:
  - Spinal muscular atrophy/Werdnig–Hoffmann (see below).
- Peripheral nerve roots:
  - Congenital polyneuropathies.
- Muscle:
  - Congenital myotonic dystrophy/dystrophia myotonica (see below).
  - Congenital muscular dystrophy.
  - Congenital myopathies:
    Central core disease.
    Nemaline rod myopathy.
  - Glycogen storage disorders.
  - Mitochondrial myopathies.
- Neuromuscular junction:
  - Neonatal myasthenia gravis: transient in babies born to mothers with myasthenia gravis who have acetylcholine receptor antibodies which cross the placenta.
  - Congenital myasthenia.
  - Infantile botulism.
  - Aminoglycoside toxicity.

Other causes

- Neonatal bacterial sepsis, especially meningitis.

General points to establish in the antenatal history

- Positive family history, e.g. dystrophia myotonica/Duchenne muscular dystrophy/maternal myasthenia gravis.
- Repeated early fetal losses: may be associated with chromosomal/neuromuscular abnormalities.
- Maternal insulin-dependent diabetes: babies may have isolated transient hypotonia.
- Strength of fetal movements: always/often poor.*
- Polyhydramnios.*
- Breech position.*
- Short umbilical cord (<40 cm).*

*Consider neuromuscular or chromosomal causes.

Specific abnormalities found on antenatal ultrasound scan?

- Nuchal translucency/absent nasal bone = trisomy 21.
- Limb contractures: consider neuromuscular causes.
- Brain abnormalities, e.g. lissencephaly.

Evidence of possible uteroplacental insufficiency?

- Sudden episode of poor fetal movements (might be caused by an acute episode of hypoperfusion between mother and fetus).*
- Chronic placental insufficiency/IUGR.*
- Pregnancy-induced hypertension.*
- Non-immune hydrops.*
- Maternal ill health, e.g. cyanotic heart disease, poorly controlled epilepsy.

*May be manifested by a neonatal encephalopathy.

Perinatal/delivery

- True knot in cord.*
- Placental abruption/ruptured uterus.*
- Cord prolapse.*

- Evidence of fetal compromise:*†
  - Abnormalities of cardiotocograph.
  - Scalp pH below 7.0 (limited value).
  - In utero passage/aspiration of meconium.
- Evidence of depression at birth†/need for sustained resuscitation/5 min Apgar ≦ 5 in term baby.*
- Prolonged rupture of membranes/known carriage of group B streptococci or other pathogens.

May be manifested by a neonatal encephalopathy.

†*NB. Babies with an underlying abnormality may well tolerate the normal rigours of delivery less well and show features of fetal compromise/depression at birth without there having been a hypoxic–ischaemic event.*

General points to establish in the postnatal history

- Was there a need for prolonged resuscitation, and how did the baby respond to these resuscitative efforts?

Ascertain the Apgar scores and, if initially abnormal, find out when they became normal. Although a 5-minute Apgar score of <5 *if associated with* signs of neonatal encephalopathy can be a predictor of long-term morbidity/mortality, if there are no later signs of encephalopathy the neurodevelopmental outcome is likely to be good. Likewise in isolation, low cord pH measurements are poorly predictive of outcome

- Was the baby admitted to the NICU and if so at what age?

A baby who was discharged home after several days without apparently having any problems is not likely to have HIE as a cause for its hypotonia at 1 month of age.

- If the baby needed prolonged ventilation, why was this? Was it as part of the general supportive care of a baby with multi-organ disease, or was it because of general inanition? Did the baby fail trials of extubation? Multi-organ failure may be a feature of HIE or generalized sepsis. An otherwise systemically 'well' near-term neonate who needs ventilatory support may need evaluation for neuromuscular disease. A baby who fails extubation after an appropriate weaning period may have a neuromuscular problem, but may also have a metabolic condition. Consider this as a possibility in any infant who was initially ventilated because of surfactant deficiency and prematurity who fails extubation and who is receiving enteral feeds.

- Were there any early seizures? Although seizures make HIE more likely, they can also occur in metabolic conditions. Middle cerebral artery infarction may present with focal or generalized seizures.

- If the baby was offered oral feeds initially, how did he or she cope with them?

Obtain any speech and language therapy assessments, if made.

- If problems occurred at any stage, ensure you know whether the baby had received significant volumes of milk feeds by that time; consider metabolic disease. A normal pH, blood sugar and ammonia are very reassuring, but if all are normal a metabolic condition has *not* been completely excluded. Serum amino and urine amino and organic acids will need to be obtained if suspicion is high; ideally discuss the patient in detail with your nearest metabolic laboratory and clinical team.

General points in the examination

- Birth weight/length/head circumference values and centiles at birth and subsequent values. Severely symmetrically small babies are more likely to have a chromosomal abnormality, whereas a very large baby may encounter difficulties due to cephalopelvic disproportion. A macrosomic baby's mother may have diabetes; these babies may also demonstrate isolated, transient hypotonia. A baby with relative microcephaly may have abnormal findings on cranial imaging. A baby who suffers a hypoxic–ischaemic event perinatally, or who had neonatal bacterial meningitis, may have a normal head circumference at birth but may develop progressive microcephaly, as may infants with neuronal migration disorders and other structural brain abnormalities.

- General state: babies whose hypotonia is caused by a myopathy are often alert and responsive; they do not have brainstem depression, unlike a baby with grade III HIE.

- Are there any obvious dysmorphic features? Dysmorphology databases have made our lives easier, but remember to take samples for chromosomes and DNA in any very sick baby, especially if blood transfusion is likely. Clinical geneticists often like to be clinically involved; liaise with your local team.

- Assess tone:
  - At rest.
  - During spontaneous movements.
  - During provoked movements.
  - Under different gravitational conditions.

A term baby or infant who is very hypotonic will adopt a 'frog posture' when supine, with hips abducted and externally rotated. Another commonly used description is that of a 'rag doll', i.e. the baby will flop and assume whatever position he is placed in. Placing the infant in ventral suspension with the examiner's hand supporting the chest will allow easy assessment of head and limb control and any abnormal spinal curvature. In central causes of hypotonia only axial (head/neck) tone is low; in neuromuscular diseases tone is low in head and neck and limbs.

- Assessment of muscle strength. This can often be made through a careful observation of posture and spontaneous movements. The baby may well make movements against gravity; if not a well-timed tickle or other stimulus may suffice!
- Assess reflexes: primitive and peripheral. Depression of the Moro reflex in a term baby is associated with severe illness of any kind. Normal reflexes in a floppy baby almost completely exclude a severe peripheral neuropathy, motor neurone disorder or severe myopathy.
- Fasciculation of tongue or respiratory muscles, if seen, is almost pathognomonic of spinal muscular atrophy.
- Skeletal abnormalities such as kyphoscoliosis, congenital hip dislocation and foot deformities are more common in dystrophia myotonica or central core disease.
- Contractures, skin dimpling, high arched palate and poor dermatoglyphic patterns are compatible with poor fetal movements and make a neuromuscular problem more likely.

Investigations

- Exclude sepsis if suspected; blood culture/FBC and film/CRP ± lumbar puncture.
  Never perform a lumbar puncture if there is any possible bleeding diathesis.
  Blood in the CSF would point to a previous haemorrhage/trauma. Stool cultures may be helpful in isolating viral pathogens.
- Ensure no electrolyte imbalance: glucose, sodium, potassium and calcium (ionized) and assess acid–base balance.
- Normal hepatic (including coagulation profile) and renal function make grade III HIE less likely.
- Ensure no large drop in haemoglobin has occurred (a large IVH in a preterm baby may cause this).
- Serum lactate may be raised in congenital sepsis or HIE; it merely reflects poor tissue perfusion and not causation.
- Raised immature red blood cells (nucleated RBCs) at birth have been cited as supporting the occurrence of an intrapartum hypoxic event.
- The baby's first urine sample or a sample of meconium can be processed for toxicology if maternal drug misuse is suspected.
- Cranial ultrasound scan, the investigation of choice in preterm infants, will pick up periventricular leukomalacia and multifocal leukomalacia.
- Cranial CT is better at detecting peripheral lesions such as subarachnoid and subdural haemorrhages than cranial ultrasound scan.
- MRI is probably the modality of choice in mature babies, especially if attempting to gauge long-term outcome. Its main disadvantage is access and the need for specialist equipment, especially if the baby is ventilated.
- EEG/modified EEG: these can allow confirmation/repudiation of any associated seizure activity. The appearance of the EEG may be of use in the management of HIE, but may also be abnormal in babies affected by inborn errors of metabolism.
- EMG/nerve conduction studies: pathognomonic in dystrophia myotonica. The myotonic discharge is described as a 'dive-bomber' discharge. Testing the mother is an alternative to testing the baby. All other muscle disorders will show abnormal EMG findings, but they may not be specific. Sensory and motor conduction studies will be normal in muscular problems. In spinal muscular atrophies, the nerve action potentials are normal but with evidence of reduced muscle mass as shown by decreased compound muscle action potentials with large-amplitude motor unit potentials.
- Creatine kinase: this will be normal in spinal muscular atrophies. It may be in the normal range or only mildly elevated in most congenital myopathies. If the CK is high, Duchenne–Becker dystrophy should be considered. Obviously, it will be 'falsely' elevated if muscle trauma has occurred.

- Muscle biopsy (light and electron microscopy): remember the risks of a general anaesthetic to any infant with a possible myopathy. In central core disease, malignant hyperthermia may be precipitated. However, it may be the only way to diagnose a congenital myopathy.
- Edrophonium test for myasthenia gravis.

Down's syndrome

Incidence increases with increasing maternal (and paternal age) but the majority of babies with Down's syndrome are born to younger mothers. Age-adjusted risk varies from 1 in 1600 at 20 years of age to 1 in 30 at 45 years. The genetic cause is trisomy 21; the gene DSCR1 (21q22.1–22.2) is highly expressed in the brain and heart and is the candidate for the pathogenesis of many of the features of Down's syndrome. However, there are at least 16 genes on chromosome 21 that are involved in mitochondrial energy pathways. Mosaic forms account for ~2.5% of cases and translocations for another 3% and recurrence risks are higher. Neonatal hypotonia is said to be pathognomonic of Down's syndrome; however, the author has personal experience that initial hypotonia is often absent in babies of African descent.

Presentation

Antenatal
Increased nuchal translucency/absent nasal bone/ evidence of associated congenital abnormalities, i.e. duodenal atresia/congenital heart disease/ oesophageal atresia on antenatal ultrasound.

Neonatal
Small for gestational age/hypotonia/brachycephaly/flat occiput/upslanting palpebral fissures/ epicanthic folds/Brushfield spots/small ears/single palmar creases/clinodactyly. Look for symptoms of Hirschsprung's. Congenital heart disease in 40–50% of children – all babies should have an echocardiograph in the first 6 months of life and some authorities suggest in teenage years too; valvular prolapse is common. Cardiac lesions include AVSD = 40%, VSD = 30%, ASD = 10%, TOF 5% and PDA = 5%. Primary hypothyroidism is present in 1 in 400 (compared to 1 in 4000 ordinary children).

Infant/childhood
Delayed motor and developmental milestones/ screen for hearing loss – both conductive and sensorineural. Screen for acquired hypothyroidism regularly and also be aware of symptoms of atlantoaxial instability. People with Down's syndrome are more prone to bacterial infections/ leukaemia (10–15 times risk) and Alzheimer's disease (75% >60 years). Coeliac disease is also more common (~5%) and should be screened for.

Prader–Willi syndrome

This syndrome is caused by a deletion or disruption of genes located in the proximal arm of chromosome 15 (15q11–13). The disorder was the first to be attributed to 'genomic imprinting'. This is when genes are expressed differently based upon parental origin. The syndrome results from the loss of paternal material or uniparental disomy of maternal genes; Angelman's syndrome results from loss of maternal genes at the same locus.

International prevalence rates vary between 1 in 8000 (Sweden) and 1 in 25 000 (USA).

Presentation

Neonatal
Hypotonia, poor feeding, weak cry, genital hypoplasia.

Toddler
Delayed motor milestones, e.g. sitting by 12 months.

Childhood
Hyperphagia and obesity (may lead to sleep apnoea/cor pulmonale/diabetes/atherosclerosis/ osteoporosis), short stature (with associated growth hormone deficiency); may develop pubic hair early, but in general puberty is grossly delayed; there are behavioural difficulties, which include temper tantrums, obsessive–compulsive behaviour, sleep disturbance and a high pain tolerance. Small hands and feet are also features.

Spinal muscular atrophy

SMA is caused by a mutation in the survival motor neurone gene SMN1. In its absence, programmed cell death of the alpha motor neurones in the anterior horn cells continues after birth. The SMN1 gene is located on the long arm of chromosome 5 (q11.2–13.3). The incidence of this autosomal recessive condition varies between nations: in Slovakia SMA affects 1 in 6000 live births, in comparison to approximately 1 in 15000 in the USA. The incidence is low in black Africans. Male : female ratio = 2 : 1.

Death occurs due to embarrassment of respiratory muscles. Sensation as well as intelligence is spared. Sometimes cranial nerves V–XII can also be affected.

There are three types, which present at different ages: Type I (Werdnig–Hoffmann) presents between birth and 6 months, Type II between 6 and 12 months and Type III (Kugelberg–Welander) after 2 years of age. Most children with Type I SMA die by 2 years of age.

Type I SMA

Mothers may report decreased fetal movements. The paucity of intrauterine fetal breathing may be revealed by thin ribs on a chest X-ray. An affected baby may be floppy and inactive but will be alert. The distal musculature is usually spared. Tongue fasciculation is pathognomonic but only apparent in approximately 50% of affected babies. Paradoxical diaphragmatic breathing may be seen and tendon reflexes will be absent. Serum creatine kinase and aldolase findings are within normal limits. Electromyography reveals a myopathic picture with normal nerve conduction velocities. Muscle biopsy shows uniformly small muscle fibres throughout.

Dystrophia myotonica

Congenital DM manifests itself as the classical 'floppy baby'. Myotonia is not usually present at this age. Talipes, congenital dislocation of the hips and other joint deformities are typical, along with a facial diplegia (flat, immobile face with triangular, open mouth). There may be a delay in establishing adequate respiration at birth, and cyanotic episodes and poor feeding are features.

This autosomal dominant disease is the commonest muscular dystrophy in adult life; incidence varies between 1 in 500 in a region of Canada to 1 in 25000 in Europe. It is very unusual in African families. The gene is located at 19q13.3 and is an example of the phenomenon of anticipation. This is when a genetic mutation causes an unstable trinucleotide repeat (CTG) and the repeat increases in length in each subsequent generation; hence the clinical 'phenotype' becomes progressive more severe from parent to child.

Adult symptoms/signs include myotonia, muscle wasting in distal extremities, cataracts, hypogonadism, frontal balding, ECG changes and impaired intestinal motility. If an affected baby survives the neonatal period, most will eventually walk, but 60–70% will suffer from learning difficulties. Diagnosis can be made on EMG (see above). 60–70% of affected babies will have ventricular dilatation on cranial ultrasound scan.

Clinical problem

A term baby was born with Apgar scores of 2 at 1 minute and 3 at 5 minutes following a placental abruption. The baby required endotracheal intubation at 2 minutes, with a heart rate above 100 and centrally pink by 5 minutes. The baby remained ventilated for 4 days because of poor respiratory effort and was not given enteral feeds until 7 days old, nutrition having been provided parenterally.

The baby was hypotonic from birth and had several generalized convulsions, each lasting between 1 and 5 minutes during the first 5 days of life. Phenobarbital was started on the second day.

During the first month, spent in hospital, the baby remained hypotonic with symmetrically decreased power and reflexes. He slowly developed a suck and was able to feed by bottle at 1 month of age. Seizures no longer occurred. His head circumference fell from the 50th centile at birth to the 10th centile. He showed no signs of being able to fix or follow visually and was generally hypotonic.

Questions

1. What is the diagnosis?

2. What investigations would you perform to confirm this?

3. What is the prognosis for the hypotonia?

Answers

1. This history is typical of hypoxic–ischaemic encephalopathy (HIE). Metabolic disease and chromosomal abnormalities should be excluded.

2. A head ultrasound scan is conveniently performed in the immediate neonatal period in an intensive care unit with minimal disruption to the baby, but is often normal; CT and MRI scans are better at revealing ischaemic damage. Typically changes are observed in the basal ganglia but may be much more widespread. A metabolic screen and chromosomal analysis should be performed.

3. The hypotonia is usually a phase in the child's response to the insult and may resolve or progress to hypertonia or other forms of cerebral palsy. Infants with HIE are particularly at risk of quadriplegia or dyskinetic cerebral palsy.

CHAPTER 14

HEADACHE IN CHILDREN
Andrew Kornberg

Introduction

The major concern for parents, and for the treating physician, when a child presents with headache is the possibility that it is caused by a tumour. A detailed history and examination will be able to alleviate this anxiety in the majority of cases and provide the child and family with a specific diagnosis and appropriate therapy.

Headache is a frequent symptom in children and adolescents. Studies of childhood headache have shown that the frequency of recurrent headache in childhood may be as high as 23%. Other studies have demonstrated that headache prevalence ranges from 57% to 82% in 7- to 15-year-olds. Migraine in childhood has been well studied and may have prevalence rates as high as 11%. Of the different types of headache encountered in childhood, migraine is the most common. Diagnostic criteria exist for migraine and other types of headaches that occur in childhood.

Headaches are caused by the involvement of the pain-sensitive structures, which include vascular and meningeal structures, cranial nerves (particularly those with sensory fibres: V, IX, X) and some structures surrounding the skull.

In the evaluation of a child with headache it is important to make a specific diagnosis, as this is the key to providing the most appropriate therapy.

Outline

The history and examination is the most important part of the evaluation of children presenting with headache. 'Routine' laboratory and imaging studies have no place, because these investigations should be used in a focused manner, depending on the differential diagnosis obtained from history and examination. The following details the important aspects of the history and examination that should be considered.

History

In the evaluation of a child with headache, a full developmental and medical history should be obtained. Previous medications for headache and other disorders should be detailed with particular attention to any drug and alcohol use. The parents and patients should be asked about anxiety and depressive symptoms. A careful family history of headache or psychiatric illnesses should be detailed. The next part of the evaluation is detailing the headache history. This should be thorough and include the questions detailed in Table 14.1. These questions may allow the clinician to make a diagnosis based on the headache type and to plan further management. Finally, a thorough systematic review is performed, concentrating on questions related to symptoms of raised intracranial pressure (ICP) or progressive neurological disease, such as ataxia, lethargy, seizures, visual disturbances, focal signs, personality change or intellectual change. Warning symptoms may include:

- Increased severity of headaches.
- Awakening from sleep.
- Change in headache pattern.

Examination

A general physical examination should include careful blood pressure measurement and examination of the skin for neurocutaneous stigmata of neurofibromatosis. Signs of trauma should be specifically sought. The head circumference should be measured, plotted and compared to previous measurements. The neck and skull should be auscultated for bruits and the sinuses should be palpated for tenderness. A careful neurological examination is performed, looking specifically for focal neurological findings. Eye movements and the optic fundi should be carefully examined.

Any abnormality in the neurological examination requires further evaluation as this is normal in between attacks in individuals with migraine.

Pattern of headache

In the evaluation of a child with headache it is useful to classify headache clinically using a temporal pattern. Based on this, a number of patterns can be identified and used in the further delineation of the likely diagnosis. Patterns which are commonly encountered include:

- Acute.
- Acute recurrent.
- Chronic progressive.
- Chronic non-progressive.
- Mixed pattern.

The various patterns are shown in Figure 14.1.

Acute headaches are single events without a previous history of headache. Acute headaches are commonly associated with systemic illnesses such as viral illnesses. If an acute headache is associated with focal neurological findings or raised intracranial pressure one may need to consider an acute intracranial haemorrhage. Other causes of acute headache are listed in Table 14.2.

Acute recurrent headaches are usually migrainous and are described in more detail below.

Chronic progressive headaches worsen in frequency and severity over time. They are usually associated with symptoms of raised intracranial pressure, such as

---

Table 14.1   Headache history questions

How long ago did the headaches start?

Are the headaches the same, better or worse overall?

How often are the headaches occurring?

Do the headaches occur at any special time, or under any special circumstance?

Are the headaches related to any triggers you are aware of?

Are there any warning symptoms?

Where is the pain located?

What is the quality of the pain?

Are there any associated symptoms?

How long does it take from the onset of the headache to the peak of the headache?

How long does the headache last?

What do you do during the headache?

What makes the headache better?

What makes the headache worse?

Between headaches are you well?

Are you on any other medications?

Have you ever been treated for headaches before?

What do you think could be causing your headaches?

Is there a family history of headaches?

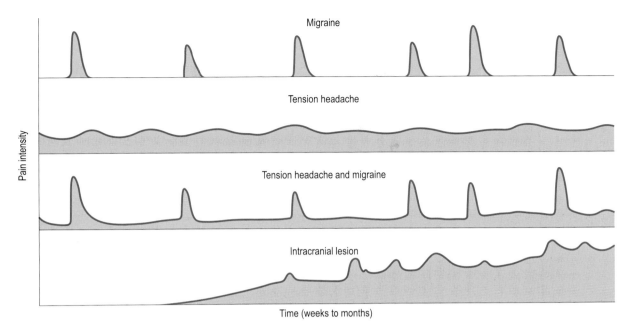

Fig 14.1   Headache patterns.

Table 14.2   Acute headache
Infections including meningitis
Sinusitis
Postictal
Acute hypertension
Hypoglycaemia
Trauma
Haemorrhage
Exertion
Dehydration

early-morning headache, vomiting and signs of papilloedema or focal neurological findings. The main differential diagnosis of this pattern of headache includes brain tumours, hydrocephalus, subdural hemorrhage and benign intracranial hypertension (BIH).

Chronic non-progressive headaches are often called tension-type headaches. They are not associated with symptoms of raised intracranial pressure or progressive neurological findings.

Mixed-pattern headaches are a combination of migraine or chronic, non-progressive headaches.

Investigations

Headaches are frequently over-investigated. As discussed earlier, investigations should only be performed after a careful history and examination. Most children with headache will not require investigation.

Laboratory tests yield little and are rarely necessary.

Skull X-rays have little or no place in the investigation of headache.

Imaging studies such as computed tomography (CT) of the brain or magnetic resonance imaging (MRI) have revolutionized the investigation of CNS disorders. Both modalities can be used to diagnose many congenital malformations, neoplasms, hydrocephalus, haemorrhage, vascular malformations or sinus pathology. However, MRI is more sensitive, particularly in the posterior fossa and in the area of the craniocervical junction.

Lumbar puncture for CSF pressure measurement is necessary for the diagnosis of BIH.

Acute recurrent

Migraine

Migraine is an acute recurrent headache characterized by episodic, periodic and paroxysmal attacks of pain, separated by pain-free periods. Migraine is often triggered by stress, anxiety, fatigue, lack of sleep, certain foods, exercise and sunlight. A family history of migraine is common.

Prior to the onset of the headache there may be an aura, which may consist of visual symptoms such as bright flashing lights, fortification spectra or an alteration of perception, the so-called 'Alice in Wonderland' syndrome. Neurological symptoms such as dysphasia, paraesthesia and hemiparesis may also begin at this stage. The headache then begins, usually frontal, lateralized, throbbing in quality, and gradually spreading. The child is often very pale and may be nauseous and begin to vomit. The child is usually photophobic and needs to go to sleep in a dark room. After sleep the child improves. Between headaches the child is normal, as is the child's examination, thus excluding organic disease. Obviously, there are less severe headaches, and many children do not have an aura.

It is important to obtain from the history and examination the following aspects:

- Aura.
- Lateralized.
- Throbbing.
- Nausea/vomiting.
- Photophobia.
- Normal intra-attack history and examination with no evidence of organic disease.

These features essentially form the basis of the diagnostic criteria for migraine.

Migraine is common in childhood and has similar manifestations in childhood as it does in adults. The various complicated migraine syndromes described in adults, such as hemiplegic migraine, occur in childhood but other migraine syndromes appear to be seen exclusively in childhood. These include:

- Benign paroxysmal vertigo.
- Cyclic vomiting.

- Paroxysmal torticollis.

Management of migraine in childhood includes:

- Identifying triggers and removing them.
- Aborting attacks by taking analgesia as early as possible into the attack (and at the onset of any aura).
- Using non-pharmacological relaxation techniques.
- Taking prophylactic agents to prevent frequent disabling events.

As the remission rate of migraine is high, prophylaxis should not be used for long periods.

Chronic progressive headaches

Chronic progressive headaches suggest that there is an ongoing pathological process occurring within the skull. It is usually associated with raised ICP, and symptoms and signs are progressive over time. The symptoms (headache) typically worsen by becoming more frequent, more severe, associated with early-morning wakening, a change in character or associated with other neurological symptoms. The headaches may worsen with coughing, bending over or sneezing. Other symptoms will suggest an ongoing neurological process. Symptoms may include a change in personality, focal weakness, ataxia, diplopia, visual loss, seizures or lethargy. Between headaches the child will have ongoing symptoms. The general or neurological examination will usually be abnormal or, if normal, will show signs of raised ICP with evidence of cranial nerve palsies or papilloedema.

Brain tumours are the second most common childhood malignancy after leukaemia and are a common cause of this pattern of headache. Other causes include hydrocephalus from congenital anomalies.

In this scenario, imaging is mandatory and diagnostic. Lumbar puncture is contraindicated if a mass lesion is considered and should only be performed after imaging.

Benign intracranial hypertension (BIH)

This condition is relatively common and presents with symptoms suggestive of raised ICP. It is termed 'benign' because the clinical features mimic a cerebral tumour, but no tumour is found.

An imaging study is required to exclude a tumour or hydrocephalus, and by definition no evidence for hydrocephalus or tumour is found on imaging.

However, this disorder is not necessarily 'benign', as it is potentially associated with permanent and disabling visual loss. The pathogenesis has not been clearly elucidated. The next step to confirm the diagnosis is a CSF pressure measurement, which will demonstrate a grossly elevated CSF pressure.

The disorder is associated with a number of risk factors including:

- Adolescence, female sex and obesity.
- Recurrent otitis media.
- Medications: steroid withdrawal, oral contraceptives, tetracyclines, vitamin A, growth hormone treatment.

Management involves close monitoring of vision, withdrawal of risk factors (drugs), lowering of ICP by lumbar puncture and the use of drugs to decrease CSF production (acetazolamide). If vision is deteriorating despite active management, neurosurgical procedures such as lumboperitoneal shunting and optic nerve fenestration is necessary.

The protection of vision is the mainstay of therapy.

The prognosis for this disorder is generally good.

Chronic non-progressive headaches

'Tension' headaches

There is a broad spectrum of headache types that fall into this group, many in some way associated with emotional factors. These types of headache appear to be more common in older children and adolescents.

The clinical features of these headaches have not been well defined. The headaches are commonly described as being frontal and pressure-like, or band-like. Unlike migraine headaches, they are not associated with a throbbing quality (although the mixed-pattern headache has features of both types). There is no preceding aura, the headache may be present on a daily basis and be present throughout the day. Many adolescents will continue their activities. There may be a myriad of other symptoms such as fatigue, dizziness and blurred vision. There may be some evidence of stressors, depressive symptoms and other issues in the individual's life.

Neurological examination and investigation are normal.

Treatment can be difficult and is best managed in a multidisciplinary manner with support, psychological intervention and occasionally tricyclic antidepressant medications such as amitriptyline.

Other headaches

Headache can be seen as part of a variety of other systemic illnesses, including:

- Connective tissue disease, e.g. systemic lupus erythematosus.
- Systemic hypertension.
- Hypoglycaemia.
- Sleep and obstructive apnoea.

These should be considered in an individual where they have the above risk factors or alternatively no other cause is found.

Clinical problem

Helen is a 15-year-old girl who had developed daily headaches over a 6-month period. These were present on wakening and on occasion were associated with vomiting without nausea. Recently, she had complained of intermittent double vision and transient episodes of loss of vision lasting seconds only.

On examination she was moderately obese, she was afebrile, and had no abnormal neurocutaneous stigmata. She had a moderate amount of acne over her face. Her blood pressure was 105/65. There were no bruits heard. Her general physical and neurological examinations were normal and there were no focal neurological findings. Her extraocular movements showed a partial left VI nerve palsy and she had gross papilloedema.

Questions

1. What is the differential diagnosis?

2. What investigations are required?

3. What other questions should be asked?

4. What is the management?

Discussion

The headache pattern is consistent with chronic progressive and the history is very suggestive of raised intracranial pressure (ICP). The child has focal neurological findings in that she has a partial VI nerve palsy. In addition, the papilloedema confirms the suspicion of raised ICP. Based on this synthesis, the differential diagnosis is between a mass such as a tumour, hydrocephalus and its causes, or benign intracranial hypertension (BIH) or pseudotumour cerebri. The obesity and the adolescent onset are risk factors for BIH, as are some therapies for acne (see below).

An imaging study is required immediately. MRI scan is the investigation of choice, but if this cannot be obtained rapidly an urgent CT scan is indicated. Although a CT scan will be able to demonstrate a mass or hydrocephalus if present, an MRI may be required to more clearly define an abnormality in the posterior fossa. CT scanning through the posterior fossa can be associated with significant artefact while MRI provides wonderful anatomical detail. If the MRI scan is normal, then the diagnosis is most likely to be BIH and a lumbar puncture with confirmatory CSF pressure measurement is necessary.

BIH can be associated with a number of risk factors including being female, adolescence, obesity, recurrent otitis media, steroid withdrawal, oral contraceptives, tetracycline use, vitamin A overuse and growth hormone treatment. Tetracyclines are used for acne. The major questions to be asked in this case are to ascertain whether any of the medications listed are being used, as withdrawal may be helpful in management.

Even though this disorder is named 'benign', it is potentially serious with the potential for permanent visual loss. Management involves close monitoring of vision, withdrawal of risk factors (drugs), lowering of ICP by lumbar puncture, and the use of drugs to decrease CSF production (acetazolamide). If vision is deteriorating despite active management, neurosurgical procedures such as lumboperitoneal shunting and optic nerve fenestration are necessary.

This patient had a normal MRI scan of the brain. Lumbar puncture confirmed a diagnosis of benign intracranial hypertension.

FITS AND FAINTS

Andrew Kornberg

Introduction

There are few events more frightening to parents than their child having a seizure. Seizures are common in childhood, with about 7% of children having a seizure of some type. Epilepsy is defined as recurrent unprovoked *afebrile seizures*. Epilepsy has a prevalence of approximately 0.5% in childhood. Seizures are classified on clinical and EEG grounds into two main groups: partial seizures and generalized seizures (Table 15.1). Partial seizures originate in a localized part of the brain, whereas generalized seizures commence synchronously from both hemispheres. A partial seizure may become secondarily generalized. In addition to the classification of seizure types, there is a classification of epilepsies or epileptic syndromes. An epilepsy syndrome includes seizure type, possible aetiology, associated clinical features (such as intellectual disability), EEG and imaging findings, prognosis and therapy (Table 15.2).

Outline

There are a number of steps in the assessment of a child with suspected seizures. The steps include:

- Distinguish epileptic seizures from non-epileptic attacks.
- Determine the types of epileptic seizures the child is having.
- If possible, try to make an epilepsy syndrome diagnosis.

The diagnosis of epileptic seizures is a *clinical* one with investigations used to confirm the diagnosis, help characterize the seizure disorder and determine the underlying cause. Hypoglycaemia and hypocalcaemia should always be considered as possible causes of the seizures, especially in infancy. EEG is seldom of value in the assessment of febrile convulsions but in other seizure disorders it may be helpful in distinguishing

Table 15.1   Classification of seizure type

Partial (focal)

Simple partial: consciousness preserved. Event consists of focal motor or sensory disturbance

Complex partial: consciousness impaired. Event may consist of staring with automatisms

Secondarily generalized

Generalized

Tonic–clonic

Absence

Myoclonic

Clonic

Tonic

Atonic

Table 15.2   Common epilepsy syndromes in childhood

Neonate

Symptomatic neonatal seizures

Benign neonatal convulsions (familial and non-familial)

Infancy

Febrile convulsions

Infantile spasms

Childhood

Myoclonic epilepsies, including Lennox–Gastaut syndrome

Typical absence epilepsy of childhood (petit mal epilepsy)

Benign (idiopathic) partial epilepsies of childhood (benign partial epilepsy of Childhood with centrotemporal spikes)

Temporal lobe epilepsy and other partial epilepsies

Adolescence

Juvenile myoclonic epilepsy

Juvenile absence epilepsy

Temporal lobe epilepsy and other partial epilepsies

partial from generalized seizures and in distinguishing various epilepsy syndromes. Video-EEG monitoring during a seizure may be useful in diagnosis and treatment, and brain imaging, usually with MRI, is indicated in children with seizures that are partial, have focal EEG abnormalities, evidence of neurological impairment or uncontrolled seizures. Brain imaging is rarely necessary in the idiopathic seizure syndromes such as typical absence epilepsy and benign partial epilepsy of childhood.

Many children referred for assessment of epilepsy do not have epilepsy, but some other paroxysmal non-epileptic disorder. In differentiating epileptic from non-epileptic events the description of the event and the surrounding circumstances of the event are very important. The history obtained may be sufficient to diagnose a non-epileptic basis to the events; however, in some cases more detailed investigations such as video-EEG monitoring may be necessary to make a specific diagnosis.

This chapter will review the most common types of seizures, seizure syndromes and non-epileptic events that may be confused with epilepsy.

Neonatal seizures

Neonatal seizures are different from seizures occurring in older children because of the different aetiologies involved as well as the varied, and often subtle, clinical manifestations. A variety of neonatal seizure types have been described and include:

- Subtle.
- Generalized tonic.
- Multifocal clonic.
- Focal clonic.
- Myoclonic.

Subtle seizures include eye, orofacial or limb movements and may be missed without video-EEG monitoring. Tonic events consist of a generalized extensor spasm and are usually associated with a severe brain insult. Clonic seizures (which may be generalized, focal or multifocal) involve the jerking of a limb. Classical tonic–clonic seizures are rarely seen in the newborn. Myoclonic seizures consist of a sudden contraction of a muscle or group of muscles, causing symptoms from jerking of a limb to massive flexion of the body. Unlike in older infants and children, neonatal seizures are not always accompanied by EEG changes.

There are varied aetiologies associated with neonatal seizures. These include:

- *Hypoxic–ischaemic encephalopathy.* Various abnormalities of the pregnancy, labour and delivery may be present on historical grounds. Fetal distress, evidence for asphyxia (poor feeding, decreased alertness) and other organ dysfunction are clinical pointers.
- *Metabolic disturbance.* Hypoglycaemia and hypocalcaemia are the most common metabolic causes of neonatal convulsions. Various inborn errors of metabolism are associated with neonatal seizures but form a rare group of causes.
- *Infections.* These may be acquired in utero: for example, cytomegalovirus (CMV) and toxoplasmosis; or acquired postnatally: for example, bacterial infections such as meningitis (group B streptococcus) or septicaemia, or viral such as herpes simplex virus infections.
- *Developmental structural anomalies of the brain.* Disorders of cerebral cortical development are being increasingly recognized as important causes of seizures in early infancy and childhood, mainly through improvements in MRI.
- *Benign familial neonatal convulsions.* This dominantly inherited disorder of familial seizures occurs in otherwise normal neonates. A family history is mandatory.

Phenomena confused with neonatal seizures include jitteriness. This is a coarse tremulousness that can be seen in any infant, but can be associated with hypoglycaemia or hypothermia. Jitteriness is usually associated with stimulation and can be abolished by holding the limb (a clonic seizure will continue) or swaddling the infant. Primitive reflexes such as the Moro reflex may also be interpreted as seizures. The circumstance associated with the event and the observation of it will allow a proper diagnosis to be made.

West syndrome (infantile spasms)

This type of epilepsy occurs in the first year of life. The seizures are often difficult to control, and children frequently develop severe intellectual disability. Other seizure types may occur later. The EEG is disorganized, with a pattern of generalized high-voltage slow wave, sharp wave and spike activity called hypsarrhythmia. The terms salaam spasms and jack-knife seizures are also sometimes used synonymously with the term 'infantile spasms'.

The onset is usually between 3 and 8 months of age, with males affected more commonly. Individual attacks usually consist of a flexor or 'salaam' spasm, with the sudden drawing up of the legs on the abdomen and hunching forward of the neck and shoulders. The arms are often flung out in extension. The events are commonly accompanied by a cry and are occasionally misdiagnosed as colic. The events typically occur in clusters soon after wakening. In many children, with the onset of spasms, there may be a sudden regression of social and motor skills. This regression of skills can be helpful in differentiating this syndrome from colic and the Moro reflex, which are occasionally misdiagnosed.

Infantile spasms have many different causes and are the product of a severe insult to the immature nervous system. In about half the infants no cause is found, with development being normal until the onset of the spasms. This group is called cryptogenic. In about one-third there is a history of an abnormal event in the prenatal or perinatal periods (symptomatic). One of the most common underlying causes is tuberous sclerosis, with depigmented patches found on examination of the skin. Other causes include a cerebral malformation, and metabolic disorders such as phenylketonuria. Pertussis immunization was suggested as a possible cause of infantile spasms, but epidemiological studies have refuted the association.

Febrile convulsions

Fever and convulsions may be present, with CNS infections such as meningitis or encephalitis. However, most commonly fever and convulsions occur together in the syndrome of febrile convulsions (FC), where there is a lowered threshold to seizures in the presence of fever. Studies have shown that FC occur in approximately 3–5% of the population, and that in approximately one-third of cases the FC are recurrent. Approximately 3% of children with FC go on to epilepsy.

An FC is defined as a seizure in which:

- There is neither clinical nor laboratory evidence of an infective process directly involving the central nervous system.
- The temperature is 38°C or higher, in a child who has not had convulsions in the absence of fever.
- Onset is between 5 months and 5 years of age.

The convulsions are usually generalized tonic–clonic in nature, although any type of seizure can occur. The majority of seizures are brief, although some children may have prolonged events. Even with prolonged seizures, large epidemiological studies have shown that the prognosis for normal development in children is excellent. Recurrence of FC is more likely if the first seizure occurs in early infancy or if there is a family history of FC. Although only a small proportion of children who have FC will develop epilepsy in later life, the prevalence of epilepsy is increased in patients who have had febrile convulsions compared with those who have not (3% vs 0.5%).

The following have been shown to be associated with an increased risk for the later development of epilepsy:

- Abnormal development or neurological status.
- Focal features present during the febrile convulsion or in the post-ictal period.
- Prolonged febrile convulsions (more than 15 minutes duration).
- Recurrent febrile convulsions within the one febrile illness.
- A positive family history of epilepsy in first-degree relatives.

The long-term use of anti-epileptic medications to prevent recurrence of FC is rarely used:

- Because of the benign nature of the great majority of febrile convulsions.
- Because there is no evidence that anticonvulsant medication diminishes the likelihood of later epilepsy.
- Because of the potential adverse effects of treatment.

Typical absence (petit mal) seizures

Absence seizures usually commence between 5 and 10 years of age, and are rare under the age of 3 years. A typical absence consists of the sudden cessation of activity with staring, usually lasting only 5–10 seconds. Blinking, upward deviation of the eyes, slight mouthing movements and some fumbling hand movements may occur (automatisms). The child does not fall with an absence event although there may be some loss of postural tone. The event is rarely associated with incontinence and is not associated with post-episode drowsiness. Many attacks usually occur

in a day. Attacks are accompanied by a characteristic EEG pattern of three-per-second generalized spike and wave activity, which can be induced by hyperventilation. The prognosis is good.

The main differentials of absence epilepsy are 'daydreaming' and complex partial seizures of temporal lobe type (see below). Daydreaming episodes can be diagnosed by the situations in which they occur, and the response to verbal or physical stimulation.

Benign partial epilepsy of childhood with centrotemporal spikes

Benign partial epilepsy of childhood with centrotemporal spikes is one of the most common forms of epilepsy in childhood. It is also known as benign focal epilepsy of childhood. The onset is usually between 5 and 10 years of age, with the seizures most commonly involving the mouth, tongue and face. At times, the seizure may be limited to a 'fuzzy' feeling of the side of the face, mouth and tongue. Other manifestations include twitching of one side of the face, gurgling and choking noises, with salivation being a prominent finding. Consciousness can be preserved but there is often an inability to speak during an attack. The event may spread from the face and involve the arm and leg and then it may secondarily generalize. The clinical events are commonly nocturnal. The seizure focus is in the central sulcus region on one or both sides. Although the seizures are partial in nature, focal cerebral pathology is not present.

The prognosis is excellent.

Temporal lobe epilepsy

Scarring of the medial temporal lobe structures (mesial temporal sclerosis) commonly causes temporal lobe epilepsy, although developmental malformations of the temporal lobe and tumours are relatively common causes as well.

Seizures may commence at any age, but usually begin during the first decade of life. The seizure often begins with the cessation of activity, and an expression of 'fear'. During this phase, the child is usually described as staring and unresponsive. Although this phase may be similar to that of children with absence seizures, temporal lobe seizures are usually of longer duration with a less abrupt onset and offset. Post-episode drowsiness is the norm. Automatisms are common and autonomic disturbance (flushing, pallor, salivation) may be evident. There may be a preceding aura of abdominal discomfort, a feeling of familiarity (déja vu), fear, and unusual smells (olfactory hallucinations). The prognosis for temporal lobe seizures is poor, with many children not obtaining complete seizure control. Spontaneous remission is rare.

Non-epileptic phenomena (Table 15.3)

Breath-holding attacks

Attacks usually commence in the first or second year of life, but occasionally from the earliest months of age. Recognition that the attacks are precipitated by either physical trauma (a minor knock to the head or other injury) or emotional trauma (fright, anger or frustration) is important in making the diagnosis. The attack usually commences with crying, but this may be brief or inconspicuous. The child takes a deep breath but during inspiration stops breathing. Cyanosis occurs, and then after an interval the child may become limp and unconscious. Rarely, the child may have some brief tonic stiffening or clonic jerking in response to the cerebral hypoxia. Incontinence may occur. Recovery is usually rapid, although some children are drowsy and lethargic if they have had an anoxic seizure. Many a parent has initially thought that their child had died during a breath-holding attack and it is important that the family is reassured that the events are benign and will abate in time.

Reflex anoxic seizures

With reflex anoxic attacks, marked bradycardia or asystole of brief duration occurs. These children have been shown to have an abnormally sensitive response to carotid sinus and eyeball pressure, with the production of marked bradycardia or asystole. The events begin in a similar fashion to breath-holding spells with an acute precipitating event such as physical or emotional trauma. The child then becomes profoundly pale, with marked bradycardia or asystole. The resulting cerebral anoxia leads to a brief tonic or tonic–clonic seizure. Recognition that the attacks are precipitated by either physical or emotional trauma will allow correct diagnosis. Atropine may be useful to prevent the profound bradycardia during episodes.

Syncope

Syncope or fainting is common in childhood. The decreased cerebral perfusion leads to loss of consciousness and collapse. Brief tonic stiffening, clonic jerking and incontinence can follow the loss of consciousness and may lead to misdiagnosis as an epileptic seizure unless a careful history is obtained. The diagnosis of syncopal attacks can usually be made on clinical grounds, as follows:

- *Posture*. Faints commonly occur while standing for long periods, or when suddenly moving from a supine to upright posture.
- *Recall*. An awareness of light-headedness, visual loss and a cold sweat prior to the event are clues to the diagnosis.
- *Situation*. Situations that are frequently associated with syncope in children are vomiting illnesses, prolonged standing, venipuncture, or sustaining or witnessing an injury.

Syncope without an obvious precipitant or syncope during exercise should prompt concern about a cardiac cause (e.g. prolonged QTc syndrome or aortic stenosis) and cardiac evaluation is indicated.

Table 15.3 Non-epileptic paroxysmal events

	Breath-holding attacks	Shuddering	Benign paroxysmal vertigo	Infantile self-stimulation	'Daydreams'	Night terrors	Nightmares	Syncope
Age	Infancy	Infancy	Preschool	Preschool	School	Preschool/school age	All ages	All ages
Circumstances	Always upset or a trigger is identified	Anytime/anywhere	Anytime/anywhere	Anytime/anywhere	Commonly school, watching TV, or at other times of inactivity	First third of sleep (non-REM)	Second half of sleep (REM)	Triggering factor or situation
Frequency	Varies	Sometimes many per day	1 per month or less	Daily or less often	Varies but not large numbers in a day	Nightly or less	Nightly or less	Occasional
Onset	Sudden, with or without crying	Sudden	Sudden	Sudden	Vague	Sudden	Sudden	Gradual or sudden
Recovery	Slow if anoxic seizure occurs	Rapid	Rapid	Rapid	Vague. May be snapped out of event	Returns to sleep	Remains asleep	Gradual
Duration	Seconds to minutes	Seconds	1–5 minutes	Minutes to hours	Seconds to minutes	Minutes	Minutes	Seconds to minutes
Impairment of consciousness	Usually	None	None	None	Apparent but not real	Apparently awake but does not respond	Asleep	Yes
Observations	Cyanotic or pale, limp, may have a seizure	Rapid shivering movements maximal in head, trunk and arms. Some relationship to excitement	Frightened, pale, holds onto objects to maintain balance. Nystagmus may be noted	Posturing with stiffening while lying on side. Irregular breathing, flushing, sweating	Blank staring but no motor automatisms or blinking. Not precipitated by hyperventilation	Screaming, crying inconsolably. Appears terrified	Nil	May describe light-headedness, dizziness or loss of vision. Seizure may occur at end of event
Post-event impairment	Mild unless anoxic seizure occurs	None	None	None	None	No recollection of event	Good recall of event	Minimal
Main differential diagnosis	Epilepsy	Epilepsy	Epilepsy	Seizures/abdominal pain, movement disorder	Absence seizures	Frontal lobe epilepsy	Night terrors	Epilepsy/Cardiac

Clinical problem

Peter, an 8-year-old boy, was referred for assessment of events that occurred four times over the previous 3 months. Each episode occurred around 6 a.m. The episodes were witnessed by an elder brother, who slept in the same room. The events consisted of Peter gagging and choking, without loss of consciousness. Peter was unable to speak. His brother had noticed that there was some jerking of Peter's jaw, with profuse salivation. One of the episodes progressed to a tonic–clonic seizure. The other three episodes were short lived and ceased spontaneously. His development and examination were normal.

Questions

1. What is the most likely diagnosis?

2. Should he have further investigations such as brain imaging?

Discussion

The nocturnal occurrence of seizures in a child of primary school age, with symptoms referrable to the orofacial region, strongly suggests the diagnosis is benign partial epilepsy of childhood with centrotemporal spikes.

In any child presenting with recurrent seizures, an EEG should be performed. This may confirm the clinical diagnosis and provide further supporting evidence for the seizure disorder being partial or generalized, or consistent with a specific epilepsy syndrome. An EEG in Peter's case showed typical focal epileptiform activity in the left central sulcus region. In view of the very typical clinical story and EEG findings, an imaging study was not performed, although close clinical follow-up is necessary.

HEARING PROBLEMS
Adrian Brooke

Introduction

Hearing problems occur when the normal functioning of either the aural apparatus or the central components of the auditory pathway are disrupted. As the intensity of sound is measured in decibels, hearing losses can be quantified and conventionally a hearing threshold of 25 dB or less is considered normal. The ear as an organ of special sense and the rest of the auditory pathway develops sensibility to a wide variety of sound stimuli; this includes a wide range of frequencies (high tones and low tones) as well as a wide range of sound intensities (from whispering to disco music). Because of the organ's function in detecting speech sounds for the developing brain to decode during language acquisition, hearing difficulties in early childhood can affect the emergence of speech and language skills. Problems in communicating can cause great frustration to the young child, which can then manifest in a range of difficult behaviours.

In childhood, the mechanical and neural parts of the ear and auditory pathway can be affected by a wide range of congenital and acquired pathologies that in turn interfere with normal functioning. The resultant hearing impairment can vary from mild and transient through to severe and persistent. One or both ears can be affected. Mild hearing difficulties in childhood are common, and approximately 1 child per 10 000 is affected by moderate hearing loss.[1,2] Temporary hearing loss is very common in young children during upper respiratory tract infections and during acute otitis media.[3] Otitis media with effusion (secretory otitis media) that can follow these episodes can cause fluctuating hearing loss but nonetheless this type of loss may interfere with language acquisition during this period of developmental vulnerability.[4]

Outline

When approaching the problem of hearing difficulties, one has to differentiate between conductive and sensorineural hearing loss to determine the degree of hearing loss and the extent (frequency range affected). A search for the aetiological causes of both forms of hearing loss should include consideration of associated congenital or inherited syndromes. Some children behave as though hearing impairment is present although formal testing shows normal aural acuity. These children may have functional hearing loss, or a central pathology causing difficulty with the processing of auditory stimuli, e.g. Landau–Kleffner syndrome.

The principal causes of hearing impairment are:

- Chromosomal abnormalities causing non-syndromic sensorineural deafness; for example:
  - Connexin 26 gene deletions.
- Inherited disorders resulting in structural problems; for example:
  - Down's syndrome.
  - Treacher Collins' syndrome.
  - Goldenhar's syndrome.
  - Pendred's syndrome (with Mondini malformation of the inner ear).
  - Osteogenesis imperfecta.
  - Cleft palate.
  - CHARGE syndrome.
- Other inherited causes:
  - Usher's syndrome.
  - Alport's syndrome.
  - Waardenburg's syndrome.
  - DIDMOAD.
  - Albinism.
  - Mucopolysaccharidosis.
- Damage to the auditory system during pregnancy or the perinatal period:
  - Intrauterine infection, e.g. rubella, CMV.
  - Perinatal asphyxia.
  - Meningitis.
  - Kernicterus.
  - Ototoxic drugs.
  - Persistent pulmonary hypertension of the newborn (PPHN).
- Damage to the auditory system acquired after the perinatal period:
  - Otitis media with effusion (secretory otitis media; glue ear).
  - Otosclerosis.
  - Trauma.
  - Infection (meningitis).
  - Ototoxic drugs.

History

The history of the hearing problem should concentrate on the duration of symptoms, carers' perception of its severity and an idea of its course. It should be established whether the hearing problems are apparently new, steadily worsening, fluctuating, if they are associated with upper respiratory tract infections (suggesting otitis media with effusion) or related to other symptoms (e.g. haematuria in Alport's syndrome, whereas night blindness or apparent increasing clumsiness may point to Usher's syndrome). Enquiry should also focus on the child's speech and behaviour. The effect on speech development, quality of speech production and clarity should be sought and any behaviour changes or difficulties should be noted. Some parents of children with hearing loss may report that the child starts to shout when speaking, sits close to the television or turns up the volume. Some children may not respond to quiet verbal cues, or to those that are delivered out of the line of sight of the child. Others may be noted to look intently at the lips of the speaker. Symptoms directly attributable to the ear should be enquired about, such as painful or discharging ears.

A developmental history should also be taken to see if any other domains are affected. Past history should begin with pregnancy, including:

- Maternal health during pregnancy, including medications.
- Rash, fever, in pregnancy (intrauterine infection).
- Length of gestation.
- Delivery.
- Postnatal course (kernicterus, PPHN, meningitis, exposure to ototoxic drugs, asphyxia or complications of prematurity).

Any significant postnatal history of chronic ear infections or other middle ear disease should be noted, as should any history of meningitis or significant head injury. The presence of congenital malformations giving rise to obvious dysmorphic syndromes is usually obvious to families early on and should be noted.

Any family history of early hearing loss, renal problems, thyroid disease or deafness should be recorded as each may point to a syndrome associated with deafness. Early fetal losses in the extended family may point to a possible metabolic cause. A family history of unexplained sudden death may suggest syndromes that combine deafness with abnormalities of cardiac rhythm (Jervell's and Lange–Nielson syndromes).

Examination

Initial observation should concentrate on identifying any obvious dysmorphism (Down's, Treacher Collins', Goldenhar's, etc.). A hypopigmented forelock and heterochromia may indicate Waardenburg's syndrome. The configuration, position and orientation of the pinnae should be noted and may point to specific diagnoses (Down's, Goldenhar's, etc.). General habitus and thyroid state should be assessed (Pendred's syndrome).

The pinnae and ear canals should be scrutinized to check for the presence of otitis externa. It is wise to delay examination of painful ears until the assessment of the child has been otherwise completed. Even when not painful, inspection of the tympanic membrane is usually one of the last parts of the examination of a younger child, as it seldom engenders full cooperation during the rest of the examination. The drum should be examined to assess size, presence of dullness, scarring or evidence of recent or past perforation (including presence of grommets). The drum may be dull or retracted; a fluid level or air bubble may be visible through the drum, indicating the presence of middle ear inflammation (otitis media). A bulging reddened drum may indicate an active infection, such as acute otitis media.

Assessment of hearing should be done formally, when indicated, but the precise modality of testing depends upon the age and degree of cooperation of the child. Pure tone audiometry is possible in children with cognitive attainments of 5 years or older; babies who are able to turn their heads to sound (i.e. at least 7 months of age) may be suitable for distraction testing, although this is a skilled activity that requires two operators and is itself heavily operator dependent. Most other modalities of testing (free field testing, performance testing, warble or chime bar, McCormick toy discrimination test) require specific training. The other cranial nerves should be tested, including fundoscopy (Usher's syndrome; cataracts, retinitis and microphthalmia of congenital rubella syndrome). The presence of neurocutaneous stigmata should be sought (neurofibromatosis).

Investigations

Problem	Investigation		Possible diagnosis
Any type	Age-appropriate audiometry; other family members may need to be screened		
Conductive loss	Tympanometry		Serous otitis media
			Otosclerosis
Sensorineural	Urinalysis: blood		Alport's
	Urinalysis: glucose		DIDMOAD
	Urinalysis: glycosaminoglycans		Mucopolysaccharidoses
	Urinalysis: cytomegalovirus	Up to day 7	Congenital CMV infection
	Blood	Viral serology	Congenital infection
		VDRL	Congenital syphilis
		Thyroid function tests	Pendred's
		Perchlorate test	Pendred's
		Karyotype	Down's
		deletion studies	Connexin 26 gene deletion

Problem	Investigation		Possible diagnosis
Sensorineural (cont'd)	ECG	Looking for prolonged Q–T interval	Jervell and Lange–Nielson syndromes
	MRI/CT	Looking for abnormalities of inner ear/focal cerebral deficits	Pendred's toxoplasmosis/ CMV
	Visual acuity testing and fundoscopy		Usher's
	ERG		Usher's

References

1. Martin JAM, Moore WJ. Childhood deafness in the European Community. Brussels/Luxembourg: Commission of the European communities (EUR 6413)
2. Van Naarden KMPH, Decoufle PScD, Caldwell KMD. Prevalence and characteristics of children with serious hearing impairment in metropolitan Atlanta, 1991–1993. Pediatrics 1999; 103(3):570–575
3. Hendly JO. Otitis media [clinical practice], N Engl J Med 2002; 347(15):1169–1174
4. Sudhakar-Krishnan V, Rudolf M. Do grommets prevent language delay? Arch Dis Child 2002; 87(3):260–262

Clinical problem

An 8-month-old boy was referred by the health visitor following a failed distraction test. The test was made difficult by the fact that the boy was delayed in his development and had only just attained sitting and still had imperfect head control. An audiologist rechecked the infant's hearing using free-field testing and obtained the following result:

Free-field audiometer	Without aids		
	Bilateral	R	L
250 Hz		90/95 dB	90/95 dB
500 Hz		90/95 dB	90/95 dB
1000 Hz			
2000 Hz			
4000 Hz		90 dB	90 dB
6000 Hz			

Questions

1. How would you describe his hearing problems on the basis of the free-field testing?

2. What problems may have influenced the results of the initial distraction testing?

Answers

1. The results demonstrate severe bilateral hearing loss but they must be interpreted with great caution.

2. There are major problems in jumping to the conclusion that this child has severe hearing loss. His general delay may mean that he has not yet reached the developmental age of being able to localize sound. Even if this has been acquired his motor problems are such that it may not be possible for him to respond appropriately. Clearly the test will need to be repeated, if he fails again, and supplemented with more sophisticated tests, such as auditory evoked brainstem potentials. However, of equal importance is to consider the extent and possible cause of his delayed development, since if his hearing loss is genuine it is important to try and understand whether this is part of a pattern of deficits or if the hearing loss is responsible for the delay in other areas.

NOISY BREATHING
Elaine Carter

Introduction

Breathing should be a silent process and noisy breathing, in general, indicates an abnormality in the upper or lower respiratory tract. Noises may arise from a variety of causes and a variety of sites; for example:

■ An abnormally narrowed airway. This is the cause in snoring (blocked nose and/or pharynx), stridor (narrowed extra thoracic airway) and wheeze (narrowed intrathoracic airways).
■ Movement of secretions. For example, 'rattles' in the upper airway and crepitations from fluid filled alveoli.
■ A noise is also produced when a child tries to increase his or her end expiratory pressure in order to keep open alveoli. This is achieved by partially closing the larynx during expiration and results in a grunt.

Outline

Noises can be considered in two groups: those heard without a stethoscope, and those heard only with a stethoscope.

■ Audible without a stethoscope:
  – Stridor.
  – Snore.
  – Wheeze (sometimes *not* audible without a stethoscope).
  – Rattle.
  – Grunt.
■ Audible with a stethoscope:
  – Altered character of breath sounds, such as bronchial breathing.
  – Added sounds, including wheezes, rubs and crepitations.
  – Transmitted sounds.

Noises audible without a stethoscope

Stridor

This is a continuous harsh sound that arises in either the larynx or the extrathoracic trachea. Narrowing of these structures, from whatever cause, leads to increased airflow velocity and turbulence. During inspiration the larynx and extrathoracic trachea, which is relatively compliant in children, undergo dynamic compression and this leads to further reduction in the airway. For this reason stridor is heard more commonly in inspiration. The obstruction to airflow causes increased respiratory effort and a large negative pleural pressure. In turn, this causes signs of respiratory distress, such as intercostal and subcostal recession, tachypnoea and use of accessory muscles of respiration. There are several important causes of stridor, the main ones being congenital laryngomalacia, croup, epiglottitis, foreign body and bacterial tracheitis.

Laryngomalacia

This presents soon after birth but it is unusual for there to be any accompanying respiratory distress. It is caused by laxity of the laryngeal tissues and adjacent structures such as the epiglottis. Characteristically the severity of the stridor varies with activity and position. The condition improves with age.

Croup

Caused by para-influenza virus, it is the commonest cause of stridor. After a mild cold, the child develops stridor, with a low-grade temperature, a hoarse voice and a harsh, barking cough. It affects children aged 6 months to 6 years. Most children recover with no problems, but 1% have severe obstruction and require intubation. Signs of obstruction must therefore be monitored closely. This is by clinical means, including pulse rate, respiratory rate, degree of recession, oxygen saturation and signs of exhaustion.

Epiglottitis

The commonest cause was *Haemophilus influenzae* but this is now less common following the introduction of HIB vaccine. There is typically sudden onset of severe stridor, with drooling, toxic appearance and very high temperature. Children often sit forward and look anxious but some may have difficulty breathing and swallowing, with very little stridor. It is important that a tongue depressor is not used during the examination as the change in posture and pain produced may provoke a respiratory arrest. There is usually shock and septicaemia. Rapid progression of obstruction occurs in 80% of cases, hence all suspected cases should be transferred to intensive care with minimal disturbance, examined under anaesthetic, and intubated. An ENT surgeon should be present to perform a tracheostomy in the event of failed intubation.

Bacterial tracheitis

This condition is usually caused by *Staphylococcus aureus* and presents with a similar clinical picture to epiglottitis. It affects a slightly older age group. The trachea is inflamed and copious pus is produced.

Foreign body

Stridor is acute in onset in an afebrile child. Obstruction may be complete or partial, and may be at laryngeal level, or bronchial, if the foreign body passes through the larynx. There may or may not have been a history of choking on a foreign body.

Diphtheria

A rare but serious cause of stridor. There is a grey mucosal slough on the larynx, causing severe obstruction.

Vascular ring

Another rare cause of stridor which is typically present consistently in affected children. However, the degree of obstruction will usually increase during intercurrent upper airway infections and this may cause diagnostic confusion.

Snoring

This is a coarse, continuous noise that occurs during sleep but does not necessarily imply serious obstruction. It arises from pharyngeal structures. In some cases it is associated with other signs of respiratory distress such as recession and apnoea, indicating that significant obstruction is occurring. The commonest cause is adenotonsillar hypertrophy. Mild obstruction may cause frequent sleep disturbance, while in severe cases hypoxia, hypercarbia and secondary cor pulmonale may result.

Rattle

Small children with upper respiratory tract infections often have a 'rattle'. This is a coarse, irregular sound produced by the movement of excess mucus in the airway during the respiratory cycle. It does not usually indicate significant pathology. However, it is also likely to be present in children who have conditions that result in hypersecretion such as asthma, cystic fibrosis, abnormal ciliary clearance of mucus and recurrent aspiration.

Grunting

This is produced by partial glottic closure during expiration in an attempt to raise alveolar pressure. It characteristically occurs in neonates with respiratory distress, and older children with pneumonia.

Wheeze

This is a common problem in childhood: 20% of children under 5 years wheeze at some time. The wheezing noise probably results from narrowing of the major bronchi. When expiration becomes an active process (perhaps as a result of narrowing in adjacent smaller airways) dynamic compression of major airways occurs. This results in turbulent high-velocity flow and hence noise.

Asthma is the commonest cause of wheezing. Symptoms are caused by increased responsiveness of the patient's airways to a variety of stimuli, including upper respiratory infection, change of temperature, exercise, environmental pollutants and exposure to allergens such as pollens and moulds. The history is usually of recurrent episodes of difficulty breathing with wheeze, and on examination during an attack there is respiratory distress. There may be a history of atopy in the child or family. Wheeze is the typical finding and is often heard even without the help of a stethoscope. Obstruction may be so severe that the chest is silent and this is a very serious sign. The chest may be hyperinflated and there may be a Harrison's sulcus, which indicates chronic airway obstruction. An exercise tolerance test will induce wheeze in 95% of asthmatics, and is a good diagnostic test. The wheeze thus produced is reversible with a beta-2 agonist inhaler.

Preschool children often have wheeze and breathlessness but only in response to upper respiratory tract infections. This is thought to constitute a different disease entity from classical asthma, and the problem frequently resolves as the child grows older. These children are less likely to respond to inhaled (preventive) steroids.

Babies under a year who contract respiratory syncytial virus infection characteristically have wheeze and features of airway obstruction, with crepitations in the inspiratory phase of respiration. This condition, termed bronchiolitis, occurs in the winter season, and affects large numbers of babies. Babies who contract it have an increased tendency to recurrent wheeze in later years.

Noises heard with a stethoscope only

Altered quality of breath sounds

The normal quality of breath sounds is termed vesicular, and is typically low pitched and heard throughout inspiration; expiration follows without a distinct pause. Expiratory breath sounds are heard only in the first part of expiration, causing a quiet phase before the onset of the next inspiration. The inspiratory breath sound is therefore longer than the expiratory breath sound; however, this should not be confused with the duration of the inspiratory and expiratory phases of respiration. During normal breathing the inspiratory phase is shorter than the expiratory.

Bronchial breathing is harsher than normal, more intense, and there is a pause between inspiration and expiration. The inspiratory breath sound and expiratory breath sound are heard for approximately equal lengths of time. Bronchial breathing occurs when underlying consolidation enhances the conduction of sound.

Added sounds

These are of three types:

- Continuous whistling sounds, caused by airways obstruction. They are called rhonchi or wheeze.
- Interrupted crackling sounds, which generally occur with alveolar pathology. They are called crackles or crepitations. They may be fine, for

example in pulmonary oedema, or coarse, as in pneumonia and bronchiolitis.

■ A rub is a coarse, rasping sound, arising from inflamed pleural surfaces, and is in time with respiration.

Transmitted sounds

Frequently, coarse rattles are heard in an infant's chest in both phases of respiration. These represent sounds conducted from the upper airways, and do not signify significant pathology; however, their presence makes auscultation of the lower respiratory tract difficult to interpret.

History

A description of the noise is needed. Ask particularly about:

■ The quality of the noise, e.g. musical as in wheeze or harsh as in stridor, or crackly and palpable as produced by an upper airway rattle?
■ The timing of the noise. Is the noise predominantly inspiratory as in stridor, or predominantly expiratory, as in wheeze, or does it occur in both phases of respiration, as produced by an upper airway rattle?

The timing of onset of the noise is important. For example, in acute stridor, did the stridor come on very suddenly as in inhaled foreign body or epiglottitis, or did the stridor develop more gradually over a few days, following on from a simple upper respiratory tract infection (more typical of croup)? Similarly, viral-induced wheeze and asthma are often preceded by an upper respiratory tract infection.

It is important to establish whether there have been features of respiratory distress, such as rapid breathing. This is common in all lower respiratory tract infections and obstructed airways.

Information about other features of respiratory disease, such as cough, is helpful. If the child does have a cough ask about the nature of the cough. A barking cough suggests croup, while a prolonged and repeated cough ending in a whoop suggests whooping cough. In older children the parents may have seen sputum produced by the child and, if purulent, this provides further evidence of lower respiratory infection.

It is important to establish if the child has had a fever. In bacterial infections such as epiglottitis and pneumonia the fever is usually high, while in croup and bronchiolitis it is rarely above 38°C.

In some cases it will be important to try and establish whether the child could have aspirated a foreign body. There may be an obvious history in which the child was seen playing with peanuts or other small objects, followed by sudden onset of stridor or wheeze. However, most children with a foreign body do not have a clear history of this type.

Past medical history can be very helpful since wheezy children have often experienced previous episodes. Similarly, children who suffer bronchiolitis as an infant often go on to develop recurrent wheeze. In other children there may be a history of previous problems which cause them to respond atypically to subsequent respiratory insults. For example:

■ Preterm infants who required respiratory support after birth may be left with chronic lung disease (and hence reduced respiratory reserve) and or subglottic stenosis following prolonged intubation.
■ Children with congenital heart disease are more susceptible to recurrent respiratory infections. In addition, common conditions such as bronchiolitis often cause much more severe symptoms in such children.
■ Children with laryngomalacia may cope poorly with infections of the upper airway, such as croup. The dual impact of the usually mild infection and normally benign congenital anomaly can result in respiratory compromise.

Family history will help to establish the extent to which the child has a genetic predisposition for atopic disease such as asthma. Similarly, social history should establish the extent to which the child is exposed to factors known to result in wheeze in susceptible children; for example:

■ Do the parents smoke?
■ Are there any family pets?
■ Where and in what type of accommodation do the family live?
■ What type of heating is used?

Examination

The examination should always commence with a rapid assessment of the child's vital signs, that is: *Airway, Breathing and Circulation*. Clearly, any abnormality must be dealt with at once but a full description is beyond the scope of this book.

After the initial rapid assessment and any necessary resuscitation have taken place it is important to go back and re-examine the respiratory system in more detail. Observe the child:

1. If there is any respiratory noise audible (without a stethoscope) establish both its character and the

phase of respiration in which it is most prominent, e.g. stridor is usually inspiratory, wheeze is expiratory.

2. Look for signs of respiratory distress:
   a) Intercostal and or subcostal recession.
   b) Tachypnoea. The normal respiratory rates for children are:

birth–1:	30–40
2–5:	25–30
6–10:	20–25
>10:	15–20

   c) Use of accessory respiratory muscles.
   d) Tachycardia.
   e) Exhaustion. This occurs as an end phase of respiratory distress and is very important to recognize as the child is in danger of sudden apnoea.
3. Take the temperature.
4. Look for evidence of an upper respiratory infection, such as a runny nose, that may have preceded croup, or provoked wheezing.
5. Identify any features suggesting a chronic respiratory problem such as clubbing, barrel-shaped chest and/or Harrison's sulcus.

Palpation is unlikely to be helpful in the smaller child but may be important in assessing chest expansion in children old enough and well enough to respond to instructions.

Similarly *percussion* requires a certain amount of cooperation from the child. In relation to noisy breathing it is only likely to be helpful in supporting a diagnosis of pneumonia where the percussion note will be dull.

Although *auscultation* should be possible in virtually all children, the information gained will again often reflect the child's ability to cooperate. Where possible assess:

■ The character of the breath sounds: listen specifically for areas of bronchial breathing.
■ Whether there are added sounds such as a rub, crepitations or wheeze. If such findings are present try to localize both where they are best heard and their timing in relation to respiration.

Investigations

Investigations are not always indicated in acute respiratory illnesses producing noisy breathing, such as in croup and asthma. However, a number of investigations, which can be helpful in certain situations, are included in the table.

Investigation	Rationale
Chest X-ray	In relation to 'noisy breathing' the chest X-ray is most useful in examining the lung parenchyma. It is a very poor method of trying to assess the airways. It may be helpful in suspected foreign body, particularly in an older child who can cooperate for an inspiratory and expiratory film (gas trapping occurs distal to the foreign body in expiration)
Peak flow	Useful to provide objective evidence of severity of an asthma attack and also for long-term monitoring of asthma. Cooperation/skill by the child is required. This is normally achieved between 5 and 6 years of age
Full blood count	Primarily used to provide evidence of bacterial infection (neutrophilia)
Blood culture	May allow isolation of organisms causing pneumonia or epiglottitis
Nasopharyngeal aspirate	Immunofluorescence may allow rapid identification of respiratory syncytial virus (RSV) or other viral respiratory pathogens
Laryngoscopy/ bronchoscopy	The definitive tests in relations to problems of the upper airways. Can be used for acute or chronic problems of this region. Where used for acute problems (e.g. severe croup) provision for tracheostomy must always be available
CT scan	Can be useful in a variety of 'non-acute' conditions, e.g. delineating a mass-causing obstruction to one or more major bronchi resulting in persistent but localized wheeze. Spiral CT can allow additional information to be gained about the airways

Clinical problem

In November, a 6-month-old baby was admitted with wheeze and difficulty in breathing. This illness had begun with a cold and cough, and had progressed over 2 days, with rapid, noisy breathing and difficulty in feeding. The child had been born at 32 weeks gestation and had had respiratory distress syndrome. He had required a period on CPAP but had run into no other significant problems from his prematurity. Since then he has been well, and gaining weight.

On examination, he has respiratory rate of 60, recession and wheezing respirations heard both with and without a stethoscope. His saturation in air is 88%.

Questions

1. What is the most likely diagnosis?

2. What tests would you do and why?

3. Name three important management issues.

He initially responds well to oxygen therapy and nasogastric feeding, but the next day he has a sudden deterioration, with a respiratory rate of 80, marked recession, increased oxygen requirement and grunting respiration.

4. What is the likely cause for his deterioration?

5. What further management would you perform?

Answers

1. RSV bronchiolitis is the most likely diagnosis but the child could have viral-induced wheeze or be a newly presenting asthmatic. His future behaviour will be important in confirming or refuting these latter two diagnoses. It is unlikely that his prematurity is of any relevance given his mild respiratory course at that time.

2. A nasopharyngeal aspirate sent for RSV immunofluorescence and viral culture is all that is necessary at this stage to confirm the diagnosis.

3. Important points in management include:
   a) *Maintain fluids.* This can be by mouth provided the course is mild but he may need tube feeds and, if very distressed, intravenous fluids.
   b) *Maintain oxygenation.* Many infants will manage the entire course of bronchiolitis in air but where physical signs or saturation monitoring suggest it would be appropriate the child should be given oxygen.
   c) *Observe.* Most children make a speedy recovery from bronchiolitis but where the course is more severe (e.g. sufficient to require admission) it is important to ensure that the child is closely monitored.

4. Aspiration of feed is the most likely diagnosis although other possibilities include pneumothorax.

5. In relation to aspiration management includes:
   a) Stop feeds.
   b) Perform a chest X-ray.
   c) Give antibiotics.
   d) Give intravenous fluids.
   e) Check blood gases.
   f) Give oxygen/other respiratory support as indicated.

CHAPTER 18

COUGH

Kate Wheeler

Introduction

Cough is a very common symptom in children. It is an expiratory noise with an explosive start arising from the larynx. A cough has two functions:

1. To expel secretions and other material from the airway.
2. To protect against aspiration.

It is generally a reflex action with some voluntary control.

The reflex action consists of several components.

Cough receptors sensitive to mechanical and chemical stimuli are present throughout the lung but especially in the larynx and large airways:

- Slowly adapting tactile receptors.
- Rapidly adapting tactile receptors (present in the carina and the large bronchi).
- C fibre endings (present from the larynx to the alveoli).
- Pulmonary stretch receptors in the smooth muscle of the respiratory tube which respond to mechanical forces in the airway.

These receptors are stimulated by chemicals, mechanical stimulants, e.g. mucus in the airway and physical irritants, e.g. smoke, cold air. Sensitivity of the receptors is increased by inflammatory mediators and viruses, which damage the mucosal epithelium.

Afferent nerves in the vagus and laryngeal nerves carry impulses to the pons and midbrain to a *central cough centre* (not specifically identified); *efferent nerves* return impulses to the muscles of respiration.

The cough mechanism involves:

- Rapid inspiration.
- Closure of vocal cords (glottis).
- Forceful constriction of chest wall, diaphragm and abdominal muscles, i.e. expiration against the closed glottis.

■ Raised intrathoracic pressure initially against the closed glottis.

■ Opening of glottis and rapid expulsions of air.

The sudden acceleration of air out of the airways causes the characteristic noise of the cough. The respiratory tract is lined with a thin film of mucus and any inhaled particles tend to be held in the mucus. During a cough the high linear acceleration of the air column either pushes the particles up towards the glottis within the mucous film or, if they are a suitable size, they are pulled into the air column and expectorated. Large objects in the airways may be difficult to cough up. Cough is only useful at removing objects in the first few branches of the airways. Below that other mechanisms are needed, e.g. cilial movements.

A cough is a natural response to an insult. It is always important to diagnose the primary insult and then direct treatment against the primary pathological process, rather than attempt to treat the cough by altering the physiological cough response with 'cough mixture'.

A depressed or absent cough reflex is always a worry as it leaves the airway unprotected.

Causes of depressed cough reflex

■ Afferent nerves:
  – Local anaesthetics.
  – Trauma to vagus nerve (postoperative).
■ Central:
  – Depressed conscious level from any cause including anaesthetic drugs.
  – Congenital or acquired CNS damage.
  – Preterm babies (<32 weeks).

Diagnoses to consider

■ Acute cough:
  – Acute infection: bacterial or viral, upper or lower respiratory tract infection.
  – Foreign body including aspiration.
  – Exposure to irritant, e.g. fog, smoke, solvents.
■ Chronic cough:
  – Asthma.
  – Infections: viral, URTI – especially adenovirus, influenza virus.
  – Sinusitis.
  – Rhinitis.
  – Pertussis, chlamydia, mycoplasma, TB.
  – Foreign body.
  – Aspiration, gastro-oesophageal reflux, hiatus hernia.
  – Cystic fibrosis.
  – Bronchiectasis.
  – Immobile cilia syndrome.
  – Immune deficiency state.
  – Congenital abnormalities: tracheo-oesophageal fistula, laryngotracheomalacia, vascular ring.
  – Tumours of the respiratory tract, e.g. bronchogenic cyst.
  – Lymphoma with mediastinal mass.
  – Irritants: passive smoking, cigarette smoking, solvent abuse, chemicals, e.g. ammonia.
  – Habit cough.

History

■ *Age of child*. Symptoms from early infancy suggest a congenital abnormality, such as laryngotracheomalacia or an H type tracheo-oesophageal fistula. A staccato cough in infancy if associated with a persisting conjunctivitis may be from chlamydial pneumonitis.

■ *Associated symptoms*:
  – *Acute*. Fever suggests an acute upper respiratory tract infection. If there is pleuritic pain and shortness of breath an acute bacterial (or viral) pneumonia must be considered. Often the cough is not a very marked feature in the initial stages of pneumonia.
  – *Chronic*. Nasal discharge, snoring, mouth breathing may indicate sinusitus or rhinitis. Vomiting and regurgitation suggest recurrent aspiration secondary to gastro-oesophageal reflux.

■ *Type of cough*:
  – Nocturnal, or exercise induced, suggests asthma. A family history of atopy should be explored.
  – Paroxysmal cough especially if associated with an inspiratory 'whoop', apnoea, cyanosis or vomiting is typical of pertussis. The typical 'whoop' is often absent in infants less than 6 months of age. CMV and pneumocystis can also produce a paroxysmal cough.
  – Productive cough is consistent with bronchiectasis which may be secondary to cystic fibrosis or immotile cilia syndrome. In both of these conditions there is often associated failure to thrive.

- *Family history of TB or TB exposure.* Although TB is not a common cause of a chronic cough in children a diagnosis of TB must be considered.
- *Foreign body ingestion.* May be recent or in the past with a history of subsequent coughing and respiratory infections.

- *Family history of atopy, pets at home.* Diagnosis of asthma should be considered.
- *History of smoking at home.* Cough may be secondary to irritants.

Investigations

Investigation	Finding	Possible diagnosis
Chest X-ray	Over-inflated lung fields	Asthma
	Inflammatory changes	Cystic fibrosis
	Upper lobe changes	Aspiration secondary to GOR
	Situs inversus	Kartagener's syndrome
	Asymmetrical lung fields	Inhaled foreign body
	Mediastinal mass	Lymphoma
Full blood count	Neutrophilia	Bacterial pneumonia
	Lymphocytosis	Pertussis
	Eosinophilia	Atopy, parasitic infection
	Neutropenia	Immune deficiency
		Viral infection
ESR, CRP	If raised	Infection
Sputum culture	If positive	Bacterial pneumonia
Immunoglobulins	Immunodeficiency	Congenital
	Raised IgE	Atopy
Nasopharyngeal aspirate	Positive	RSV
Pernasal swab	Positive	Pertussis
Mantoux	Positive	TB
Lung function tests	Air trapping	Asthma
Sinus X-ray		Sinusitis
Barium swallow		TOF, aspiration, vascular ring
Oesophageal pH study		Gastro-oesophageal reflux
Bronchoscopy		Congenital abnormalities
		Foreign body

Differential diagnosis of chronic productive cough (bronchiectasis)

Cause of underlying abnormality	Diagnosis	Features
Airway lumen	Inhaled foreign body	Choking at start of symptoms, vomiting,
	Recurrent aspiration	choking on feeding, depressed cough reflex
Airway mucus	Cystic fibrosis	Loose stools, failure to thrive
Cilia dysfunction	Ciliary dyskinesia	ENT problems, dextrocardia
Airway immune deficiency	Variety of congenital or acquired problems	Recurrent proven chest infections, infection at other sites
Abnormal airway architecture	Congenital	?Other congenital lesions
	Post-infective	Previous whooping cough or measles

Clinical problem

A 3-month-old baby was brought to the hospital A&E department by ambulance after his mother found him cyanosed and gasping for breath 30 minutes after a feed. In the previous 2 weeks he had developed a cough which had been unassociated with infection, fever or feeds. The mother started basic cardiopulmonary resuscitation and the baby stared to breathe again, and was pink and breathing normally on arrival in hospital.

On examination, the baby had a slight inspiratory stridor and subcostal recession; the respiratory rate was 40 per minute and the O_2 saturation in air was 89%. There were no other abnormal chest signs but there was a flow murmur in the pulmonary area with normal heart sounds. The chest X-ray and ECG were normal.

Questions

1. What are the three most likely diagnoses?

2. What three investigations would differentiate these diagnoses?

Answers

This is an ALTE (see Ch. 37, SIDS); as the cough is not associated with an URTI, it is reasonable to conclude that it is directly related to this acute episode. The baby has developed stridor and moderate breathing difficulties, suggesting pulmonary involvement. Gastro-oesophageal reflux is common and may not always be associated with overt vomiting or difficulty in feeding but may cause aspiration. A normal chest X-ray taken soon after the event does not rule out aspiration, however. Stridor is not typical of simple aspiration and suggests an underlying abnormality of the airway such as laryngo- or tracheo-malacia; these abnormalities may be associated with a vascular ring or sling.

Appropriate investigations would include:

- Upper GI contrast study.
- pH probe.
- Echocardiography.
- Bronchoscopy.
- Upper GI endoscopy.

CYANOSIS

John Stroobant

Introduction

Cyanosis, a dusky blue discoloration of skin and mucous membranes, is a variable clinical sign which may indicate a significant pathophysiological problem. If detected, it is essential to determine its cause. The degree of cyanosis may not reflect the severity of the underlying abnormality; subtle changes in colour may occur in serious disease. The development of a differential diagnosis must take into account an understanding of the pathophysiology of cyanosis, the age of the child, include a comprehensive physical examination and may require several straightforward investigations.

Pathophysiology

Deoxygenated blood appears dark red. Cyanosis, the dusky blue discoloration of skin and mucous membranes is produced by the presence of at least 5 g/dL of deoxygenated haemoglobin (Hb). Its presence therefore depends on the total amount of circulating Hb as well as the degree of Hb saturation. Cyanosis may be central or peripheral. Central cyanosis results from incomplete saturation of arterial blood leaving the heart and is caused by either or both cardiac and pulmonary abnormalities. Peripheral cyanosis is due to increased O_2 uptake by peripheral tissues in situations of increased peripheral metabolic activity or where there is slower blood flow when peripheral cutaneous arterioles are constricted by cold, shock or changes in neurovascular tone. It is usually benign and may therefore occur when central arterial saturation is normal, but will be present if there is central cyanosis.

Cyanosis does not always indicate hypoxia, which is a condition where there is an inadequate O_2 supply for normal metabolic activity. If the Hb level is higher than normal (polycythaemia), there may be more than 5 g/dL which is desaturated and cyanosis will occur, although the oxygen content will be sufficient not to cause hypoxia. Conversely, if anaemia is present, all Hb will be saturated but there may be insufficient Hb present to carry enough O_2 for normal metabolism and hypoxia will occur, although the blood will appear bright red.

Gas transport

Transport of O_2 and CO_2 by red blood cells forms part of a critical physiological system to provide O_2 for cellular aerobic metabolism and for the removal of CO_2 from this process. Other important components of this system include delivery of O_2 to the lungs, efficient pulmonary gas exchange and an adequate blood supply to the body. Any disruption of this system will result in tissue hypoxia. Although both O_2 and CO_2 are dissolved in plasma, the amount carried in this way under normal conditions is inefficient; thus, most O_2 and CO_2 is combined with Hb, an iron-containing molecule whose properties are uniquely suitable for this function. In air, the concentration of O_2 is 21% and at normal atmospheric pressure (760 mmHg) the partial pressure of O_2 (pO_2) is therefore 160 mmHg. In blood, when the Hb is fully saturated, which occurs when breathing air at atmospheric pressure, the partial pressure of O_2 is about 100 mmHg or 12.9 kPa.

If the partial pressure of inspired O_2 is increased either by raising the concentration of O_2 or by increasing the pressure of the inspired O_2 (e.g. in a hyperbaric O_2 chamber), more O_2 can be carried, but only dissolved in solution. This increase is directly related to the increase in pressure or O_2 concentration. However, at partial pressures of O_2 below 12.9 kPa, which occur physiologically, the relationship of partial pressure to O_2 concentration is non-linear because of the particular properties of the Hb molecule.

The oxygen–haemoglobin dissociation curve

The manner in which Hb binds to O_2 at tensions less than 12.9 kPa is shown in the characteristic sigmoidal O_2–Hb dissociation curve (Fig. 19.1). Hb remains almost fully saturated until a pO_2 of about 12.0 kPa because of a high affinity for O_2 above this partial pressure. Once the O_2 tension of surrounding tissue falls below this, there is an initially gradual fall in O_2 saturation until about 7.0 kPa. The physiological implications of this are that O_2 will be readily taken up by the

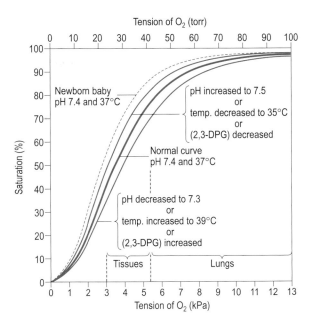

Fig 19.1   Oxygen–haemoglobin dissociation curve.

Hb molecule even if breathing air at higher altitudes. At lower tensions than 7.0 kPa , the dissociation curve becomes steeper. This reflects a physical change in the shape of the Hb molecule, changing its affinity for O_2, allowing O_2 to be released more readily to the relatively hypoxic surrounding tissues which are metabolically active and utilizing O_2.

Furthermore, the O_2 dissociation curve will be influenced by other factors such as acidosis, pCO_2 and temperature. A decrease in pH (acidosis), an increase in pCO_2 or an increase in temperature shifts the curve to the right. The physiological advantage of this effect is that O_2 is more efficiently released to metabolizing tissues which are producing CO_2, lactic acid and heat, and have an increased O_2 requirement. Conversely, as occurs in the lung where the pH is higher, the pCO_2 lower and the surrounding tissue cooler, O_2 will be taken up from inspired air more readily.

Release and uptake of O_2 is further influenced by the concentration of 2,3-diphosphoglycerate (2,3-DPG) in the red cell. The interaction between this molecule and Hb influences the configuration of Hb; the concentration of 2,3-DPG increases in anaemia, acidosis and hypoxia, shifting the O_2 dissociation curve to the right, further facilitating the release of O_2 to tissues where these conditions are present (see Fig. 19.1).

Differences between fetal and adult oxygen dissociation curves

Further differences occur between the dissociation curves of fetal Hb (HbF) and adult Hb. Physiologically, because it binds less readily to 2,3-DPG, the dissociation curve for HbF is to the left of the normal adult curve. Therefore, for a given pO_2, HbF has a greater affinity for O_2 than maternal blood, an advantage for the fetus in utero. However, because the amount of desaturated Hb is less than would occur in adult Hb, a baby will not appear cyanosed until a lower pO_2. After birth, HbF is gradually replaced by adult Hb, the concentration of 2,3-DPG rises and by 4–6 months of age the dissociation has become adult type.

Effect of drugs on binding to Hb

Some drugs may oxidize the iron (Fe) molecule in Hb, forming methaemoglobin (metHb), a compound which is dark blue. Its presence may mimic cyanosis and may reduce effective transport of O_2. Such drugs include nitrites, sulphonamides and aniline. Congenital absence of the enzyme Hb reductase, which normally reduces any metHb produced, is associated with marked methaemoglobinaemia.

CO_2-carrying capacity of Hb

CO_2 is also carried by Hb, although some remains in solution after diffusion from tissue cells. Some is attached to Hb, displacing O_2 to be taken up by metabolizing cells but most combines with H_2O to form carbonic acid, the process requiring the enzyme carbonic anhydrase. Bicarbonate produced from the reaction diffuses along a concentration gradient into the plasma and Cl^- is actively pumped into the cell to maintain electrical neutrality (the chloride shift). Once in the lung, CO_2 rapidly diffuses into the alveoli. Unlike O_2, the CO_2 dissociation is linear and CO_2 will diffuse in proportion to its partial pressure. This process is rarely compromised even in pulmonary disease, while O_2 uptake is more affected by abnormalities in the lung.

Ventilation/perfusion inequality

An imbalance between ventilation (V) and perfusion (P) is the usual cause of central cyanosis. A model of normal and abnormal ventilation/perfusion balance is shown in Figure 19.2.

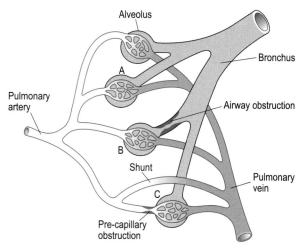

Fig 19.2 Normal and abnormal ventilation/ perfusion balance.

Example (A) shows the physiological situation with the pulmonary artery from the right side of the heart perfusing an alveolus in normal lung and oxygenated blood returning to the left side in the pulmonary veins. The alveolus exchanges CO_2 from blood for O_2 from inspired air.

Example (B) shows an abnormal situation where the ventilation to the alveoli is decreased either segmentally (e.g. asthma, bronchiolitis, bronchopneumonia or bronchiectasis) or to one or more lobes (e.g. lobar pneumonia or emphysema). The normal blood supply will pass through those non-ventilated areas, remain desaturated and cause cyanosis, although normal areas of lung may compensate to allow complete elimination of CO_2.

In example (C) there is normal ventilation but abnormal perfusion. This may be due to obstructed or abnormal pulmonary arterial flow (e.g. pulmonary embolism or an A–V malformation) bypassing (a shunt) the aerated alveoli, the blood remaining deoxygenated. On a larger scale, there may be an intra- or extra-cardiac shunt in congenital heart disease, with blood crossing from the right to the left side of the heart (e.g. transposition of the great arteries), bypassing the lungs completely. Cyanosis will be profound and will remain uncorrected even if the concentration of inspired O_2 is increased.

Hypoxia and its causes

When cyanosis is associated with hypoxia, cellular metabolism may be compromised. If there is insufficient O_2 for normal aerobic metabolism this will activate the anaerobic pathways, resulting in less efficient metabolic activity, lactic acid production and clinical manifestations such as:

- Cyanosis.
- Breathlessness.
- Tachycardia.
- Tachypnoea.
- Decreased consciousness.
- Seizures.

These symptoms, in conjunction with physical examination findings and investigations, will help determine the underlying pathophysiological process.

Hypoxaemia

1. Low inspired O_2 concentration. Usually arises when breathing air at high altitudes. Physiological adaptation may occur.
2. Pulmonary causes:
   a) Hypoventilation:
      i) Depressed respiratory centre: drugs, head trauma, raised intracerebral pressure, central alveolar hypoventilation (Ondine's curse).
      ii) Airway obstruction: foreign body, large tonsils or adenoids, upper airway stenosis, croup, tumours, asthma, bronchiolitis.
      iii) Chest abnormalities: asthma, respiratory muscle disease or paralysis, kyphoscoliosis.
   b) Loss of functioning alveoli:
      - Pneumonia.
      - Atelectasis.
      - Cystic fibrosis.
      - Pulmonary fibrosis.
      - Bronchiectasis.
      - Diffusion impairment.
      - Pulmonary oedema.
   c) Uneven distribution of perfusion and/or ventilation.
3. Cardiac causes:
   i) Congenital heart disease with left-to-right shunt.
   ii) Cardiac failure.

Abnormal O_2-carrying capacity of blood

- Anaemia.
- Methaemoglobinaemia.
- Carboxyhaemoglobinaemia (CO_2 poisoning).

Ischaemic hypoxia

- Distributive shock (circulatory failure from sepsis or blood loss).
- Peripheral oedema.
- Cold.
- Increased peripheral utilization of O_2.

Histotoxic hypoxia

- Ingestion of tissue poisons (e.g. cyanide).

Investigations

Physical examination:
- Effort of breathing:
  – Rate.
  – Muscle activity.
  – Intercostal recession.
- Effect of breathing:
  – Chest wall movement.
  – Chest air entry.
- Efficacy of breathing:
  – Cyanosis.
  – Conscious level.
- Heart rate.

Arterial blood gases:
It is essential to determine levels of O_2 and CO_2, pH, acidosis, O_2 saturation and HCO_3^-. A further blood gas analysis following several minutes breathing 100% O_2 will help distinguish between a right-to-left shunt and primary pulmonary disease as the cause for the cyanosis: in pulmonary disease the pO_2 will rise, at least partly, while this will not occur in a fixed right-to-left shunt.

Echocardiography:
The definitive test to determine abnormal cardiac anatomy.

Chest X-ray:
Will determine the characteristics of the lung, including vascular supply, airway outline, patterns in the lung parenchyma, congenital abnormalities.

Blood tests:
Blood count, haematocrit, electrolytes, blood culture, blood sugar.

ECG.

Clinically important diagnoses

The age of presentation of symptoms is important in determining the cause of cyanosis; most congenital heart disease presents in the first few days of life. Other important diagnoses that present at this age include sepsis, pneumonia and the respiratory distress syndrome (RDS).

In the older infant or child, other respiratory causes and sepsis are more likely, although some congenital cardiac abnormalities may take several years to become evident. Nevertheless, the diagnostic process as indicated above is similar. Patterns of clinical presentation may be identified and the following outlines include those signs, symptoms and investigations that are clinically useful.

Congenital heart disease

1. Diminished pulmonary blood flow, without failure, and a right-to-left shunt:
   - Pulmonary atresia.
   - Tricuspid atresia.
   - Critical pulmonary stenosis.
   - Tetralogy of Fallot.
   - Ebstein's anomaly.
   - Eisenmenger's syndrome.

   Clinically there is:
   - Modest increase in respiratory rate and tidal volume.
   - No response to inhaling 100% O_2.
   - Normal blood count, sugar, electrolytes.
   - Low pO_2.
   - Low or normal pCO_2.
   - Normal pH.
   - Chest X-ray has decreased pulmonary markings.
   - ECG varies.

2. Increased pulmonary blood flow, without heart failure, and a right-to-left shunt.
   - Hypoplastic left heart syndrome.
   - Total anomalous pulmonary venous drainage (TAPVD).
   - Truncus arteriosus.
   - Atrioventricular septal defect.

   Clinical signs include:
   - Increased respiratory rate.
   - Absent response to 100% inhalation.
   - Chest X-ray shows increased pulmonary markings.
   - Low pO_2.

- Normal pCO_2 and pH.
- ECG variable.

3. Heart failure with or without shunt.
   - Patent ductus arteriosus.
   - Ventricular septal defect.
   - Severe aortic stenosis.
   - Cardiomyopathies.
   - Coarctation.
   - Some conditions in groups 1 and 2.

   Clinical signs:
   - Because of cardiac failure there is associated pulmonary oedema and consequently there is associated impairment of gas exchange.
   - Moderate cyanosis.
   - Increased respiratory rate.
   - Crepitations throughout the lungs.
   - Intercostal and sternal recession.
   - Inhalation of 100% may produce an increase in pO_2.
   - Blood count and electrolytes normal.
   - Frequent acidosis and elevated pCO_2.
   - Low blood sugar.
   - Chest X-ray shows a large heart, pulmonary oedema and increased vascular markings.
   - Variably abnormal ECG.

Primary lung disease

- RDS.
- Pneumonia.
- Asthma.
- Aspiration syndromes.
- Pulmonary haemorrhage.
- Lymphangiectasia.
- Bronchopulmonary dysplasia.
- Cystic adenomatoid malformation.
- Atelectasis.

Clinical findings:

- Response to inhalation of 100% O_2 (varies but pO_2 usually rises significantly).
- Raised pCO_2.
- Variable acidosis.
- Normal blood count and electrolytes.
- Chest X-ray often abnormal.
- ECG usually normal.

Airway obstruction

- Mucous plugs.
- Lobar emphysema.

- Diaphragmatic hernia.
- Pneumothorax.
- Chylothorax.
- Thoracic cage abnormalities.
- Vascular rings.
- Tracheo-oesophageal fistula.
- Choanal atresia.
- Pierre Robin syndrome.
- Mediastinal masses.

Clinical signs include:

- Increased respiratory rate.
- Intercostal and subcostal recession.
- Stridor.
- Other signs of respiratory distress.
- Normal response to inhaled 100% O_2.
- Variable cyanosis and low pO_2.
- Low pH.
- Raised pCO_2.
- Chest X-ray often characteristically abnormal.
- ECG either normal or may show right ventricular hypertrophy.

Pulmonary hypertension

- Persistent pulmonary hypertension of the newborn.
- Primary pulmonary hypertension.
- Hyperviscosity.
- Alveolar proteinosis.
- Multiple pulmonary thromboses.

Clinical signs:

- Hyperventilation.
- Variable response to inhaled 100% O_2.
- Cyanosis, often profound.
- Normal blood count, electrolytes and sugar.
- Elevated pCO_2.
- Chest X-ray will show oligaemic lung fields; the heart may be normal or enlarged.
- ECG may show right ventricular hypertrophy.
- May be an associated cardiac murmur.

Central hypoventilation

- Respiratory centre abnormality due to:
  - Intracerebral haemorrhage.
  - Meningitis.
  - Encephalitis.
  - Major intracerebral congenital abnormalities.

- Convulsions.
- Ondine's curse.

Clinical findings:

- Periodic breathing.
- Apnoea.
- Variable tidal volumes.
- Lethargy.
- Seizures.
- Normal response to inhaled 100% O_2.
- Low pO_2 and cyanosis.
- Raised pCO_2.
- Combined respiratory and metabolic acidosis.
- Normal chest X-ray and ECG.

Methaemoglobinaemia

- Methaemoglobin reductase deficiency.
- Ingestion of nitrates and aniline dyes.

Clinical findings:

- Often minimal.
- Cyanosis.
- Increased respiratory and heart rate.
- No response to inhaled 100% O_2.
- Normal or low pH.
- Normal or low pCO_2.
- Normal chest X-ray and ECG.

Polycythaemia

- Twin–twin transfusions.
- Chronic cyanotic heart disease.
- Growth retarded babies.
- Infants of diabetic mothers.

Clinical findings:

- Apparent cyanosis.
- Normal blood gases except for decreased O_2 saturation.
- Increased respiratory rate.
- Apnoea.
- High haematocrit.
- Normal chest X-ray and ECG.

Shock and sepsis

- Many causes of shock and sepsis:
  - Blood loss, primary myocardial disease and septicaemia may produce similar symptoms.

Clinical findings:

- Cyanosis.
- Lethargy.
- Apnoea.
- Shallow respiration.
- Decreased peripheral perfusion.
- Tachycardia.
- Tachypnoea.
- Decreased conscious level.
- Some improvement with 100% inhaled O_2.
- Low Hb with decreased platelet count.
- Acidosis and variable pCO_2.
- Chest X-ray may show cardiomegaly and pneumonia.
- ECG may be normal or show myocardial dysfunction.

Respiratory muscle abnormalities

- Muscular dystrophy

Clinical findings:

- Normal blood count.
- Normal response to inhaled 100% O_2.
- Normal pO_2.
- Raised or normal pCO_2.
- Normal chest X-ray.
- ECG may show associated cardiac muscle abnormalities.

Clinical problem

A 4-year-old boy who had recently arrived from Somalia was brought to the emergency department by his parents because of increasing breathlessness, which has been developing over several months. They said he had had a heart murmur detected before but had not been investigated. He was treated for tuberculosis at 3 years of age but was no longer on treatment, which was thought to be successful.

On examination he was cyanosed, clubbed, his O₂ saturation was 85% and he had normal pulses.

His respiratory rate was 30 per minute and pulse 110 beats per minute.

There was no thrill, the apex beat was in the 5th intercostal space in the midclavicular line, the pulmonary component of the second heart sound was loud and there was a decrescendo systolic murmur at the left sternal edge. There were no signs of cardiac failure.

His height and weight were on the 25% centile.

There were no abnormal pulmonary findings, no lymphadenopathy and the remainder of the examination was also normal.

Questions

- What are the possible causes for his cyanosis and murmur?
- What are the appropriate investigations?

Discussion

- Important features in the history include:
  - Cyanosis and O₂ desaturation.
  - Chronic history.
  - An otherwise well child.
  - Normal pulmonary signs.
  - Clubbing, suggestive of a long-standing abnormality.
  - Tachypnoea.
  - Decrescendo systolic murmur in association with a loud P2, which is suggestive of pulmonary hypertension.
- The differential diagnosis in this case, given the features above, include:
  - Congenital heart disease:
    - Tetralogy of Fallot.
    - Ebstein's anomaly.
    - Eisenmenger's syndrome.
  - Primary pulmonary hypertension.
  - Chronic pulmonary disease e.g. TB.

TB is unlikely as he is otherwise well, his nutritional status is within normal limits and he has no pulmonary symptoms.

Primary pulmonary hypertension would have produced symptoms at a much earlier age.

Undiagnosed congenital heart disease is the most likely group of conditions. Ebstein's anomaly would usually have become symptomatic at an earlier age, and tetralogy of Fallot, which may present late, is associated with a soft P2 and decreased pulmonary blood flow rather than pulmonary hypertension, suggested by the loud P2. An undetected left-to-right shunt such as a large VSD would produce eventual pulmonary hypertension, reversal of the left-to-right shunt, causing an Eisenmenger's syndrome.

Appropriate investigations include:

- Echocardiography with Doppler studies.
- Chest X-ray.
- CT and V/Q lung scans.

Conclusion: this boy had an uncorrected VSD with reversal of the shunt (Eisenmenger's syndrome).

HEART MURMURS

John Stroobant

Introduction

Cardiac murmurs are a common finding in children; they may be detected during routine examination or during the formal assessment of the cardiovascular system because of the presence of other signs or symptoms. It is essential to determine accurately the cause of the murmur, either to diagnose an abnormality that will require further investigation and treatment, or to exclude a pathological cause for the murmur; even non-organic or functional murmurs may cause considerable anxiety in parents and therefore it is important to be confident about its origin. Some functional murmurs can be diagnosed accurately on clinical findings alone but others, particularly if there are associated clinical abnormalities, will need investigation.

Pathophysiology

Murmurs are sounds, usually audible only with a stethoscope, that arise from either turbulence of blood flow through vessels, valves and heart chambers, or from vibrations in valves, vessels or adjacent structures. Usually, the narrower the structure and the more turbulent the flow, the louder the murmur. Furthermore, in younger children, as the heart is closer to the chest wall, which is itself thinner, the murmur may be more easily heard. Murmurs occur in systole or diastole or both (Tables 20.1 and 20.2).

Systolic murmurs

These are classified in two ways:

- Pansystolic murmur:
  - Occurs throughout systole at the same intensity.
  - Usually due to a shunt through a ventricular septal defect (VSD), a patent ductus arteriosus or an incompetent tricuspid or mitral valve.

Table 20.1   Systolic murmurs

Character and site of murmur	Diagnosis
Systolic ejection	
2nd right intercostal space	Aortic stenosis
2nd left intercostal space	Coarctation Pulmonary stenosis Atrial septal defect
Pansystolic	
3rd to 5th left intercostal space	Ventricular septal defect
Apex	Patent ductus arteriosus
4th right intercostal space	Mitral incompetence Tricuspid incompetence

Table 20.2   Diastolic murmurs

Site	Diagnosis
2nd right intercostal space	Aortic incompetence
2nd left intercostal space	Pulmonary incompetence
3rd to 5th right intercostal space	Tricuspid stenosis
Apex	Mitral stenosis

- Ejection murmur:
  - May not occur throughout systole.
  - Rises to a crescendo in mid-systole.
  - Usually coarse.
  - Due to flow through aortic or pulmonary valves, or a small VSD.

The intensity of the murmur is usually graded into six levels:

- *Grade I*. The faintest murmur, requiring very careful auscultation.
- *Grade II*. A slightly louder murmur.
- *Grade III*. Moderate intensity, but without a thrill.
- *Grade IV*. A loud murmur with a thrill.
- *Grade V*. A very loud murmur, with a thrill but still requiring a stethoscope.
- *Grade VI*. The loudest murmur; can be heard without a stethoscope in contact with the chest wall.

Diastolic murmurs

There are three groups:

- Ventricular filling murmurs:
  - Audible in early diastole.
  - Decrease in intensity during diastole.
  - Usually due to narrow or high flow rate across tricuspid or mitral valves.
- Atrial systolic murmurs:
  - Late diastole.
  - Increase in intensity towards second sound.
  - Usually caused by mitral stenosis.
- Regurgitant:
  - Occur throughout diastole.
  - Decrease in intensity.
  - Due to incompetent aortic or pulmonary valves.

Clinical examination

A suggested system for clinical assessment of murmurs is given in Table 20.3.

Some aspects of the clinical examination require further discussion:

- Auscultation requires practice and should be performed carefully; there may be an advantage in making it the first part of an examination before a baby or young child becomes restless or upset.
- Auscultation should always be performed in the:
  - Upper praecordium.
  - Left and right sternal border.
  - Apex.
  - Left and right axillae.
  - Back.
- Murmurs should be assessed for intensity (and variation), pitch, timing, area of maximal intensity and radiation.
- Heart sounds also provide vital information and should be listened for carefully (Table 20.4).
- Clicks also need to be specifically sought; they are usually present in valvular aortic and pulmonary stenosis.
- It is preferable to spend time assessing each component rather than trying to gather information about murmurs, sounds and clicks at the same time.
- Mild cyanosis is often difficult to detect; it may be best noted in the fingernails.
- Pulses may be difficult to feel in chubby babies; the brachial pulse is often the most accessible.

Table 20.3   Clinical cardiac assessment

1. History including birth and family and birth details
2. Exercise tolerance
3. Dyspnoea
4. Infections
5. Squatting
6. Cyanosis
7. Physical examination
   - Height and weight
   - Heart and respiratory rate
   - Blood pressure in right and left arms and leg
   - Cyanosis
   - Clubbing
   - Chest deformity
   - Recession
   - Thrills
   - Pulmonary sounds
   - Abdominal examination
8. Heart assessment
   - Rhythm
   - Cardiac impulse and thrills
   - Position of apex beat
   - Heart sounds
   - Clicks
   - Murmurs
   - Pulses

- It is crucial to make a determined search for the femoral pulses; this may require patience and persistence.
- External abnormalities of the chest wall should be noted. Kyphoscoliosis or pectus carinatum may distort the mediastinum and make subsequent interpretation of the chest X-ray more difficult.
- Careful examination of the abdomen will show an enlarged liver or spleen. A large liver is a sign of cardiac failure in an infant.
- A thrill is usually associated with a grade IV or louder murmur; it is associated with valvular disease, a shunt but not coarctation.

Investigations

Physical findings must be assessed in conjunction with investigations which might include:

- Chest X-ray.
- ECG.
- Echocardiogram.
- Cardiac catheterization.
- Blood count.
- Blood gas analysis (with and without 100% O_2 inhalation; see Ch. 19 Cyanosis).
- Electrolyte assay.

Diagnoses

'Innocent' or functional murmurs

These are common, have no diagnostic significance and no anatomical abnormality. They are usually quiet systolic murmurs, localized to a small area, and brief. There are several recognized:

- Systolic ejection murmur at the left sternal edge, quiet to moderate and not audible at the back; it may be transmitted into the neck. They are often more apparent with fever or anaemia. Probably due to flow through a normal aortic valve.
- Systolic ejection murmur at the upper left sternal edge, well transmitted to the neck; due to flow through a normal pulmonary valve.
- A venous hum heard in the sitting position in the neck; it has a diastolic component and may sound continuous. It is diminished by pressure on the jugular vein

Systolic murmurs

Ejection

1. Aortic stenosis:
   - Palpable abnormal left ventricular impulse.
   - Suprasternal and carotid thrill.
   - Normal first sound.
   - Ejection click after the first sound in the left praecordium in valvular stenosis.
   - Second sound often normal; in severe stenosis the second sound may appear single or even paradoxical, with the aortic component closing after the pulmonary valve.
   - Systolic murmur at the upper right sternal border, usually with a thrill and radiating to the neck.
   - ECG may show left ventricular hypertrophy or strain.

Table 20.4   Pathological heart sounds

A. **1st sound**

  1. *Accentuated*
     Tachycardia
     Mitral stenosis
     Hyperdynamic circulation
     Tricuspid stenosis

  2. *Soft*
     Myocarditis
     Mitral incompetence

  3. *Split*
     Physiological
     Bundle branch block

B. **2nd sound**

  1. *Loud A2*
     Coarctation
     Hypertension

  2. *Soft A2*
     Aortic stenosis
     Aortic incompetence

  3. *Loud P2*
     Pulmonary hypertension
     Pulmonary artery stenosis

  4. *Soft P2*
     Pulmonary stenosis
     Pulmonary incompetence
     Tetralogy of Fallot

  5. *Widely split*
     Atrial septal defect
     Right bundle branch block
     Pulmonary stenosis
     Tetralogy of Fallot

  6. *Absent split*
     Left bundle branch block
     Hypertension
     Aortic incompetence
     Aortic stenosis
     Left-to-right shunts

C. **3rd sound**
     Physiological
     Myocardial disease
     Cardiac failure

D. **4th sound**
     Pulmonary or systemic hypertension
     Valvular stenosis

- Chest X-ray may show cardiomegaly.
- Most aortic stenosis is valvular but occasionally subvalvular and supravalvular stenosis also occurs.
- Symptoms may be minimal but can also include chest pain and syncope.

2. Coarctation of the aorta:
   - May occur proximal or distal to the site of the ductus arteriosus.
   - Preductal coarctation presents in infancy with heart failure but postductal coarctation may remain asymptomatic for many years.
   - Typically there are decreased or absent pulses in the femoral and left brachial arteries.
   - The cardiac impulse is left ventricular in type.
   - There may be an associated bicuspid aortic valve with an aortic ejection click.
   - The murmur of coarctation is variable, but there is usually a systolic ejection murmur from the aortic valve or segment of coarctation, and collateral vessels produce systolic murmurs across the praecordium.

- ECG shows left ventricular hypertrophy.
- Chest X-ray may show cardiac enlargement and rib notching produced by enlarged intercostal vessels eroding the bone.

3. Pulmonary stenosis:
   - Usually valvular but may be infundibular, peripheral or atretic.
   - In mild stenosis there may be no symptoms, a murmur often being detected coincidentally.
   - There is a right ventricular impulse and occasionally a suprasternal thrill.
   - The second sound is more widely split and the intensity of the pulmonary component decreases with increasing stenosis; it may be absent in severe stenosis, producing a single second sound.
   - An ejection click occurs in moderate stenosis.
   - Loud systolic murmur maximal in the second or third left intercostal space at the sternal edge.
   - ECG shows right ventricular hypertrophy.
   - Mild cardiomegaly on Chest X-ray.

4. Atrial septal defect:
   - May occur in two positions: the commonest is an ostium secundum defect, high on the atrial wall; the less common defect – an ostium primum – is situated lower. The clinical signs are similar, but the ECG pattern is frequently different: in an ostium primum there is left axis deviation and right bundle branch block (RBBB); in a secundum defect there is partial RBBB and right axis deviation.
   - The soft systolic murmur at the upper left sternal edge does not arise from flow through the defect but from increased flow through the (normal) pulmonary valve.
   - There is an abnormal right ventricular impulse.
   - There is a widely split second sound which characteristically does not vary with respiration.
   - Increased flow through the tricuspid valve may produce a soft mid-diastolic murmur at the left lower sternal edge.

Pansystolic

1. Ventricular septal defect:
   - This is the commonest cardiac anomaly in children.
   - Position of the defect varies; either high in the upper membranous septum or lower in the muscular septum.
   - There may be more than one defect present.
   - If the defect is large cardiac failure may appear early in infancy; however, if the defect is small the murmur may be asymptomatic and detected accidentally.
   - The intensity of the murmur varies considerably but does not always reflect the size of the defect; pulmonary vascular resistance also varies and will influence flow across the VSD.
   - In a large defect with high flow, there will be evidence of a hyperdynamic circulation.
   - The first and second sounds are usually normal.
   - If there is high pulmonary flow in a large defect, there will be a loud pulmonary component of the second sound.
   - There may be an associated pulmonary flow murmur because of increased flow across the pulmonary valve.
   - Similarly there may be a mitral valve flow murmur: a mid-diastolic murmur at the apex.
   - ECG is variable; it may be normal or evidence of left and/or right ventricular hypertrophy.

   - Chest X-ray usually shows cardiomegaly and increased pulmonary vascular markings.
2. Mitral incompetence:
   - This may be congenital or, more rarely, due to rheumatic heart disease.
   - Pansystolic murmur at the apex radiating to the axilla and back.
   - Soft first heart sound and normal second sound.
   - ECG shows wide bifid P waves (P mitrale) and possible left ventricular hypertrophy.
   - Chest X-ray may confirm the left ventricular hypertrophy.
3. Tricuspid incompetence:
   - Usually asymptomatic.
   - Pansystolic murmur in the fourth intercostal space on the right.
   - Usually associated with right heart failure and right ventricular dilatation.
   - ECG and Chest X-ray usually reflect this ventricular enlargement.
   - May be associated with a pulsatile liver.

Diastolic murmurs

1. Patent ductus arteriosus:
   - May be asymptomatic or associated with heart failure, full bounding pulses and a thrill.
   - Classically there is a continuous murmur throughout systole and diastole.
   - May be localized to the second left intercostal space or radiate more widely.
   - Diastolic component is less apparent if there is high pulmonary vascular resistance.
   - ECG reflects left or biventricular hypertrophy.
   - Chest X-ray shows ventricular enlargement and increased pulmonary vascular markings.
2. Aortic incompetence:
   - Usually associated with other valvular defects.
   - May be asymptomatic.
   - Collapsing pulse.
   - Soft blowing murmur occurs in early diastole at the second right intercostal space.
   - ECG and chest X-ray show evidence of left ventricular hypertrophy.
3. Pulmonary incompetence:
   - Usually occurs following endocarditis or surgery for pulmonary valve stenosis; it is rarely congenital.
   - Soft pulmonary component of the second heart sound.
   - Decrescendo diastolic murmur at the second left intercostal space.

- ECG shows right ventricular hypertrophy.
- Chest X-ray confirms this and will also have dilated pulmonary vessels.

4. Tricuspid stenosis:
  - Diastolic murmur in the third to fifth right intercostal space.
  - ECG shows right atrial hypertrophy with tall, wide P waves.
  - Chest X-ray may be normal or show evidence of right atrial hypertrophy.

5. Mitral stenosis:
  - Usually occurs as a complication of rheumatic fever, although may be congenital.
  - The murmur is at the end of diastole and is heard over the apex.
  - Loud pulmonary component of the second sound.
  - ECG shows wide notched P waves.
  - Chest X-ray shows pulmonary congestion and left atrial enlargement.

Clinical problem

A 3-year-old girl from Colombia was referred to the paediatric clinic after the family doctor heard a systolic murmur.

During assessment in the clinic a decrescendo pansystolic murmur, grade 3/6, was heard at the left sternal edge radiating to the axilla. There was no thrill and no signs of cardiac failure. There were no other abnormalities.

A year previously she had experienced an episode of arthritis which had resolved after several days and had not been investigated. She was now well and has had no other illnesses.

Questions

1. What is the differential diagnosis of this murmur?

2. What investigations should be performed?

Discussion

The causes of a pansystolic murmurs include:

- VSD.
- Mitral incompetence.
- Tricuspid incompetence.

In this case the murmur is decrescendo and radiates to the axilla, both characteristics of mitral incompetence (MI).

While this may be due to a congenital VSD or tricuspid incompetence, rheumatic mitral incompetence is more likely because of the history of an arthropathy, consistent with an episode of rheumatic fever. While congenital MI is more common, the history is an important factor in making the diagnosis. Rheumatic MI is often asymptomatic and the signs may resolve after months or years. Long-term penicillin prophylaxis is indicated as well as regular clinical review.

Investigations indicated here are:

- ECG.
- Chest X-ray.
- Echocardiography.
- ASOT.

PAINFUL JOINTS

Peter Houtman

Aches and pains in the limbs in childhood are both very common, and often difficult to characterize. The likelihood of relatively non-specific symptoms being related to a definable condition is fairly low, but at the other end of the spectrum such problems may be the presenting feature of serious systemic illness, when early recognition is vital.

In children it is often very difficult to localize pain. Thus it is not just diseases of joints that need to be considered in this context. When a joint is acutely inflamed, the pain experienced is due to stretching of the fibrous joint capsule. The joint capsule is supplied by two major branches of each articular nerve and pain is therefore often poorly localized.

There are no pain fibres to the synovial membrane, whose only innervation is to the vasculature. Inflammation within the joint elicits an axon reflex that causes vasodilatation and warmth over the joint.

Acute arthritis

There is a formidable differential diagnosis of acute arthritis (see below), although this is not as large as that of 'arthralgia', when the joints are aching but there is no actual primary joint inflammation. The distinction between arthritis, when there is objective clinical evidence of inflammation (red, hot and/or swollen joint), and arthralgia, when there is no inflammation, is important. Arthralgia is much less likely to herald a serious underlying cause, and is usually just the non-specific accompaniment to a viral illness. It is also commonly found in 'functional' illness.

Causes of acute arthritis

Trauma

In cases of primary inflammatory mono-arthritis, a history of minor trauma to the joint is commonly given by parents as a possible explanation.

Reactive

Reactive arthritis, defined as a sterile synovitis occurring in association with an infection elsewhere in the body, is probably the commonest cause of acute arthritis. In children this may be seen following upper respiratory infection. The classical presentation following genitourinary infection is rare except in sexually active adolescents.

Gastrointestinal infection is a not uncommon precipitant, the usual organisms being *Yersinia enterocolitica*, *Shigella*, *Salmonella* and *Campylobacter* infections.

Viral infection

Many viruses are capable of causing reactive arthritis as above and in most cases the difference between the terms 'viral', 'reactive' and 'post-infectious' arthritis is academic. Viruses such as rubella, herpes simplex, varicella-zoster and cytomegalovirus have been isolated from the joint space, but in other cases the pathogenesis may be immune mediated.

The arthritis associated with rubella typically affects the small joints, but is rarely seen before puberty. A pauci-articular (fewer than five joints involved) arthritis may occur in chickenpox and a migratory large joint arthritis with mumps. Parvovirus B19 has been implicated in other children, often following a febrile illness and 'slapped cheek' rash ('fifth disease'). Worldwide, both HIV and hepatitis B cause arthritis in a significant minority of patients.

Bacterial infection

Septic arthritis usually affects a single joint, but may be multifocal. Children are typically toxic, febrile and have severe limitation of movement of the affected joints, which are red, hot and swollen. However, in infants and particularly in neonates, the signs may be far less obvious. If the diagnosis is suspected a needle aspiration or exploration of affected joints (or both) should be performed.

In children under 4 years of age *Haemophilus influenzae* type b is an important cause of septic arthritis, both primary and complicating meningitis. Group B streptococcus is a frequent cause in neonates, but *Staphylococcus aureus* should be considered in children of all ages. Rarely, arthritis may arise from gonococcal infection, and an immune complex arthritis occasionally occurs in meningococcal bacteraemia. Tuberculosis causes a more indolent arthritis, typically a monoarthritis of knee, hip or wrist, associated with pain, swelling, muscle wasting and low-grade fever.

Rheumatic fever

Rheumatic fever is now rare in the developed world, but is still a major cause of morbidity, in particular through acquired heart disease, in the developing world. The condition results from an aberrant immune response to infection with Lancefield group A beta-haemolytic streptococcus, but in individual cases there may no clear historical evidence to suggest a preceding infection. It is most common between 5 and 15 years of age.

Malignancy

Leukaemia may present with hip or knee pain, or more rarely with hand and wrist involvement. Arthritis may also result from uricaemia caused by rapid turnover of leukaemic cells, especially at the onset of treatment. In metastatic neuroblastoma the fever and irritability, together with bone or joint pains and swelling, may be mistaken for systemic-onset juvenile arthritis.

Haemoglobinopathies

Pre-school children with sickle-cell anaemia typically present with tender swelling of the hands or feet (or both), the so-called 'hand–foot syndrome'. Older children may have recurrent episodes of severe bone or joint pain from infarction, and these may mimic septic arthritis or osteomyelitis. The incidence of both septic arthritis and osteomyelitis, particularly with *Streptococcus pneumoniae* and *Salmonella,* is increased in sickle-cell anaemia, and the differential diagnosis between a bone infarct and osteomyelitis is often difficult. Joint pain, swelling and stiffness may occasionally occur episodically in beta-thalassaemia major and in patients with sickle thalassaemia.

Immune deficiency

Children with immune deficiency may present with a pauci-articular arthritis, which is of non-infectious origin and particularly affects the knee joints. Immune-deficient children are also at increased risk for septic arthritis, often with unusual organisms. Signs may be few, and the distinction between the associated arthritis and septic arthritis in a patient with known immune deficiency may not be easy.

Vasculitis

In Henoch–Schönlein purpura (HSP) the arthritis may precede the characteristic rash and other features, making diagnosis obscure. Joint involvement is often symmetrical and non-migratory, affecting elbows, wrists, knees or ankles. True arthritis, usually of large joints, may occur in Kawasaki disease, as well as painful oedema of the hands and feet, which can mimic arthritis.

Stevens–Johnson syndrome

Polyarthritis can accompany the other features. Of the infective associations, *Mycoplasma pneumoniae* is the most commonly implicated organism.

Connective tissue disorders

Occasionally, arthritis may be the first presenting feature of such diseases as systemic lupus erythematosus (SLE) or dermatomyositis, but usually other features predominate.

Acute presentation of chronic inflammatory arthritis

See below.

Chronic arthritis

Most of the conditions listed above can continue chronically. However, it is unusual for primary inflammation of a joint to persist continuously for more than a few weeks. Notable exceptions to this include the joint inflammation in connective tissue diseases such as SLE and dermatomyositis. Although these conditions are rare in childhood, they should be considered particularly in older children and adolescents when there are systemic features including fever and rash.

Juvenile idiopathic arthritis (JIA)

Formerly variably referred to as juvenile chronic arthritis (JCA) or juvenile rheumatoid arthritis (JRA), this disease is now defined internationally simply as joint inflammation ('arthritis') persisting for 6 weeks or more, with initial onset in a person under 16 years, in the absence of another specific cause. The definition is crucial because it is entirely clinical, and is a diagnosis of exclusion of other causes (see above). Thus it cannot be diagnosed definitively before 6 weeks even if the features are clear without worrying alternatives. The condition can, of course, be actively managed during this period, but prognosis cannot be predicted. Reactive or viral arthritides can persist continuously beyond 6 weeks, and are in practice the most common differential diagnoses.

The incidence of JIA is approximately 1 in 10 000 with a prevalence of about 1 in 1000. At one end of the spectrum it can be a chronic disabling condition complicated by joint destruction, loss of function and impaired growth, but in other cases it is a self-limiting disease with no sequelae. Within the international definition are several subtypes encompassing the range of clinical presentations (see Table 21.1). It should be emphasized, however, that this classification is primarily for epidemiological purposes, and in clinical practice children do not necessarily fall neatly into a particular category.

History

Because of the wide range of conditions associated with painful joints, history taking should be focused towards the likely conditions in individual cases, but be broad-based enough to cover unexpected symptoms. Certain points in the history are particularly pertinent:

- *Joints.* A history of swelling as well as pain is important to distinguish arthralgia from arthritis, but beware that parents often mention 'swelling' when this has not been objectively observed.
- A short history consistent with joint inflammation is often more worrying than a longer one. This is particularly true when septic arthritis is considered to be part of the differential diagnosis.
- Morning stiffness is worth asking about specifically, and is a marker of inflammatory rather than mechanical conditions.
- *Associated symptoms.* Always ask directly about rashes and bruising. For example, in HSP, a preceding rash may well have appeared trivial but may be the only specific clue to the diagnosis. Similarly, the pattern of a fever or preceding systemic illness

Table 21.1 Subclassification of JIA

Systemic arthritis	This is commonest in children under 5 years of age but it may occur at any age. The sexes are equally affected. Toddlers are often toxic, listless and miserable, but older children only appear unwell during bouts of fever, which is the hallmark of the disease. Rash is almost invariable and is usually a pink, macular eruption with the small macules being discrete or becoming confluent. The rash is evanescent and tends to appear when the child is febrile and where the skin has been rubbed by clothes; it appears most commonly on the trunk and limbs.
	Of the other systemic features of the disease, lymphadenopathy is the commonest, but hepatosplenomegaly and abdominal distension may also occur. Symptomatic pericarditis is rare but may be life-threatening. Myocarditis, pleurisy and pneumonitis are rare. Hepatitis may occur early.
	Joint manifestations at the onset of the disease vary in severity, and may even be absent. The arthropathy is usually symmetrical, with knees, wrists and carpal joints most commonly involved in the early stages. After a few weeks, involvement of the flexor tendons in the hand causes swelling of the proximal phalanges and palm and limitation of movement at the proximal interphalangeal joints. Neck involvement presents as pain and loss of extension, which may mimic meningitis; torticollis can occur and may be the presenting complaint.
	At a later stage hip involvement may occur. Cervical spine involvement may result in a fixed flexion deformity of the neck, and bilateral temporomandibular joint involvement can lead to failure of development of the mandible
Oligo-arthritis Persistent Extended	By definition, this indicates involvement of fewer than five joints at onset. It is the commonest presentation of JIA, being responsible for about 50% of cases, and is primarily a disease of young children, particularly girls. Knees and ankles are most commonly affected, and usually in an asymmetric pattern.
	There is a group of children in whom arthritis is associated with chronic anterior uveitis and this is strongly correlated to the presence of a positive antinuclear factor. The onset of the uveitis is usually insidious and asymptomatic and, if left untreated, leads to blindness. It is essential, therefore, to get an expert ophthalmological opinion including a slit-lamp examination on every child.
	The new classification includes two subtypes: in the 'persistent' type there is no progression to polyarthritis, but in 'extended' there is progression after the first 6 months. The prognosis is worse in the extended type
Polyarthritis RhF negative RhF positive	This term is reserved for children with more than four joints involved within the first 6 months of disease and with little or no systemic upset. Both large and small joints are involved. In general, the condition can begin at any age within childhood, but there is a small group (less than 5% of JIA) of older children and adolescents who have an erosive arthritis and positive rheumatoid factor. This disease is analogous to rheumatoid arthritis in adults and is much more common in girls
Enthesitis-related	Enthesitis refers to inflammation of ligamentous and tendon insertions, both spinal and peripheral. Most cases are in older children, with a male preponderance. It includes those with juvenile ankylosing spondylitis, but not all cases are HLA-B27 related
Psoriatic	This may occur in the absence of the typical rash. Nail changes, dactylitis or a positive family history of psoriasis may suggest the diagnosis. Usually large joints in particular are involved
Other	This category is really to acknowledge that not all children fall neatly into particular subtypes and may, in particular, present with a combination of the clinical pictures described above

such as gastroenteritis may give valuable clues. Other features suggesting significant inflammatory or generalized conditions include weight loss, mouth ulcers and bowel disturbance.

- *Past history*. A history of even mild joint involvement in the past may be relevant in distinguishing a purely acute condition from a relapsing chronic disease. Indeed a history of seemingly trivial joint swelling some time previously may focus attention on that joint, in which significant limitation of movement is to be found.
- *Family history*. Most often this provides an opportunity to reassure the family that a history of rheumatoid arthritis in adult relatives is not a predisposition to childhood arthritis. However, a family history of psoriasis or psoriatic arthropathy is relevant to children with appropriate symptoms and signs.

Examination

Clinical examination of joints is, unfortunately, on the whole poorly performed, as it does not seem to be a routine clinical tool. When joint swelling, redness, heat and limitation of movement are obvious there is no difficulty, but more subtle degrees of arthritis require more definite observational skills. Do not be tempted to diagnose joint swelling, particularly in young children, unless you are sure that the joint itself is swollen, when compared carefully with the other side. Demonstrating a full range of movements in children is often difficult, and it is usually best for children themselves to demonstrate such movement (such as kneeling on the floor for knees and ankles) rather than the examiner moving the joints passively. Do not forget the spine and jaw as important joints often involved in chronic arthritides.

Wasting around a joint is a sign of significant problems, and takes a comparatively short time to appear in otherwise active young children.

The skin can give valuable clues to diagnosis. Rashes can be characteristic, such as the 'butterfly' facial distribution in SLE, or heliotrope (mauvish) discoloration of the upper eyelids in dermatomyositis. Nail-pitting may be the only superficial marker of psoriasis in the absence of a typical rash.

Although uveitis is usually clinically silent at first, it is worth looking for irregularity of the pupil. However, formal ophthalmological assessment is always indicated in cases of JIA.

It is often a cliché that a full systematic examination is indicated in a patient, but in this area it really is imperative that a thorough check is done, given the wide range of possible associated problems.

Investigation

The most important aspect of investigation for 'painful joints' concerns the exclusion of serious conditions, usually involving the joints secondarily. The combination of tests to be performed depends very much on the type of clinical presentation, and the degree of concern.

Tests	Uses
Inflammatory markers	ESR and plasma viscosity can be valuable in distinguishing significant disease from mechanical or functional problems. However, they are relatively poor in providing clues to more specific diagnoses. These markers may also be helpful in gauging disease activity, and in vasculopathies the platelet count (usually raised in active disease) can be just as helpful in this respect. C-reactive protein is usually raised in bacterial infections, but can be raised in non-infective inflammation
Haematology Full blood count	Can be helpful in relation to the investigation of an acute arthritis (e.g. raised white count in septic arthritis; a variety of abnormalities such as leucocytosis and/or thrombocytopenia are possible in leukaemia). Anaemia is a feature of systemic JIA. White count can be raised, or depressed (particularly in SLE), in inflammatory conditions. Thrombocytosis is common in inflammatory conditions
Blood film	If leukaemia is suspected

Tests	Uses
Coagulation screen	Helpful where arthritis is associated with suspected bleeding problems. Also, lupus anticoagulant may be present in cases of SLE. (Note that the presence of this substance usually has no clinical anticoagulant (or thrombotic) effect)
Biochemistry	Not usually helpful unless there are secondary features to a rheumatological condition, e.g. renal involvement in autoimmune disease. Possible proteinuria should be monitored in such circumstances. However, liver function tests become very important as part of monitoring in patients on methotrexate, commonly used to treat JIA
Immunology	
Antinuclear antibodies	Useful in JIA for predicting the likelihood of uveitis, particularly in girls with oligo-articular JIA. Can be helpful for the diagnosis SLE, but anti-double-stranded DNA antibodies are more specific for this disease
Rh factor	Only useful in a small subset of older girls with polyarthritis
Bacteriology	The only reliable test for acute septic arthritis is microscopy and culture of joint aspirate. Blood culture is also indicated. If chronic infection is suspected, specific tests are indicated, such as tuberculin sensitivity in TB. Specific serology can be helpful in certain conditions such as Lyme disease (*Borrelia burgdorferi*), but this is primarily a clinical diagnosis. In rheumatic fever, a throat swab should be taken in suspected cases, or skin swabs when impetigo or infected eczema is the presumed source of

Tests	Uses
	infection. Additionally, anti-streptolysin O titres (ASOT) should be measured, as should anti-deoxyribonuclease B (DNase B) titres. The latter are particularly associated with streptococcal skin infections and may then be elevated despite a normal ASOT
Virology	Useful, if available, for cases of reactive arthritis (e.g. rise in antibody titres to parvovirus B19); viral isolation from joint aspirate in primary viral arthritis
Radiology	In infection X-rays of suspect joints, including the opposite limb for comparison, may show swelling of the joint capsule, although early bony changes only occur in the neonatal period. Ultrasound scan of suspect joints is being used increasingly to assess joint swelling, especially of relatively inaccessible joints such as the hip. A technetium bone scan may show increased uptake. In inflammatory arthritis X-rays may be helpful to gauge the severity of chronic damage, but are not usually helpful for diagnosis. However, MRI scanning may be indicated in enthesitis, looking at the sacroiliac joints in particular. In sickle-cell disease, X-rays may show periosteal elevation due to dactylitis, and later show infarction
Ophthalmic	As indicated in the text above, ophthalmological examination, particularly with slit-lamp, is indicated in children with JIA. There are protocols for the follow-up of such children depending on the relative risk to the eyes, and this may mean regular slit-lamp exam for 7 years following onset of JIA, even if the joints have been quiescent for some time

Clinical problem

A 7-year-old girl presented with a 2-month history of joint pain and swelling. Initially her parents noticed her limping and the right knee looked swollen. She had fallen off her bicycle the day before. An X-ray of the joint was normal. About 3 weeks later she also began to complain of pains in the ankles and wrists. She was not otherwise unwell, and continued to go to school. She had no fever or rash, and no preceding illness.

General examination was unremarkable. Her right knee was warm and slightly tender laterally.

There was soft-tissue swelling around the joint and signs of a moderate effusion. She could not straighten the knee completely. There was anterior thigh muscle wasting on that side. Her left ankle was also slightly swollen anteriorly and there was pain on full dorsiflexion. Her left wrist was limited in extension to 45° beyond neutral. She had a full and painless range of movements of other joints, including lower spine, neck and jaw. There was no eye redness and the pupils were equal.

Questions

1. What is the diagnosis?

2. What investigations would you perform?

Answers

1. From the history and examination, she has had inflammation of at least one joint for more than 6 weeks. In the absence of any suggestion of other underlying disease, the most likely diagnosis is *juvenile idiopathic arthritis*. It is likely to be oligo-articular (fewer than five joints involved) although such categorization should wait until the first 6 months have elapsed. The main differential diagnosis is a reactive arthritis, which may rarely persist for more than 6 weeks.

2. A full blood count should be performed, along with inflammatory markers (see above), mainly as a baseline. Measurement of her antinuclear antibody status would also be appropriate, but would not influence initial management. Rheumatoid factor is likely to be irrelevant in a child. She should be reviewed by a paediatric ophthalmologist, in particular for first slit-lamp examination, and thereafter for regular follow-up. This is because of the association between pauci-articular JIA (often ANA positive) and chronic iridocyclitis.

CHAPTER 22

ABDOMINAL PAIN IN CHILDREN

Tina Sajjanhar

Introduction

Children commonly present with acute abdominal pain and the clinician should distinguish cases requiring surgery from those that require non-operative intervention. A knowledge of the potential differential diagnosis is essential, as pain may be due to localized gastrointestinal disease, but may occur as a symptom of systemic disease.

Recurrent abdominal pain may in unusual cases have a surgical cause, but medical causes are more likely, although in many children there is no pathology. The clinician needs to decide how intensively to investigate a child to exclude organic disease, and how best to manage the child with non-organic abdominal pain.

A careful history and examination will help distinguish the possible causes of the pain, so that investigations may be tailored appropriately.

Causes of abdominal pain in children

Surgical	Non-surgical abdomen	Systemic
Acute		
Appendicitis	Gastroenteritis	Pneumonia
Bowel	Urinary tract	Sickle-cell
obstruction	infection	disease
Intussusception	Pyelonephritis	Diabetes
Volvulus	Renal stones	Henoch–
Strangulated	Gallstones	Schönlein
hernia	Cholecystitis	purpura
Trauma	Reflux	Nephrotic
Gastrointestinal	oesophagitis	syndrome
bleeding	Colic	Migraine
Ectopic	Pancreatitis	
pregnancy	Hepatitis	
Testicular		
torsion		

Surgical	Non-surgical abdomen	Systemic
Recurrent		
Adhesions	Obstructed	Sexual abuse
Malrotation	renal system	Porphyria
	Irritable bowel	Hereditary
	Helicobacter	angio-
	infection	oedema
	Mesenteric	Migraine
	adenitis	Familial
	Functional	Mediterranean
	abdominal	fever
	pain	
	Crohn's disease	
	Constipation	
	Coeliac disease	
	Dietary	
	intolerance	
	(lactose,	
	fructose)	
	Giardiasis	
	Dysmenorrhoea	
	Pelvic	
	inflammatory	
	disease	

Acute abdominal pain

In children who present with acute abdominal pain, acute surgical causes should be considered where pain has lasted 3–4 hours or more.

There is some crossover as chronic conditions may also present with acute episodes of abdominal pain. Some children with stress-related abdominal pain may develop an organic cause such as acute appendicitis.

There are particular features in the history and examination that should be sought:

- The age of the child may be a pointer to a diagnosis, but the younger the child, the more difficulty there is in localizing the site of the pain.
- Abdominal pain originating from abdominal viscera will often localize to a particular site. However, it is important to remember that abdominal pain may be referred, e.g. from the pleura, or the testes in boys.

- Colicky pain may predominate in renal colic, or intussusception.
- Bilious vomiting in babies is strongly suggestive of obstruction, but persistent vomiting may be a feature of obstruction at any age, or can occur as part of gastroenteritis, infections of the urinary tract, hepatitis or migraine headaches.
- Diarrhoea is a common symptom of gastroenteritis and may be bloody with *Campylobacter*, and very profuse with *Salmonella*. However, bloody diarrhoea may also occur during intussusception, in association with other features of an acute abdomen.
- Fever can occur in appendicitis, urinary tract infections, gastroenteritis and cholecystitis, but may also indicate a systemic disease process such as pneumonia.
- Look for pointers of systemic disease:
  - Respiratory symptoms of cough and shortness of breath in pneumonia.
  - Ethnic origin may alert the clinician to look for sickle-cell disease.
  - Kussmaul's breathing with ketotic breath in diabetes.
  - Typical purpuric rash of HSP (although the rash may also be urticarial).
  - Periorbital swelling in nephrotic syndrome.
- Systemic diseases may present with features of an acute abdomen, and operative intervention sought unless these conditions are actively considered and excluded.
- Pubertal girls should be asked about the date of their last period and sexual history.
- Known conditions:
  - History of sickle-cell disease which may predispose to gallstones.
  - Known diabetic.
  - Previous surgery.

During examination, the following particular points should be looked for:

- Abdominal distension is suggestive of obstruction, but may not be present in high small bowel obstructions.
- The presence of rebound and guarding indicates an acute surgical abdomen.
- Jaundice may be present in conditions obstructing the gall bladder and hepatitis:
  - However, abdominal pain, nausea and vomiting may precede jaundice in hepatitis A by many days.

- Gallstones may present with:
  - Cholecystitis.
  - Biliary colic.
  - Pancreatitis.
- A mass may be palpable in cases of intussusception; however, a mass may also prove to be a tumour such as Wilms' or neuroblastoma, with abdominal pain an incidental symptom in many cases.
- Presence of bronchial breathing may be the only indicator of pneumonia.
- Ketotic breath in diabetes.
- Rash of HSP on extensor surfaces of the lower and upper limbs; the intussusception can precede rash in some cases by up to a week.
- Testes must be examined in boys:
  - If the scrotum is red, swollen and painful, suspect torsion of the testis, which is more common around puberty.
  - In the prepubertal child these findings may be due to torsion of the testicular appendages and surgical opinion should be sought.
- Look for presence of strangulated hernia.
- Look for bruising associated with trauma, and ensure that the history is consistent and there are no features to suggest non-accidental injury.
  - Trauma can also lead to pancreatitis.

Investigations

- Straight abdominal X-ray may show fluid levels in obstruction.
- Urinalysis for:
  - Proteinuria – large amount in nephrotic syndrome.
  - Leucocytes and nitrites indicating possible UTI.
  - However, the absence of one of these does not exclude UTI but presence of both has high positive predictive value in presence of abdominal pain.
- Urine for microscopy, culture and sensitivities (MC&S) where urinalysis positive or there is clinical suspicion.
- Stool for MC&S.
- 'Hot stool' for *Giardia*.
- FBC for:
  - High WCC indicating infective cause.
  - Low Hb.
  - Sickle-cell status.
- CRP useful only if high, indicating significant infection.

- BMstix, and if abnormal there must be formal laboratory blood sugar.
- Liver function tests, albumin, amylase.
- Chest X-ray to look for pneumonia.
- Ultrasound can help in detection of free peritoneal fluid, appendix mass, gallstones (although this may be an incidental finding as it is quite common), pyelonephritis, ectopic pregnancy (must be specifically looked for if requested).
- May require endoscopy in acute gastrointestinal bleed.

Recurrent abdominal pain

Recurrent abdominal pain may be defined as pain that occurs on at least three occasions over 3 months and interferes with normal activities.

Previous studies of recurrent abdominal pain in childhood have shown quite clearly that most cases, i.e. up to 90%, have no demonstrable organic cause. However, with the advent of new approaches to diagnosis, e.g. small bowel biopsy, dysmotility studies, endoscopy and 24-hour pH monitoring, in parallel with the growth of paediatric gastroenterology as a subspecialty, this is likely to be an underestimate and the prevalence of organic disease may well be higher.

Recurrent abdominal pain is a spectrum of clinical disease from a relatively well-defined process such as irritable bowel to functional abdominal pain which may be more poorly defined.

Incidence

Recurrent abdominal pain (RAP) is extremely common in childhood, with an incidence of 10–15% in school children. The proportion of these with organic disorders has varied from 5% to 20% in different studies.

Pathophysiology

The gut and nervous system are derived from the same tissues embryologically. Neuropeptides and neuro-transmitters produced in the gastrointestinal tract regulate gastrointestinal motility, blood flow, secretion and absorption. The enteric nervous system and central nervous system have direct effects on each other, e.g. stress is known to aggravate the gastro-intestinal tract by release of neuropeptides and neurotransmitters, leading to various gastrointestinal responses. The brain–gut connection links the psychological state to gastrointestinal disorders and to functional bowel disorders.

It is important to remember the term 'functional' may imply that symptoms are psychological or imagined. However, the child genuinely feels pain although there is no obvious organic basis and all investigations are negative. A number of children are thought to have gastrointestinal dysmotility or visceral hypersensitivity.

Predisposing factors are:

- Underlying anxious personality.
- Inappropriate parental response to illness.
- Previous illness experience in the family.
- Family stress, death, separation, school problems.

The pain may have started at the time of a family upheaval such as parental discord, separation, death of a family member or birth of a sibling. Children with problems at school such as bullying, unhappiness in the class, or fear of exams may have abdominal pain in the mornings. Parents may not be aware of any problems at school and it may be necessary to write to the school for information or ask the parents to specifically ask the school. The GP may be able to provide information, as may the school nurse.

Other symptoms of anxiety may be present, such as sleep disorders, nocturnal enuresis, feeding problems and undue fears.

Typical features include:

- 4–14 years (slight female predominance after 9 years of age).
- Periumbilical.
- Difficult for child to describe.
- Interrupts normal activity.
- History of clustering of episodes.
- No symptoms of organic disease, e.g. change in bowel habit.

RAP is associated with anxiety disorders in females and ADHD in males. Girls with RAP may be at increased risk of irritable bowel disease later in life.

The diagnosis should be given a positive spin although with emphasis on lack of pathology or negative sequelae. Psychological input may be offered if there are obvious exacerbating emotional or psychological factors and, with family therapy, 30–40% may have resolution of their pain. The rest may go on to develop abdominal pain in adulthood and suffer from anxiety or other somatic disorders.

Other disorders in the spectrum have some typical features.

Abdominal migraine

There is increasing recognition that this is distinct entity with specific diagnostic criteria:

- Pain severe enough to interfere with daily activity and leading to time off school.
- Periumbilical or poorly localized pain, dull or colicky.
- Associated with two of the following:
  - Vomiting.
  - Nausea.
  - Anorexia.
  - Pallor.
- Lasts about 1 hour.
- Complete resolution between attacks.

Prevalence is 2.4–4.1%; girls are more commonly affected, with mean age of onset being 7 years. Pain is the primary symptom, but pallor is also a consistent feature.

There is evidence of overlap between abdominal migraine and migraine headaches. These children may go on to develop migraine headaches and there may be a positive family history of migraine. Children may respond to antimigraine medication.

There is also overlap with cyclical vomiting.

Cyclical vomiting

The understanding of this disorder is limited.

The main feature is explosive bouts of vomiting with medical morbidity, i.e. hospital admission, i.v. therapy, time lost from school. Prevalence is up to 2% of school-age children.

The child has abdominal pain associated with:

- Pallor.
- Lethargy.
- Anorexia.
- Nausea.
- Ketosis.
- Blood glucose level not abnormally low.

Episodes may be provoked by intercurrent infection, fasting or strenuous exercise, and begin in the second year of life until puberty.

Other causes of vomiting should be excluded such as acute surgical conditions, CNS disease and in particular metabolic disease, such as fatty acid oxidation defects, before making the diagnosis. Urinary organic acid analysis shows prominent ketosis but no pathological metabolites. The condition may be due to impaired uptake of ketones into peripheral tissues. Some patients have been shown to have deficiencies of either beta-ketothiolase or succinyl CoA:3-oxoacid CoA transferase. For most children a coherent explanation is not found, although in the future increased understanding of metabolic disease may help discover the pathogenesis.

Irritable bowel disease

This is well defined within the spectrum of recurrent abdominal pain and increasingly recognized in adolescents.

Symptoms include:

- Lower abdominal pain.
- Bloating.
- Alteration of bowel habits, alternating between periods of constipation and periods of more frequent, looser stools with passage of mucus.
- There may be a feeling of incomplete evacuation and relief of pain with passage of stool.

No anatomical or physiological markers are present and diagnosis is on clinical grounds and exclusion of any other organic pathology.

There may be altered gastrointestinal motility, associated with psychological factors.

Organic causes of recurrent abdominal pain

In many cases of organic abdominal pain there are features in the history and examination that lead the clinician to suspect an organic pathology, at which point investigations may be required to elucidate the actual cause.

The following features should be taken in the history:

- Site of the pain:
  - Generally as a rule, the further from the umbilicus the more likely the pain is to be organic.
  - Epigastric pain occurs in 50% of children with *Helicobacter* infection, and is associated with vomiting in 40% and haematemesis in 16%.
  - Periumbilical pain is typical in mesenteric adeni-

tis, and there is often an associated high fever, symptoms of intercurrent viral infection and lymphadenopathy.
  - Loin pain may be secondary to intermittent ureteric obstruction, and is often associated with nausea or vomiting, with symptoms exacerbated by a fluid load or position.
- Colicky abdominal pain is typically severe in renal colic, and can occur in cases of lactose intolerance; otherwise the type of pain is a poor discriminatory factor.
- Timing:
  - About 8% of children with non-organic pain wake at night, so although night waking suggests severe pain it is not necessarily indicative of severe disease.
  - The pain of peptic ulcer typically occurs at night.
- Diarrhoea may be present intermittently as part of inflammatory bowel disease, in association with blood and mucus.
- Giardiasis.
- Dietary intolerance.
- Bloating may be a particular feature in coeliac disease.
- Vomiting is not a good discriminator of organic causes of abdominal pain as it may occur in intermittent obstructive bowel lesions, renal tract obstruction and infections such as PID, but can also occur as part of functional bowel disease and cyclical vomiting.
- Fever occurs with pelvic inflammatory disease, but also as part of Crohn's disease, and recurrent fevers can be part of the rare familial fevers.
- Weight loss is common in inflammatory bowel disease and may be associated with anorexia, malaise and growth failure.

Examination may:

- Be helpful to elicit the site of pain.
- Indicate the presence of lymphadenopathy in mesenteric adenitis.
- Elicit the presence of a faecal mass in constipation.
- Indicate organic pathology if the child's height and weight are compromised.
- Indicate the presence of the following in Crohn's disease:
  - Mouth/perianal ulcers.
  - Anal skin tags.
  - Clubbing.
  - Iritis.
  - Arthritis.

Investigations

- In Crohn's disease the following blood test abnormalities may occur:
  - Normochromic, normocytic anaemia.
  - Iron deficiency due to malabsorption, blood loss or dietary.
  - Folate deficiency.
  - Vitamin B_{12} deficiency.
  - Leucocytosis.
  - Elevated ESR and CRP.
  - Hypoalbuminaemia.
- *Helicobacter* titres should be performed in the presence of RAP, especially associated with symptoms of dyspepsia, and a positive result treated.
- RAP may be associated with higher incidence of coeliac disease and may occur in absence of other typical features e.g. weight loss, abdominal distension, diarrhoea. Serological markers (antiendomysial, antigliadin and antireticulin antibodies) may be used as a screening test to decide which children go on to need further investigation.
- Urine dipstick and microscopy may reveal haematuria in the presence of a renal calculus, or urine infection.
- Abdominal X-ray is not routinely required in constipation but may reveal a megarectum or gross faecal loading.
- Ultrasound scan:
  - A renal ultrasound may show a dilated system but this does not prove obstruction and further renal imaging such as micturating cystourethrogram (MCUG) and Mag 3 scan may be required.
  - Also useful in diagnosis of inflammatory bowel disease.
  - Presence of mesenteric nodes may confirm diagnosis of mesenteric adenitis.
- Endoscopy: to exclude *Helicobacter* infection and look for peptic ulceration where relevant.

Key points

Helicobacter infection

- *Helicobacter pylori* is a spiral-shaped Gram-negative rod with four to six sheathed flagella. There are approximately 40 unrelated strains of *H. pylori*.
- The organism possesses a urease enzyme that allows it to catalyse urea into ammonium and bicarbonate; this alkaline microenvironment protects it from gastric acid.

- Prevalence is higher in developed countries, with a higher incidence in those of lower socio-economic class.
- There is a lower incidence of *H. pylori* in children compared to adults. It is probable that early, self-limiting infection is possible in children.
- Transmission is thought to be person-to-person via the faeco-oral route.
- *H. pylori* exclusively colonizes the gastric mucosa and normally the highest concentration is in the gastric antrum.
- *H. pylori* induces a chronic active gastroduodenitis.
- The relationship between *H. pylori* infection and gastroduodenal disease in children is not as clear cut as that in adults. Studies draw conflicting conclusions about the role of *H. pylori* and abdominal pain in children.

Urinary tract obstruction

- Obstruction of the urinary tract or dysplasia of the urinary tract can lead to an abnormal pelvicalyceal dilatation and hydronephrosis.
- Obstruction can occur at the pelviureteric junction due to stenosis, congenital kinking or a lower pole vessel crossing the ureter as it joins the renal pelvis. The obstruction may be intermittent.
- Obstruction may occur at the level of the vesicoureteric junction and cause dilatation of the ureter as well.
- Renal stones or ureteric calculus is a rare cause of acute obstruction in children, and may cause acute hydronephrosis.

Crohn's disease

- Increasingly diagnosed in childhood.
- Incidence unusual under 5 years of age.
- 4–8 new child cases per year per 1 000 000 of the population in the UK.

Periodic fevers

Diffuse abdominal pain occurs as part of the periodic fevers such as familial fever.

Associated findings are:

- Non-infective peritonitis, pericarditis, meningitis, orchitis, arthritis, erysipelas-like erythroderma, amyloidosis leading to renal failure.
- Onset in childhood occurs in the severe form.

- Common in ethnic groups such as Sephardic and Armenian Jews and some Arab communities.
- Due to defect in marenostrin (pyrin), a protein in the myelomonocytic-specific proinflammatory pathway, responsible for downregulation of inflammatory response. FMF gene has been identified to aid diagnosis.

Porphyria

- Uncommon in childhood and rare before adolescence.
- Suspected often when recurrent bouts of abdominal pain have occurred.
- May be severe enough to mistake for surgical emergency.
- Diffuse/colicky abdominal pain with constipation.
- May be suspected in the presence of personality change, and intermittent passage of burgundy-red coloured urine.
- In the commonest form, acute intermittent porphyria, episodes may be triggered by drugs or hormonal change and may present as depression, abdominal pain, peripheral neuropathy or demyelination.
- Hyperpigmentation of the skin and photosensitivity occur in other forms of porphyria.

Myths surrounding recurrent abdominal pain

Constipation

Severe constipation can cause abdominal pain due to attempted passage of stools, particularly in the acute phase.

Chronic constipation is not usually associated with abdominal pain. It is debatable what the contribution of lesser degrees of constipation is to recurrent abdominal pain.

Worms

Pinworms, *Enterobius vermicularis*, are equally common in symptomatic and normal children and are unlikely to be a cause of recurrent abdominal pain. Symptoms are more likely to be those of local irritation. In developing countries there may be other parasitic infestations such as *Ascaris lumbricoides* that can cause abdominal pain by leading to abdominal obstruction, but other symptoms would be present to raise suspicion of this.

Grumbling appendix

Occasionally RAP may be improved by removal of the appendix, but such cases are rare.

Clinical problem

A 10-year-old boy is brought to the A&E department from school accompanied by his teacher. Apparently, in the middle of his maths class he developed central abdominal pain and has been rolling about in agony for the last 40 minutes.

On examination:

Temperature 37.5°C
Respiratory rate 20
Heart rate 110

Abdominal examination is difficult as the child appears to have voluntary guarding – there is slight central abdominal tenderness.

Weight 75th centile
Height 50th centile

He is given a dose of oral morphine, which helps his pain to settle, but 2 hours later he starts vomiting and is unable to keep fluids down.

His mother arrives and gives further history. He has apparently been having abdominal pains on and off for the last few months but she has not done much about it as she has been busy with his younger brother, who has haemophilia and has required many hospital visits. In between times, his appetite has been normal and he has not lost any weight. His father suffers from severe Crohn's disease, for which he has had surgery. Parents have been separated for the last year.

Blood results:

Sodium 140
Potassium 4.3
Urea 7.5
Creatinine 70
Albumin 36
Haemoglobin 11
White cell count 7.2
Platelet count 348
Erythrocyte sedimentation rate 15
C-reactive protein 25

Urinalysis and urine microscopy are normal.
He is admitted to the ward.

Question

Which course of action is the most reasonable one to take next?

a) Barium enema.
b) Colonoscopy and biopsy.
c) Abdominal X-ray followed by abdominal ultrasound scan.
d) Referral to a clinical psychologist.
e) Observation only before any investigation or referral.
f) Urgent laparotomy.

Answer

c)

This boy has significant abdominal pain, requiring oral morphine. Although he has many risk factors for psychogenic pain, it is important to exclude an organic cause for his pain. An abdominal X-ray would show up radio-opaque renal calculi only, although there is no haematuria, which makes this unlikely. Ultrasound is a non-invasive test and would allow visualization of the kidneys to exclude pelvicalyceal dilatation, an appendix mass or free fluid indicative of appendicitis, the mesenteric nodes and the ileocaecal region for evidence of Crohn's disease. However, Crohn's disease is unlikely in the absence of anaemia, systemic features including weight loss, and low albumin levels.

If these are normal then management may be expectant. If the pain continues, further investigation may be required, although this could be done in conjunction with psychological input.

This boy's investigations were in fact normal at this stage. However, he was followed up, and his abdominal pain continued. Within the next year, he too had developed Crohn's disease.

CONSTIPATION
Elaine Carter

Introduction

Constipation may be defined as the infrequent or painful passage of hard faeces. It is a common problem in childhood.

A formed stool is produced as faecal fluid passes through the colon, and 95% of the contained water is absorbed. The stool remains in the rectum until there is sufficient to cause an urge to defaecate. The mechanism of defaecation begins with peristaltic waves in the colon which advances the faeces into the rectum. The rectum then contracts, expelling the faeces through a relaxed anal canal. The anal canal then empties by contraction of the levator ani muscles, and finally there is contraction of the voluntary external sphincter.

The normal neonate passes meconium in the first 24 hours of life. It is dark green in colour, and soft. Over the next few days, the stool becomes firmer, and changes in colour to greenish brown in the bottle-fed baby, or bright yellow in the breast-fed baby. Breast-fed babies often pass a stool with every feed, or sometimes only once daily. Constipation is unusual in breast-fed babies unless there is an organic cause. Formula-fed infants usually pass stools less frequently and sometimes only once every 2 or 3 days.

Voluntary control of defaecation is usually achieved around the second birthday, and potty training is a common time of onset for functional constipation. The rate of passage of stool varies from three times per day to three times per week in normal children.

Failure to defaecate occurs if there is a mechanical obstruction of the bowel such as an atresia or displaced anus; absence of normal peristalsis in the lower bowel (such as in Hirschsprung's disease); or where there is voluntary withholding of faeces (functional constipation).

Outline

Causes may be organic, for example intestinal obstruction, or functional, for example faulty sphincter training. The causes vary with age, and whether the onset is acute or chronic.

Onset in first week of life

While delayed passage of meconium and/or stools can occur at this time in the absence of an organic cause, it is much more likely that specific pathology will be present and that the child will also have features of intestinal obstruction. Such causes include the following.

Anal atresia

Confirming the presence of an anus is part of the routine examination of the newborn. Anal atresia is an easy diagnosis to make but is sometimes missed because the doctor performing the examination assumes that if the child has a large quantity of meconium in the nappy the anus must be normal. This is not the case as the anal atresia is often accompanied by a fistula into the vagina or urethra which allows meconium to be passed.

Abnormal position or function of anus

The anus may be displaced anteriorly and this interferes with the normal passage of meconium/stool and may lead to chronic constipation from an early age. There may be accompanying anal stenosis and/or the sphincter may be incorrectly aligned with the anal canal. These latter abnormalities are likely to require surgical correction.

Intestinal atresia

The onset of obstruction is sudden and severe. Symptoms of abdominal distension and vomiting usually dominate. The exact timing of the onset depends on the level of the atresia, a high lesion causing symptoms earlier than a lower lesion. It is important to note that some stool may be passed despite the presence of an intestinal atresia.

Meconium ileus

Almost always caused by cystic fibrosis, this condition presents with intestinal obstruction as a result of tenacious meconium occluding the bowel.

Hirschsprung's disease

This is a condition in which ganglion cells are absent from the myenteric plexus of the large bowel. The length of bowel involvement varies from short segment, where the absence is confined to the rectum, to long segment, where much or all of the colon can be involved. Ninety-five per cent of cases present in the neonatal period, but very short segment cases may present later with chronic constipation. In late-presenting cases, there is often a history of delay in passage of meconium. It is more common in boys than girls and may run in families. It is important not to miss this rare diagnosis, because late diagnosis, whether in the neonate or in cases presenting at a later age, can have serious consequences, with enterocolitis, perforation and shock.

Neonatal paralytic ileus

A number of conditions affecting neonates, especially those that produce septicaemia, induce paralytic ileus and 'constipation'. Here it is more important to deal with the underlying condition.

Acute onset in the older child

A sudden onset of constipation, associated with vomiting and abdominal pain in an unwell child, suggests intestinal obstruction. Mechanisms include:

- *Intussusception.* A length of bowel telescopes down an adjacent length of bowel, causing obstruction and necrosis of the bowel wall. It occurs mainly in preschool children.
- *Malrotation and volvulus.* Note that symptoms may be intermittent.
- *Adhesions.* As a result of previous surgery.
- *Crohn's disease.* Obstruction may be caused by an inflammatory mass or adhesions.

Chronic onset in the young child

After the neonatal period, the cause of constipation is functional (non-organic) in 90–95% of cases. The bowel itself is normal, but there is irregular and incomplete defaecation, due to voluntary withholding of faeces. Causes include the following.

Painful defaecation

An anal fissure may be produced by the passage of a hard stool, perhaps formed due to dehydration occurring during a febrile illness. The child then fears defaecation as a painful process, and avoids opening the bowels. This, in turn, results in even larger and harder stools, and further pain on defaecation, reinforcing the child's fear. This leads to a vicious cycle, and the problem can become prolonged for months or years and cause much stress in the family.

Poor potty training

Excessively coercive potty training or attempted training at too early an age results in the child becoming unwilling, and afraid of, opening their bowels.

Poor diet

Inadequate fluid intake, inadequate fibre intake and excessive milk intake can all result in the formation of hard stools that are painful to pass.

Where aspects of the history appear unusual (e.g. onset of problems in the neonatal period) it is important to consider short-segment Hirschsprung's disease, as this may present in this way.

Chronic onset in the older child

Many children presenting in later childhood will have problems that actually started in infancy and hence 'causes' are as listed above. However, when problems first arise in older childhood, psychological problems (e.g. family break-up, bullying), neglect and abuse should all be considered.

Causes that occur at any age

Neurological problems

- Spinal cord lesions: various mechanisms.
- Myotonic dystrophy.

Drugs

- Painkillers such as codeine.
- Chemotherapy agents such as vincristine.
- Antidepressants.

Rare causes

- Hypothyroidism.
- Hypercalcaemia.

History

Onset in the first week of life

In general, the primary concern in this situation is whether the child does or does not have intestinal obstruction. In this situation the presence of constipation is accompanied by other features such as bile-stained vomiting and abdominal distension. Here diagnosis will be made either by investigation (e.g. contrast study) or at surgery. A small group of mature babies will have delayed passage of stool for no discernible cause, although it is sensible to check that such infants do not have cystic fibrosis.

Acute onset in the older child

Here too the priority is to enquire whether constipation is present as a feature of intestinal obstruction by seeking other symptoms such as abdominal distension and bile-stained vomiting. Past medical history may be important in elucidating the cause of the problem, e.g. previous abdominal surgery causing adhesions.

Small children will sometimes present with severe acute problems of chronic constipation (defaecation has become too painful to bear). The preceding constipation (often unknown to the family) has usually been present to a less severe degree for some time.

Chronic constipation

In all cases the following should be ascertained:

- What does 'constipation' mean to the family? This is important, as people have different expectations, and the normal range of bowel actions in children is very variable. Passage of stools varies from three times per week to three times per day in normal children.

- How often does the child open the bowels? How much is passed? Is the consistency hard, normal or soft?
- Does the child have pain with defaecation, or pass blood?
- A dietary history is very important because preschool children are often fussy with food and frequently have an inadequate fluid or fibre intake.
- When did the problem begin, and for how long has it continued? Ask specifically about problems in the newborn period. Ask also about how potty training was managed.
- Ask if the child has been soiling. It is important to note that the retention of faeces for a long period often results in 'spurious diarrhoea' as the stools break down and leak from the distended anus. This results in soiling, which is a very common presentation for constipation in children. Parents often find it difficult to accept that diarrhoea can be caused by constipation. Soiling is sometimes associated with antisocial behaviour in the form of hiding soiled clothes and/or smearing faeces. Such behaviour clearly implies an emotional element to the problem.
- Are there urinary symptoms? Severe constipation may cause retention of urine due to obstruction of urinary flow and/or predisposition to infection.
- Enquire about motor or sensory symptoms in the legs as constipation may be due to a spinal cord lesion.

Examination

Acute onset in the first week of life

1. Assess whether resuscitation is needed and act appropriately.
2. Look for features to suggest that intestinal obstruction is present, e.g. abdominal distension with visible bowel loops and prominent bowel sounds.
3. Examine the anus to confirm it is present and correctly placed.
4. Look for other evidence of:

a) The child being generally unwell; in this case the child may have a paralytic ileus.
b) Dysmorphic features, increasing the risk of congenital anomalies being present.

Acute onset in the older child

Here the priority, as in the newborn, is to decide whether the child has acute intestinal obstruction and carry out any resuscitation. If the child is obstructed, palpation may be difficult and important signs, such as a sausage-shaped mass in intussusception, can be missed.

Growth and nutrition should be assessed since they may indicate the presence of a chronic illness such as inflammatory bowel disease.

The child may be presenting acutely after a prolonged period of constipation and therefore it is important to palpate specifically for any faecal masses (i.e. indentable abdominal masses). In the presence of severe constipation the bladder may be palpable because of obstruction to urination by a faecal mass.

Chronic constipation

Here the focus of the examination is to exclude serious underlying disease. Therefore, as well as a general examination, particular attention should be paid to the child's nutritional state, growth and whether there is evidence of anaemia.

The area of the lower spine should be inspected for any evidence of a spinal anomaly such as an overlying birthmark (e.g. a thick tuft of hair). Where such an anomaly exists, or where the history suggests a spinal lesion, motor and sensory function of the legs, together with saddle sensation and the deep reflexes of the legs, must be checked.

Investigations

These differ depending on whether the constipation is the result of an organically obstructed bowel or is due to a functional problem. Investigations also vary with the age of the child.

Acute obstruction

Investigation	Rationale
Full blood count	Used mainly as part of the preoperative assessment
Urea and electrolytes	Electrolyte abnormalities are likely in the presence of obstruction and should be assessed. The findings are also helpful in assessing the child's state of hydration
Abdominal X-ray	Very helpful in confirming the diagnosis of intestinal obstruction where distended loops of bowel, with fluid levels, are typically apparent
Abdominal ultrasound	May be diagnostic in some situations such as intussusception in the preschool child
Contrast studies	Often used to confirm the level of an atresia in a newborn, or demonstrate the presence of a malrotation, which, if present, increases the risk of volvulus. Can also be therapeutic in meconium ileus by 'washing out' the retained meconium
Air enema	Used particularly in suspected intussusception both to confirm the diagnosis and, in a proportion of cases, reduce the intussusception
Rectal biopsy	The 'gold standard' for the diagnosis of Hirschsprung's disease

Functional (non-organic)

Where the history and clinical findings support a diagnosis of functional constipation, in many cases no investigations are required. In those where there is an inadequate response to aggressive treatment, or where there are unusual features, further tests should be considered.

Investigation	Rationale
Serum calcium Thyroid function	Hypercalcaemia and hypothyroidism may cause constipation but in both conditions other features are usually present
Abdominal X-ray	It is rarely necessary to perform an X-ray to make the diagnosis. However, an X-ray can be helpful to demonstrate to parents that the child really is constipated. Parents may find it particularly difficult to accept the diagnosis and treatment with laxatives when the presentation is with diarrhoea
Rectal biopsy	The 'gold standard' for the diagnosis of Hirschsprung's disease and should certainly be considered if the child's response to treatment is poor
Manometry	Used in specialist centres, this technique can be useful in deciding whether the child's lower bowel function is normal

Clinical problem

A 3-year-old boy presented with a large, hard, craggy abdominal mass arising centrally from the pelvis, and was referred to hospital as a tumour was suspected. The child was otherwise well and his nutritional status was good. He had no pain, no vomiting, but he had been having episodes of profuse diarrhoea over the past few weeks. There was no vomiting. He was described as a fussy eater, but drank a lot of milk. He was potty trained for bowel and bladder at about $2^{1}/_{2}$ years of age. He lived with his parents and sibling, who were also well.

On examination, the mass was as described, and an ultrasound was performed, which confirmed there to be a mass and a hugely distended rectum filled with faeces. He was treated with laxatives and an enema, and the mass disappeared.

Questions

1. What is the likely cause of the faecal mass?

2. Why did he have diarrhoea?

3. Is a rectal biopsy needed?

Answers

1. Functional constipation (non-organic). He has probably been constipated for a long time, as this problem typically arises insidiously – hence the formation of the mass. This is a common age for functional constipation to present – following on soon after potty training. His diet appears to rely on a high milk intake and as a result is low in fibre. This too would support the diagnosis.

2. Spurious diarrhoea. The bowel is impacted with hard faeces distending the rectum and distorting the anus. Liquid stool arriving in the colon and old stool undergoing bacterial breakdown cannot be controlled, leading to what appears to be a diarrhoeal illness, often with soiling.

3. It is important to consider Hirschsprung's disease in all such cases, but there are no particular risk factors presented in the description. It would be helpful to know if the child had any problem passing stools in the neonatal period since this information is not provided. It would seem sensible not to proceed to rectal biopsy at this stage but instead review the child after laxative therapy. If the response to therapy is satisfactory biopsy is unlikely to be helpful.

DIARRHOEA

Kate Wheeler

Diarrhoea is one of the commonest symptoms in childhood. Because there is considerable variation in the consistency and frequency of passage of stool in healthy children, it is an *alteration* in the frequency and/or consistency of a stool which defines diarrhoea for that individual child. Furthermore the nature of a stool will vary as a child becomes older. Infants who are breast-fed will produce many watery stools in 24 hours, while a formula-fed baby may only produce one firmer stool per day. Diarrhoea results from a disruption of the normal absorptive capacity of the bowel, or a disruption of normal physiological mechanisms.

Physiology

Embryologically, the gut forms from the endodermal layer which develops into the foregut (pharynx, oesophagus, stomach and duodenum), midgut (jejunum, ileum and part of the large bowel) and hindgut (remainder of the large bowel).

The four main functions of the gastrointestinal tract involve:

- Transit.
- Digestion.
- Absorption.
- Elimination.

There is a complex integration of these functions dependent on the interrelationship between external influences (e.g. psychological factors, taste, central nervous system control), blood supply, volume of food and fluid ingested, ingested toxins and infections, intracellular factors (active and passive absorptive mechanisms, intrinsic smooth muscle contractility affecting motility), local enteric neuronal control, immune function and local and systemic hormonal control.

Diarrhoea results when there is an imbalance of some of these factors; for the purposes of evaluation and investigation, diarrhoea is conveniently divided

Table 24.1   History: children presenting with diarrhoea should be assessed for the following

Questions	Clinical implication
Duration of symptoms of diarrhoea	Determine if acute or chronic
Alteration of bowel habit	Alternating hard and liquid stool suggests constipation with overflow
Character of stool	Watery – suggests infection
	Bloody – suggests either bacterial infection, e.g. *Shigella*, *Salmonella*, *Campylobacter*, or inflammatory bowel disease, e.g. ulcerative colitis or Crohn's disease
Systemic upset with fever	Suggests infective diarrhoea or diarrhoea as part of a systemic illness
Past medical history	Establish underlying chronic disorder, e.g. cystic fibrosis
Whether thriving	Chronic weight loss suggests a long-standing symptom with malabsorption
Dietary history	Establish relationship with diarrhoea; may suggest a food intolerance, e.g. cow's milk protein intolerance or lactose intolerance
Drug treatment	Some medications produce diarrhoea, e.g. antibiotics
Family history of travel	May suggest infective diarrhoea disease, e.g. *Giardia*

into acute or chronic, determined by the period of symptoms as well as the severity of symptoms. The initial principles of assessment in a child presenting with diarrhoea are shown in Table 24.1.

Chronic diarrhoea

This is defined as the passage of watery stools for more than 2 weeks, at least four times a day. There are many causes of persistent diarrhoea, summarized in Table 24.2.

- *Non-specific toddler diarrhoea* is the commonest cause of chronic diarrhoea in a 1- to 5-year-old in developed countries. Typically the child is thriving and has diarrhoea three to five times per day, which contains mucus and undigested vegetable material – often peas and carrots. Physical examination excludes any abnormality.
- *Malabsorption*:
  - *Carbohydrate malabsorption*. This diarrhoea may be intermittent, and is often associated with abdominal pain, excessive flatus and large, sometimes frothy stools. Disaccharidase deficiency, the commonest, lactase deficiency, can occasionally be a primary condition but more commonly

follows viral gastroenteritis with damage to the brush borders of the villi lining the small intestine. Lactase is temporarily deficient. The diarrhoea resolves after the removal of lactose from the diet. There are often deficiencies of other disaccharidases. Monosaccharide intolerance probably occurs as a result of an inability to transport these molecules across the gut wall. Diarrhoea is a presenting symptom and a clear history can usually aid diagnosis. The best-documented type is glucose/galactose intolerance where fructose is the only monosaccharide that can be absorbed. Another rare condition – fructose intolerance – is caused by deficiency of the enzyme fructose 1-phosphate aldolase. It is inherited as an autosomal recessive condition and presents with symptoms of hypoglycaemia and diarrhoea after the ingestion of fructose.

  - *Protein malabsorption*. In coeliac disease there is sensitivity to the gliadin fraction of the wheat protein, causing damage to the small intestinal villi and resulting in diarrhoea. Diagnosis is made by a jejunal biopsy, which shows the intestinal villi to be flattened. Treatment is by removal of gluten from the diet. Cow's milk protein intolerance is another cause of chronic diarrhoea.

Table 24.2   Causes of chronic diarrhoea

Cause	Symptoms	Pathophysiology	Investigations
Toddler diarrhoea; Irritable bowel syndrome	Non-specific/ functional	Decreased transit time; excessive fluid intake; excessive carbohydrate intake	Exclude infection and failure to thrive
Primary lactose intolerance	Abdominal pain; bulky frothy stools	Congenital lactase deficiency	Stool chromatography; trial of lactose exclusion
Secondary lactase deficiency	Symptoms related to recent acute gastroenteritis; bulky frothy stools	Temporary damage to microvilli and loss of disaccharidases	Chromatography; lactose exclusion
Protein intolerance	May relate to recent gastroenteritis; may be damage from cow's milk protein; pale bulky stools	Temporary or permanent damage to microvilli; sensitivity of mucosa to dietary antigen	Jejunal biopsy; cow's milk protein exclusion
Fat malabsorption	Pale, fatty, offensive stools	Pancreatic insufficiency: cystic fibrosis; Shwachman's syndrome; abetalipoproteinaemia	CF: Sweat test; genotype Shwachman's syndrome: identify cyclical neutropenia; metaphyseal dysplasia; fasting lipids
Inflammatory bowel disease	Abdominal pain; bloody, mucous stools; weight loss	Crohn's disease; ulcerative colitis	Upper GI endoscopy; colonoscopy; biopsy; GI contrast studies
Intestinal infection; enteropathic bacteria (E. coli; Salmonella; Shigella); Giardia; Cryptosporidium; viruses; amoebae	Abdominal pain; watery, bloody stools; mucus	Persistent inflammation	Stool cultures
Surgical: postoperative 'short gut syndrome'; malrotation; blind loops; Hirschsprung's disease	Abdominal pain; obstruction; toxic megacolon; translocation infection	Bacterial overgrowth; reduction in absorptive area	GI contrast studies; endoscopy; biopsies
Tumours: carcinoid; VIP-oma; lymphoma;	Loose stool with increased frequency and abdominal pain	Disruption of physiological motility and absorptive mechanisms	Fasting blood hormone assays (VIP; gastrin); endoscopy; GI contrast studies; biopsies and gut enzyme assays

Table 24.2   Causes of chronic diarrhoea—cont'd

Cause	Symptoms	Pathophysiology	Investigations
Coeliac disease	Malaise; pale bulky stools; weight loss	Inflammatory immune response to gliadin	IgA and IgG antigliadin and anti-endomysial antibodies; jejunal biopsy
Immune deficiency: IgA deficiency; hypogammaglobulinaemia; HIV; severe combined immune deficiency	Loose stools; mucus; blood	Persistent bacterial overgrowth; translocation of gut organisms	Stool culture; investigation of immune deficiency
Gut biochemical dysfunction	Profuse watery stools	Electrolyte pump dysfunction; electrolyte imbalance	Stool electrolytes; biopsy and enzyme assay
Miscellaneous: drugs; Munchausen's syndrome by proxy; endocrine disease; protein-losing enteropathies	Varies	Varies	Drug and social history; endocrine evaluation; serum albumin

  - *Fat malabsorption.* Deficiency of pancreatic exocrine secretion, particularly protease and lipase, occurs in cystic fibrosis. These children have frequent loose oily stools (steatorrhoea). They may also have chronic lung disease and failure to thrive. Treatment of their fat malabsorption is by replacement of the deficient pancreatic enzymes. Shwachman's syndrome consists of exocrine pancreatic insufficiency, cyclical neutropenia and metaphysial chrondroplasia. Steatorrhoea and failure to thrive may be a presenting and ongoing feature.

- *Infections.* Giardiasis or amoebiasis can cause prolonged diarrhoea, particularly if there is a history of travel to endemic areas. Chronic bacterial infection is also associated with persistent diarrhoea.
- *Inflammatory bowel disease* presents with bloody diarrhoea, abdominal pain and weight loss, usually in older children and teenagers. Investigation would include inflammatory markers, barium meal and follow-through for suspected Crohn's disease, upper gastrointestinal endoscopy, and colonoscopy with biopsies for a definitive diagnosis. Lower gastrointestinal contrast studies are rarely performed in children.
- *Short gut syndrome.* This can occur in children who have had previous major intestinal surgery and results in catastrophic long-term diarrhoea, which may require total parenteral nutrition to maintain nutrition and normal growth.

Investigations

Table 24.3 gives an outline of appropriate investigations of chronic diarrhoea. Although the first-line investigations suggested are appropriate in most cases, subsequent investigations are dependent on the details determined in the history. Some of these tests are usually performed at a specialist gastroenterology centre.

Acute diarrhoea

Acute diarrhoea is a very common symptom in the UK (16% of medical paediatric attendances to emergency departments in the UK) and even more common worldwide. Diarrhoea occurs when the normal absorptive capacity of the bowel is exceeded or when there is an imbalance between the secretory and absorptive roles of the gut.

Acute diarrhoea is defined as watery stools of less than 7 days' duration with or without vomiting and fever. When diarrhoea has persisted for over 4 weeks it is defined as chronic.

Table 24.3   Investigations of chronic diarrhoea

First line
Full blood count
ESR, CRP
Urea and electrolytes
Liver function and clotting
Bone analysis
Ferritin
Blood gas
Urine culture pH and electrolytes
Stool
   Culture
   Microscopy
   Electrolytes
   Reducing substances
   Chromatography

Secondary tests dependent on history and results of previous investigations
Coeliac screen (anti-gliadin, endomysial and
   reticulin antibodies)
Endoscopy with jejunal biopsy
Rectal and colon biopsy
Abdominal ultrasound
Sweat test
Upper GI contrast study with follow-through
Carbohydrate breath hydrogen test
Cholesterol and triglycerides
Pancreatic function tests
   VIP
   Gastrin
   Pancreozymin-secretin test
   Stool elastase or chymotrypsin

Diarrhoea may be a non-specific presentation of a child with generalized sepsis; however, a diagnosis of gastroenteritis should always be considered, as worldwide it is the commonest cause of diarrhoea and causes 5–6 million childhood deaths per year (WHO estimation). In the UK the incidence of gastroenteritis is approximately 10% of all children under the age of 2 years. The majority of cases are viral in aetiology, 60–80% being caused by rotavirus. The major causes of acute diarrhoea are given in Table 24.4. The transmission of acute infectious diarrhoea is almost always faeco-oral. Investigations appropriate for the evaluation of acute diarrhoea are given in Table 24.5. The most serious consequence of acute viral gastroenteritis is dehydration. The successful management of acute diarrhoea depends on correction of dehydration and electrolyte losses, followed by maintenance of hydration and nutrition. See Table 24.6 for assessment of dehydration.

Practice points

- The main cause of death from acute diarrhoea worldwide is dehydration.
- In developed countries toddler diarrhoea is the most common cause of chronic diarrhoea in children aged 1–5 years.
- Food poisoning (whatever the cause) and dysentery (diarrhoea with pus) are notifiable conditions.

Table 24.4   Causes of acute diarrhoea

Cause	Epidemiological features	Clinical presentation	Laboratory diagnosis (faecal)
Viral			
Rotavirus (RNA virus)	Major cause of endemic severe diarrhoea in infants and young children worldwide. (seasonal)	Vomiting, then 5–7 days' fever and dehydration	Immunoassay, electron microscopy, polymerase chain reaction
Enteric adenoviruses (DNA virus)	Second most important cause of endemic diarrhoea among infants and young children (not seasonal)	Prolonged diarrhoea lasting 5–12 days; occasional vomiting and fever	Immunoassay, electron microscopy
Caliciviruses (e.g. Norwalk virus) (RNA virus)	Epidemics of vomiting and diarrhoea in older children and adults; often associated with shellfish, water or ice (not seasonal)	Acute vomiting, diarrhoea, fever; myalgia for 1–2 days	Immunoassay
Astroviruses (RNA virus)	Diarrhoea in children and the elderly (seasonal)	Watery diarrhoea often lasting 1–7 days, vomiting	Immunoassay, electron microscopy
Coronavirus	Few cases of neonatal enterocolitis	Necrotizing enterocolitis	Electron microscopy
Bacterial			
Salmonella (Gram-negative bacilli); uncooked eggs potent source	Sporadic and epidemic cases systemic illness. Can occur in sickle-cell disease	Diarrhoea, vomiting, fever. Only treat with antibiotics if systemic illness	Culture stool/blood
Shigella (Gram-negative bacilli)	Very infectious; causes outbreaks	Asymptomatic carriers. Diarrhoea with pus and/or blood, fever	Stool culture
E. coli (Gram-negative)		Vomiting, abdominal cramps, diarrhoea	Stool culture
Campylobacter	Ingestion of contaminated food; direct contact with lambs/puppies	Diarrhoea ± pus and blood, vomiting, fever	Stool microscopy
Other			
NEC (necrotizing enterocolitis)	Occurs in neonates, usually premature	Bloody diarrhoea; abdominal obstruction; bilious vomiting; pneumatosis intestinalis	Stool culture
HUS (haemolytic uraemic syndrome)	Epidemics follow diarrhoea (bloody) episode with verotoxic E. coli (VTEC) serotype 0157; main reservoir: cattle	Diarrhoea and clinical triad of: 1. Microangiopathic haemolytic anaemia 2. Thrombocytopenia 3. Acute renal failure	Stool culture

Table 24. 5   Investigation of diarrhoea

Investigation	Diagnosis
Stool microscopy	Giardia
Stool culture, immunoassay	Viral/bacterial agent
Electron microscopy	
FBC	Exclude haemolytic uraemic syndrome
U & Es creatinine	Monitor hydration
Inflammatory markers, ESR, CRP	Inflammatory bowel disease:
	Crohn's disease
	Ulcerative colitis
Stool electrolytes	Secretory diarrhoea
Stool-reducing substances	Post-enteritis enteropathy
Stool chromatography	Lactose intolerance
Jejunal biopsy	Coeliac disease (flat villi)
Barium meal and FT	Crohn's disease
Barium enema	Ulcerative colitis
Colonoscopy and biopsy	Crohn's/ulcerative colitis
Abdominal ultrasound	Surgical conditions, e.g. intussusception

Table 24.6   Assessment of severity of dehydration

No dehydration (<3% weight loss)	Mild–moderate dehydration (3–8% weight loss)	Severe dehydration (>9% weight loss)
No signs	Dry mucous membranes (be wary in the mouth breather)	Signs from the mild-mod group *plus*:
	Sunken eyes (and minimal or no tears)	Decreased peripheral perfusion (cool/mottled/pale peripheries; capillary refill time >2 s)
	Diminished skin turgor (pinch test >1 s)	Circulatory collapse
	Altered neurological status (drowsiness, irritability)	
	Deep (acidotic) breathing	

Signs are listed in each column in order of increasing severity.
If in doubt clinicians should err by overestimating the % dehydration.
Modified from WHO classification of dehydration.

Clinical problem

A 2-year-old boy presents with a 3-month history of intermittent passage of loose offensive stools three to five times per day. These episodes last for several days and then stool frequency lessens temporarily. In association with the diarrhoea he has had three episodes of rectal prolapse which have required reduction but he has never been constipated. There is no bleeding but he does get mild abdominal pain in association with the loose stools. His parents think he has lost 1 kg in weight over the 3 months. He has a good appetite and is otherwise asymptomatic.

On examination he is slightly pale and his abdomen is soft on palpation, although slightly distended.

His initial investigations arranged by the general practitioner are:

Hb 9.9 g/dL
WCC 5.3 × 10⁹ /L; normal differential white cell count
Stool culture negative
Ferritin 5 μg/L (N 16–300)
Urine culture negative
Thyroid function tests normal
Na 130 mmol/L
K 5.6 mmol/L
Urea 6.0 mmol/L
Creatinine 41 mmol/L

Questions

1. What is the most likely diagnosis?

2. What abnormalities in the blood tests support this diagnosis?

3. How would you establish the diagnosis?

Answers

1. The unifying diagnosis with these symptoms is cystic fibrosis. Although chest symptoms usually accompany gastrointestinal symptoms, they are not universal and depend on the associated genotype. The intermittent nature of the diarrhoea (which may reflect the fat content of the diet) and its character together with the rectal prolapse are characteristic. Although reports vary, up to 11% of rectal prolapse may be associated with cystic fibrosis. The weight loss despite a good appetite and the distended abdomen suggest the patient has malabsorption. Infection has been partly excluded by the negative cultures and chronic infection would not produce intermittent symptoms. Postenteritis enteropathy does not usually result in significant weight loss lasting this period of time. Coeliac disease might present with weight loss but rectal prolapse is not typical.

2. Cystic fibrosis and the associated malabsorption syndrome may produce a characteristic iron deficiency anaemia. There may also be hypoalbuminaemia and secondary oedema. Hyponatraemia may also be present.

3. The diagnosis is made by a positive sweat test; confirmatory tests include a CF genotype which will be identified in about 95% of cases, and by a low faecal elastase. Coeliac disease should be excluded by an antibody screen or small bowel biopsy.

VOMITING
Elaine Carter

Introduction

Vomiting is a very common symptom in many childhood illnesses, and is caused by various mechanisms:

- Incompetence of the gastro-oesophageal sphincter can lead to gastric contents refluxing up the oesophagus.
- Inflammation in the stomach (e.g. viral gastritis, stress ulceration) can cause vomiting because of the irritation.
- Obstruction of the gut prevents the free passage of stomach contents down the gastrointestinal tract and results in vomiting.
- Central nervous system problems can provoke vomiting by direct action on the vomiting centre, which is situated in the floor of the fourth ventricle. A variety of drugs and toxins can also induce vomiting in this way.

Outline

Causes are many and can be divided into groups:

- A non-specific symptom of an acute illness.
- Acute or chronic gastrointestinal tract illnesses.
- Central nervous system conditions.

Non-specific symptom of acute illnesses

A number of infections lead to vomiting by causing the child to cough (raising intra-abdominal pressure) combined with a degree of gastric irritation (e.g. viral upper airway infections and pertussis). In the case of infections such as urinary tract infections it is the general 'toxaemia' (mediated via the vomiting centre) which probably leads to vomiting. This mechanism is also important when vomiting occurs in association with metabolic derangement, e.g. during diabetic ketoacidosis.

Causes specific to the gastrointestinal tract

Acute-onset vomiting

Gastroenteritis

This condition presents at any age, but is more common, and there is more serious risk of dehydration, in infancy. It is still responsible for many childhood deaths throughout the world, especially in developing countries. In the UK there are now only about 25 deaths from gastroenteritis per year, but it is still responsible for a great deal of morbidity and a large number of hospital admissions. The commonest causes are rotavirus and the Norwalk virus (winter vomiting disease), which are very infectious, often spreading rapidly through family members, schools and nurseries. Bacterial causes include *Salmonella*, *Shigella*, *E. coli* and *Campylobacter*, where the clinical picture is often more severe and diarrhoea is typically the predominant symptom. *Giardia lamblia* enteritis occurs throughout the world, and may progress to a chronic phase resulting in malabsorption.

Pyloric stenosis

This condition is characterized by projectile vomiting in a 4- to 8-week-old baby. The vomit is never bile stained, the baby is usually hungry after the vomiting, appears alert and well, but fails to gain weight. The pyloric muscle is hypertrophied (and can often be palpated as the baby feeds), and there is hypochloraemic alkalosis.

Appendicitis

This can occur at any age, but is rare in children under 2 years of age, because of the reduced patency of the appendix at this age. However, it can occur under 2 years, when the diagnosis is easily overlooked, because of its rarity, with serious consequences. The pain is typically central during the early stages and is followed by vomiting. As the condition progresses, again in the typical case, the pain becomes localized to the right iliac fossa. In the young child presentation may simply combine non-specific abdominal pain and vomiting. This can lead to delay in diagnosis. Problems of diagnosis can also arise where the appendix is retrocaecal. Mesenteric adenitis can mimic many of the features of appendicitis but does not show the progression.

Intestinal obstruction

This clinical picture can emerge secondary to a variety of underlying conditions, e.g. duodenal or intestinal anomalies and atresias, intussusception, adhesions, volvulus, strangulated herniae and Hirschsprung's disease.

All these conditions present with varying degrees of the classic picture of vomiting, abdominal pain, abdominal distension and constipation. Atresias present in the early hours or days of life. More proximal atresias result in an earlier onset of vomiting, e.g. a duodenal atresia will present on the first day of life (with vomiting which may or may not be bile stained depending on the exact site of the atresia in relation to the ampulla of Vater), while a low ileal atresia may present with bile-stained and faeculant vomiting on day 2 or 3 of life.

Malrotation and volvulus often present in the early weeks or months of life, but in some cases the presentation may be delayed until a few years of age.

Intussusception occurs most often in the age range of 9 months to 2 years. The onset is sudden, and intermittent screaming is a prominent feature, often followed by lethargy. This combination (vomiting and lethargy) can lead to a misdiagnosis of meningitis. Intussusception is caused by a section of bowel, often with a swelling at the leading end such as a swollen Peyer's patch or a polyp, telescoping into an adjacent piece of bowel.

Hepatitis

Vomiting and non-specific abdominal pain may occur before the classic signs of jaundice and right upper quadrant pain commence. Hepatitis A and EBV virus are common causes of hepatitis in children.

Chronic GIT causes

Gastro-oesophageal reflux

This is a common problem in infancy. It results from the combination of:

- The tendency for babies to have an 'incompetent' cardiac sphincter.
- A predominantly liquid diet.
- Prolonged periods of lying flat.

Under these circumstances it is easy for semi-digested food to be refluxed up the oesophagus. The volume of vomit and its timing (i.e. pre-feed, post-feed) characteristically varies. Although common, very few children develop serious complications such as failure to gain weight, apnoea and aspiration pneumonia.

Peptic ulcers

This is an uncommon problem, occurring mainly in teenage years. There may be a family history of peptic ulcers. Pain, the most important symptom, is usually very specific to the epigastrium, and wakes the child from sleep at night.

Cyclical vomiting

This is an uncommon condition affecting school-age children. Typically the child presents with spells of uncontrollable vomiting, sufficient to become markedly dehydrated, lasting for a few hours or, occasionally, days. The vomiting is self-limiting, and the child is perfectly well between episodes. Underlying causes must be excluded. It is thought to be related to migraine, and sufferers may go on to have migraine as adults.

Food allergy

Food allergy as a cause of vomiting is probably over-diagnosed but should be considered where vomiting occurs soon after contact with a particular food.

Bulimia

This psychosomatic condition is associated with anorexia nervosa, and occurs most commonly in teenage girls but younger children and boys may be affected. Bulimia refers to self-induced vomiting perhaps after a binge of eating, with the purpose of losing weight. These children have often become emaciated before they present to health professionals and often appear unconcerned at their weight loss. It is important to exclude other causes for the weight loss.

CNS problems

Acute

Meningitis

Both the inflammation of the CNS and the toxaemia associated with meningitis produce vomiting, which is a common feature.

Cerebrovascular accidents (CVA)

Although rare in childhood, where cerebral haemorrhage or infarction does occur (perhaps as a result of a leaking vascular malformation), vomiting is common.

Sub-acute/chronic

Raised intracranial pressure

All causes of raised intracranial pressure tend to cause vomiting. This can be acute (e.g. following severe head trauma or leaking vascular malformation); however, accompanying symptoms and signs usually make the diagnosis obvious. Where the rise in intracranial pressure occurs more slowly, the diagnosis may be more difficult to make as other symptoms and signs may be sparse. Important causes include:

- *Tumours*. Early morning vomiting and headaches are characteristic in the early stages.
- *Blocked VP shunt*. This can occur insidiously after years of normal function.

Migraine

Recurrent episodes of headache, often unilateral, preceded by a prodrome of visual disturbance and vomiting, suggests a diagnosis of migraine. The onset is usually sudden, and the headache lasts for 4–72 hours, during which time the child cannot take part in normal activities. Between episodes, the child is perfectly well with no symptoms.

Rare causes

Porphyria

This is an autosomally inherited disorder of haem metabolism which causes recurrent vomiting episodes and neuropathy.

Metabolic disorders

Inborn errors of metabolism, e.g. urea cycle abnormalities and fatty acid oxidation problems, often present with vomiting, especially if there is an intercurrent infection.

Poisoning

Vomiting may be induced purposefully in a child by his/her parent or carer in factitious illness. The child may have been given a drug to make them sick, typically table salt.

History (acute)

Clarify the nature, extent and severity of the vomiting:

- When was the onset?
- How long has it been a problem?
- How often does it occur?
- How much vomit is there?
- What is the colour and content of the vomit (in particular, clarify whether it is green, indicating bile, and therefore suggestive of intestinal obstruction)?
- Is there any blood or brown streaks in the vomit, indicating bleeding?

Associated symptoms

- *Diarrhoea.* The presence of diarrhoea suggests gastroenteritis. This is a very common cause of vomiting in childhood and the diagnosis is highly likely if other family members or friends are also affected. If the child has travelled abroad recently, a wider range of organisms must be considered. Blood in the diarrhoea stool could indicate a bacterial cause such as *Salmonella*, *Shigella* or *Campylobacter*.
- *Pain.* It is important to establish whether the child has abdominal pain. If so, where is it situated, what is the severity and for how long has it been present? However, the 'typical' distribution of pain associated with certain conditions (right iliac fossa/appendicitis; right upper quadrant/hepatitis; loin and suprapubic pain/urinary tract infection; central abdominal pain/intestinal obstruction) is rarely seen in young children. Certainly under 5 years of age all children tend to localize pain to the umbilicus.
- *Fever.* If the child has been feverish it is likely that the cause is related to infection; however, such a history is unreliable unless the temperature was actually measured.

A *full systemic enquiry* is necessary to detect the many non-specific causes of vomiting; for example:

- *Upper respiratory tract infection* (URTI) (rhinitis, earache, etc.).
- *Urinary tract infection* (UTI) (dysuria, haematuria or frequency). However, fever and vomiting may be the only symptoms of a UTI in a small child.
- The first presentation of a new *diabetic* (polydipsia, polyuria, weight loss).
- Acute onset of headache and fever with vomiting may indicate *meningitis*.

Past medical history

This is vital in identifying pre-existing causes of vomiting, e.g.:

- Previous abdominal surgery: adhesions.
- Inflammatory bowel disease.
- Known metabolic disease (including diabetes).
- Regular use of steroids.
- Previous insertion of intracranial shunt.

Supplemental questions for the child with chronic problems of vomiting

In an infant, frequent effortless vomiting is likely to be due to reflux. This can occur any time but is typically worse when the child is full, i.e. after a feed or when winding. If the description is suggestive ask about other symptoms to support the diagnosis:

- Is it worse when lying flat?
- Is the baby hungry after the vomit? This is often true in simple reflux.
- Is there any history suggestive of discomfort? This is a feature of oesophagitis caused by reflux in some children.
- Was an improvement noted at the time of weaning?

Recurrent episodes of vomiting, with no symptoms in between, suggests cyclical vomiting.

Recurrent abdominal pain may be a feature of both peptic ulcer and inflammatory bowel disease, although it is likely that the latter would be accompanied by other symptoms such as weight loss.

Intermittent headache with vomiting, photophobia and visual disturbance may suggest migraine.

General examination (acute)

- *Temperature.* If raised this indicates an infective cause.
- *Hydration and circulatory state* must be assessed and any necessary resuscitation undertaken.
- *Lymphadenopathy.* If present, this raises the possibility of mesenteric adenitis.
- Look specifically for evidence of *jaundice*.

Abdomen (acute)

It is important to look for evidence of tenderness, and if present to try and localize the site. Similarly, any guarding should be noted. However, in small children this may prove impossible and more information may be obtained by observing how the child moves when they are not aware that they are being watched.

Look for the following diagnostic features:

- *Hepatitis.* Enlarged and tender liver.
- *Intestinal obstruction.* Abdominal tenderness and distension with loud bowel sounds.
- *Strangulated hernia.* Irreducible hernia present.
- *Testicular torsion.* Swollen, acutely tender testis.
- *Pyloric stenosis.* Visible peristalsis may be present and a pyloric mass may be felt during a test feed.
- *Intussusception.* A sausage-shaped mass may be present.

Other systems

A full examination of the respiratory and ENT should be performed to identify non-specific causes of vomiting such as URTI or otitis media. Look for evidence of meningism in the febrile child.

Supplemental points for the child with chronic problems of vomiting

Look for evidence of significant chronic disease, e.g. anaemia and weight loss (Crohn's). Persistent vomiting with reflux may cause failure to thrive in a baby, while bulimia may result in emaciation in a teenage child.

If CNS causes are suspected, a full examination of this system is necessary. Look for signs of raised intracranial pressure and focal neurology, including abnormalities of the pupils and fundi.

Investigations

Investigations that may be helpful in the vomiting child include:

Investigation	Rationale
Urine 'stick test'	Excludes 98% of cases of UTI if negative for nitrites, leucocytes and blood, and the protein is within normal limits.
	Absence of glycosuria largely excludes diabetes, although ketones may well be present in any child with prolonged vomiting
Full blood count	A raised neutrophil count suggests the presence of a bacterial infection
Urea and electrolytes	Rarely of diagnostic value in relation to vomiting but essential in managing fluid replacement
Blood glucose	Necessary to exclude diabetes
Liver function tests	Important if hepatitis is suspected
Acute-phase reactants	Helpful in supporting a diagnosis of inflammatory bowel disease (produces very high levels) but in general too non-specific to be useful
Abdominal X-ray	Essential in confirming a clinical diagnosis of intestinal obstruction
Abdominal ultrasound	Has a number of potential roles – particularly helpful in relation to pyloric stenosis and intussusception
Barium studies	Can be useful in diagnosing: Gastro-oesophageal reflux Intestinal obstruction Inflammatory bowel disease
pH study	The gold standard for the diagnosis of gastro-oesophageal reflux
Lumbar puncture	The gold standard for the diagnosis of meningitis
CT/MRI of the brain	Essential if any intracranial cause, other than meningitis, is considered likely

Clinical problem

A 9-year-old girl was seen in A&E having recently arrived in the UK as a refugee. She was admitted with severe vomiting for about 12 hours, which contained yellow liquid and food, but no bile. There were occasional streaks of blood. She had vomiting about 20 times. The mother explained that this had happened before, occurring about once every 4–6 weeks over the past 2 years.

Between episodes she was quite well, with no vomiting or abdominal pain or bowel symptoms. She lived with her mother and two siblings, having left their father behind in another country because he abused her mother.

On examination she was 5% dehydrated, abdomen was soft, and there were no other abnormal features on examination.

Questions

1. What is the likeliest cause for her symptoms?

2. What investigations should be undertaken?

Answers

1. A diagnosis of cyclical vomiting most closely fits the description of this child's problems over the last 2 years. However, a large variety of pathologies could present in this way and in this child it is not possible to be certain whether she is now suffering from an acute illness or, as mother suggests, a recurrence of her previous chronic symptoms. Therefore the important message from this case is that all potential organic causes must be excluded before making the diagnosis of cyclical vomiting. The streaks of blood in the vomit are common after recurrent forceful vomits.

2. In terms of investigations it is important to exclude all potential organic causes. Clearly there is little here to suggest gastro-oesophageal reflux or intracranial pathology. A reasonable initial combination would include:
   a) Serum biochemistry, because of the risk of dehydration, electrolytic disturbance and to look for evidence of metabolic derangement (as well as noting the specific measurements it is also sensible to assess the anion gap).
   b) Blood sugar to exclude diabetes.
   c) Blood gas to check for acidosis.
   d) Blood and urinary amino acid profiles.
   e) Full blood count to look for evidence of infection.
   f) MSU to exclude urinary tract infection.

Further investigation could await the results of these investigations and the child's response to rehydration – often curative in cyclical vomiting.

LUMPS

Kate Wheeler

Introduction

A lump or abnormal mass may be found by parents or detected coincidentally during physical examination, either in a routine surveillance check or during the assessment of a child with symptoms. Lumps detected in early life are more likely to caused by congenital abnormalities; occasionally they are as a result of the birth. Lumps that develop (or are discovered) after the neonatal period can still be congenital but are more likely to be infective, traumatic, functional or neoplastic. The cause of a lump is very dependent on its anatomical site (Table 26.1).

History

General points:

- Age of child.
- Length of presentation.
- Presence of associated other symptoms:
  - Pain.
  - Fever.
  - General malaise.

Head and face

Birth injuries to the head and face are common. These are usually minor and disappear within days of birth:

- *Caput succedaneum.* An oedematous swelling on the back of the head due to pressure on the scalp during delivery, this is relatively common following ventouse extraction.
- *Cephalhaematoma* caused by bleeding under the periosteum of the scalp. Characteristically the swelling does not cross the margins of the neighbouring suture line. It may take weeks to resolve, developing into a hard calcified mass before gradually being absorbed into the skull bone.

Table 26.1　Causes of lumps

Site	Congenital	Birth injury	Infective	Traumatic	Neoplastic	Obstructive	Functional
Head and Face	Plagiocephaly Encephalocele Dermoid Hydrocephalus	Cephalhaematoma Caput succedaneum Skull moulding	Orbital cellulitis Parotitis	Haematomas Skull fractures	Orbital tumours		
Neck	Cystic hygroma Bronchial cyst Torticollis Thyroglossal cyst Dermoid cyst		Lymphadenitis		Lymphoma ALL		Goitre
Thorax		Fractured ribs and clavicle	Mastitis		Sarcoma		Gynaecomastia
Abdomen	Exomphalos Gastroschisis Cystic kidneys Hydrocele Bowel duplication		Appendicitis	Haemorrhage into: Liver Spleen Kidney	Neuroblastoma Wilms' tumour Hepatoblastoma Lymphoma Testicular tumour	Choledochal cyst RV thrombosis Intussusception Pyloric stenosis Hernias	Constipation
Back	Meningocele Meningomyelocele	Fat necrosis					
Limbs	Lymphoedema		Osteomyelitis Septic arthritis	Fractures	Osteosarcoma Ewing's sarcoma		
Skin	Haemangiomas Neurofibromas Naevi		Warts Boils				

- *Plagiocephaly* (asymmetry of the head). This is not due to birth trauma. It usually results from a constricted position in utero, or rarely from premature fusion of the cranial sutures.
- *Congenital CNS lesions* may present at birth. An encephalocele is a defect occurring in the cranium, resulting in a swelling containing meninges with or without brain tissue. Headache, vomiting and neurological abnormalities suggest associated hydrocephalus.
- *Proptosis*. The presence of a fever with a swollen eye may suggest orbital cellulitis. This can occur at any age, is usually bacterial and requires prompt treatment with systemic antibiotics and, sometimes, surgical drainage. In the absence of systemic features a proptosed eye may be due to a primary tumour of the eye, a retinoblastoma (often hereditary) or from a retro-orbital mass (e.g. a primary retro-orbital rhabdomyosarcoma or metastatic neuroblastoma).

Neck

Neonatal

Swellings of the neck noted at birth are most likely to be due to a congenital abnormality of development of the lymphatic system, a cystic hygroma. Very rarely this may be due to a congenital abnormality of blood vessels, a haemangioma or a lymphangioma. These swellings, if large enough, may cause obstruction to the larynx and trachea, compromising respiration or superior mediastinal obstruction as a result of large blood vessel compression in the neck. A cystic hygroma will transilluminate and can be removed surgically.

A sternomastoid tumour is a muscular swelling within the sternomastoid muscle that develops in response to birth trauma. It usually resolves with simple physiotherapy.

Childhood

The most common causes of childhood neck lumps are lymphadenopathy and thyroid enlargement.

Lymphadenopathy

Almost all children have palpable cervical and/or inguinal lymphadenopathy. Common viral or bacterial illnesses of childhood often cause significant enlargement in lymph node size. A common clinical difficulty is to determine whether enlarged lymph nodes in children represent a normal state, a transient hyperplasia in response to a simple viral illness or more serious underlying pathology. Useful clinical guidelines include the following:

- Normal nodes should not exceed 2–3 cm in diameter.
- There should be no overlying erythema, fluctuance or tenderness.
- A supraclavicular node should not be greater than 3–5 mm.

Lymphadenopathy can be due to an increase in the normal number of lymphocytes and macrophages within a lymph node in response to an antigen (infection), actual infiltration of the lymph node by inflammatory cells in response to an infection localized to the node itself (e.g. streptococcal infection) or other inflammatory process, proliferation of malignant lymphocytes (e.g. leukaemia, lymphoma), or infiltration of lymph nodes by abnormal macrophages in a storage disease (e.g. Gaucher's disease).

Some causes of generalized lymphadenopathy are given in Table 26.2.

Thyroid enlargement

This is unusual in children; in 90% of cases it is due to auto-immune thyroid disease. The two commonest forms of this are Hashimoto's thyroiditis and Graves' disease. In Hashimoto's thyroiditis there is a defect in cell-mediated immunity, which results in lymphocytic infiltration and enlargement of the thyroid gland; these patients are usually euthyroid. This may occur alone or in association with other autoimmune endocrine disorders. In Graves' disease there is overactivity of the thyroid gland in association with signs and symptoms of hyperthyroidism. If the thyroid enlargement is not uniform other diagnoses need consideration:

- Congenital thyroglossal cyst.
- Branchial cleft.
- Thyroid adenoma.
- Thyroid carcinoma.

Chest

Lumps on the chest wall are unusual:

- *Trauma*. A fractured rib and/or clavicle can produce calluses during healing.

Table 26.2   Causes of generalized lymphadenopathy

Infections
Viral
   Upper respiratory tract infections
   EBV
   CMV
   HIV
   Rubella
   Varicella
   Measles
Bacterial
   Septicaemia
   Typhoid
   TB
Protozoal
   Toxoplasmosis

Autoimmune
Juvenile rheumatoid arthritis
SLE
Serum sickness
Drug reactions: phenytoin, isoniazid

Abnormal proliferation of cells
Acute leukaemia
Non-Hodgkin's lymphoma
Hodgkin's lymphoma
Neuroblastoma
Langerhans cell histiocytosis

Storage disorders
Gaucher's disease
Niemann–Pick disease

■ *Malignant tumours* can present as painless swellings of the chest wall. These will require full imaging and biopsy. Ewing's sarcoma, rhabdomyosarcoma and osteosarcoma can all present in this way.

■ Swelling of breast tissue in infant boys and girls is common as a result of the effect of maternal hormones and it resolves spontaneously. Gynaecomastia, the presence of excessive breast tissue in males, occurs in approximately 60% of boys going through puberty. It can be unilateral and may be painful and in most cases regresses spontaneously as puberty progresses to Tanner stage 3.

Back

Neonatal

A mass on the lower back of an infant may represent a meningocele or myelomeningocele. A *meningocele* is the herniation of the meninges without any neural tissue, which is covered by skin or a thin-walled membrane. A *myelomeningocele* results from a failure of the posterior neural tube to close. The resultant swelling contains neural tissue and the clinical features depend on the level of the lesion (usually lumbar or lumbosacral). There is usually associated limb paralysis, bladder and bowel dysfunction. Ninety per cent of these cases have associated hydrocephalus. Surgical correction of these problems is complex and in view of the varied prognosis the decision to treat the defect must be made in conjunction with the parents. Most neural tube defects can be detected antenatally, when termination may be offered.

Other back swellings include a sacrococcygeal tumour, when an elevated level of the tumour marker alpha-fetoprotein can be diagnostic.

Skin

Numerous minor lesions may develop on the skin at any time during childhood. At birth, naevus haemangiomas will be noted immediately. Most cavernous haemangiomas typically become more prominent after birth and enlarge until around 1 year. They then resolve slowly over subsequent years. Those that compromise vision or the airway are the only lesions that require treatment.

Skin infections are common in childhood. Warts can be left to resolve spontaneously or can be removed surgically by cryocautery or chemical applications. Large bacterial carbuncles may cause systemic symptoms, particularly in young children.

Abdomen

Masses can often be felt on examination of the abdomen. Many normal structures can be palpable, e.g. liver, spleen, kidneys, stool in bowel, full bladder and small inguinal lymph nodes. Other masses are from an obstructed or dysfunctional organ. Specific signs and symptoms important in determining the cause of an abdominal mass include:

- Jaundice.
- Vomiting.
- Constipation.
- Haematuria.
- Dysuria.
- Bowel obstruction.
- Ascites.
- Hypertension.

Neonatal

Many abdominal masses can be detected on antenatal ultrasound scan:

- Gastrointestinal:
  - *Gastroschisis.* An abdominal wall defect through which the gut protrudes without a covering sac.
  - *Exomphalos.* An embryological failure of the gut to return to the abdominal cavity, so the gut remains outside the abdomen in a sac formed by the umbilical cord. It is often associated with other congenital abnormalities.
  - *Intestinal duplication cysts* and *choledochal cysts* can also present in later childhood.
- Renal:
  - Dysplastic/hypoplastic kidneys.
  - Polycystic disease.
  - Obstructed renal tract.

Children

Non-malignant

- *Intussusception* (invagination of the bowel into a lower portion, causing obstruction) can present with:
  - 'Sausage'-shaped mass in the abdomen.
  - Abdominal pain.
  - Rectal bleeding.
  - Shock.

Eighty per cent of cases present before 1 year – diagnose with a barium or air enema.

- *Appendix mass.* A mass in right iliac fossa in association with pain and fever. Diagnose with ultrasound scan.
- *Pyloric stenosis.* Congenital hypertrophy of the pylorus which causes vomiting, weight loss and dehydration and a metabolic alkalosis. The enlarged pylorus can be palpated during a feed or seen on ultrasound examination. It is rarely diagnosed later than 8 weeks of age.

Malignant

Several childhood tumours present as abdominal masses. These masses may present either as a painless swelling noted by the parents, as a chance finding on routine examination or together with other signs and symptoms.

- Acute leukaemia and lymphomas may present with hepatosplenomegaly, usually in association with lymphadenopathy elsewhere and an abnormal full blood count and bone marrow examination.
- Intra-abdominal solid tumours may present as an isolated abdominal mass:
  - *Wilms' tumour.* Can present as an isolated painless abdominal swelling or there may be associated haematuria, scrotal swelling and hypertension. Wilms' tumour can be associated with congenital abnormalities such as aniridia and hemihypertrophy. It is bilateral in 5% of cases.
  - *Neuroblastoma.* Neuroblastoma tumours arise from cells that form the sympathetic ganglia and the adrenal medulla. These tumours can be very large and may extend across the midline of the abdomen. There may be associated symptoms when there is metastatic disease (present in 70% cases) weight loss, anaemia, fever and bone pain. In young infants the disease can sometimes spontaneously regress without treatment. Diagnosis is made by confirmatory histology of the primary mass or secondary deposits within the bone marrow, appropriate imaging and a positive *meta*-iodobenzylguanidine (mIBG) scan and increased urinary excretion of the catecholamine precursor vanillylmandelic acid (VMA).
  - *Hepatoblastoma.* This is a rare primary liver tumour of infancy. Most cases are diagnosed during the first year of life. Presentation is with an enlarged liver often associated with anorexia and weight loss. The serum alpha-fetoprotein (αFP) is very high.
  - *Ovarian germ cell tumour.* Can present with an abdominal mass together with abdominal pain and/or distension and symptoms related to hormonal dysfunction, vaginal bleeding, amenorrhoea or precocious puberty. Tumour markers αFP or beta-human chorionic gonadotrophin (βHCG) may be raised.

Scrotal masses (Table 26.3)

A hydrocele is common in the neonatal period and it usually resolves spontaneously in the first year of life. If it presents in later childhood with a painless, often unilateral, transilluminating scrotal swelling, surgery will be required. An indirect inguinal hernia can also present as a similar swelling but it will not transilluminate and treatment is surgical.

Inguinal masses

The most common cause of an inguinal lump is an indirect hernia. These are common in preterm infants (the incidence is 5% overall and 30% in babies under 1 kg at birth) and more common in boys. The hernia, which is caused by a persistence of the processus vaginalis, may present as an inguinal lump or may extend into the scrotum. It is painless unless obstructed. The hernia is most obvious when the infant is crying, coughing or walking. An undescended testis can be felt in the inguinal area and if palpated in the inguinal canal can usually be pulled down into the scrotum. Lymph nodes in the inguinal region can be identified as they are usually multiple and firm and may be in association with other lymphadenopathy in the body or with signs of infection (Table 26.3).

All lumps should have imaging as appropriate:

- Ultrasound.
- CT scan.
- MRI scan.

MRI is the safest three-dimensional imaging, as it does not use ionizing radiation. However, a young child will need a general anaesthetic for an MRI scan; it takes longer than a CT (approximately 30 minutes) and the scans are degraded by any movement.

Table 26.4 summarizes the investigations involved in the diagnosis of lumps.

Table 26.3 Causes of scrotal and inguinal masses

Scrotal mass	Hydrocele
	Indirect inguinal hernia
	Varicocele
	Scrotal oedema from hypoalbuminaemia, e.g. nephrotic syndrome
	Testicular tumour, e.g. germ cell tumour, rhabdomyosarcoma, leukaemia
Inguinal mass	Lymphadenopathy
	Hydrocele
	Undescended testes
	Inguinal hernia:
	Direct
	Indirect
	Femoral hernia

Table 26.4 Summary of investigations indicated in the diagnosis of lumps

Investigation	Findings	Possible diagnosis
Full blood count	Anaemia	
	Pancytopenia	Acute leukaemia
ESR/CRP	Raised	Acute infection/inflammation
LFTs	Raised	Liver dysfunction, secondary to obstruction Hepatitis, infiltration
αFP	Raised	Hepatoblastoma, germ cell tumour
βHCG	Raised	Germ cell tumour
Urinary VMA (spot value)	Raised	Neuroblastoma
Chest X-ray	Mediastinal mass	Lymphoma
	Lung metastases	Metastatic disease
Urinalysis	Haematuria	Wilms' tumour
	Infection	Pyelonephritis

Clinical problem

A 5-year-old boy presents to his general practitioner with a 3-week history of a slightly tender mass in the posterior triangle of his neck. Although he had a presumed viral upper respiratory tract infection at the time of onset, the mass has not become smaller since the infection has resolved. He is otherwise well. The GP has organized a full blood count and a Monospot test for EBV infection. The blood count is normal and the Monospot is negative.

The family is originally from West Africa and has been living in the UK for 5 years, but has returned to Africa every year for holidays. The boy has had all the appropriate immunizations, including a BCG at birth.

He is referred to a hospital clinic for further assessment.

On examination there is a 2 × 2 cm firm mobile mass which is slightly tender. There are no other cervical masses or lymphadenopathy elsewhere. Physical examination is otherwise normal.

Initial investigations, including a repeat FBC, a chest X-ray, liver function tests, urea and electrolyte analysis and thyroid function tests, are all normal. His Mantoux test is 7 mm.

Questions

1. What is the differential diagnosis?

2. How would you manage the child now?

Answers

1. Infection:
   a) Non-specific viral.
   b) Atypical mycobacterial infection.
   c) TB.

2. After 3 weeks, a viral infection remains the most likely cause; a low-grade bacterial infection is also possible. From a practical point of view most of these acute masses will resolve, sometimes with the help of antibiotics. His Mantoux response is consistent with his previous BCG and is unlikely to represent TB infection. A normal FBC does not exclude a lymphoma; this diagnosis, however, is unlikely given the short history.
   If the mass persists for a further 6 weeks, an excision biopsy is indicated. At this point an atypical mycobacterial infection is most likely. Although it is possible to perform differential Mantoux tests against atypical mycobacteria (*Mycobacterium avium-intracellulare*), this is not always practicable. Biopsy with culture and sensitivities will give the best chance of a definitive diagnosis, will exclude human TB and is also the optimal treatment of the atypical mycobacterial infection.

CHAPTER 27

BRUISING AND BLEEDING

Richard Stevens

Introduction

Evaluation of a patient with a possible bleeding tendency is a relatively common routine in paediatric practice. It requires the identification of key elements in the clinical history and physical examination and the integration of this information with the results of laboratory investigations.

Outline

Clinical evaluation of a bleeding child can be considered under five categories:

1. *Platelet problem.* Thrombocytopenia or platelet functional defect.
2. *Single coagulation factor deficiency.* Factor VIII, IX, XI, VII, V, fibrinogen deficiency.
3. *Multiple factor deficiency.* Vitamin K deficiency, liver disease, warfarin.
4. *Circulating anticoagulant.* Heparin, factor VIII or factor IX antibody, lupus anticoagulant.
5. *Consumptive coagulopathy.* Haemolytic uraemic syndrome, malignancy, hypoxia/acidosis etc.

History and examination

Important diagnostic information is provided by the clinical setting because of the associations between bleeding abnormalities and certain disease states. The following points need consideration:

- *Who?* The child's age at diagnosis (possible congenital defect), sex (e.g. haemophilia), racial background (e.g. factor XI deficiency in Jews), and family history (e.g. haemophilia and von Willebrand's disease).
- *When?* Any association with a disease state, surgery, trauma, dental extractions or drug ingestion.

Where? The site(s) of the bleeding. Is it skin, mucous membranes, gastrointestinal, joint, muscle or solid organ?

What? The characteristics of the bleeding. Is it petechial (capillary) haemorrhage or purpuric? Bruises (ecchymoses) and haematomas are usually seen with larger vessel bleeding. Has the bleeding followed surgery, dental extraction, trauma or immunization?

Platelet (and small vessel) disorders are usually associated with:

- Petechiae and ecchymoses.
- Small haematomas.
- Mucous membrane bleeding.
- Short-lived bleeding after trauma.

A plasma coagulation defect is suggested by:

- Large, deep haematomas.
- Haemarthroses, either spontaneous or after minimal trauma.
- Persistent and recurrent oozing after trauma or surgery

Absence of bleeding after surgery or dental extraction argues against a major haemostatic defect, although the patient may be mildly affected. However, a normal response to trauma (e.g. circumcision or intramuscular injection) in a neonate does not necessarily exclude a plasma coagulation defect.

Bleeding that is excessive for the degree of trauma is an important observation. On the other hand, bleeding is a natural consequence of abnormal stress on the vasculature, e.g. bleeding in the distribution of the superior vena cava due to prolonged coughing, vomiting or seizures, physical abuse or self-inflicted injury.

The presence of a petechial rash is suggestive of a platelet abnormality either in number or function. The coexistence of anaemia, lymphadenopathy and/or hepatosplenomegaly is suggestive of associated disease (e.g. leukaemia or malignancy) and not just an isolated platelet disorder.

Investigation

There are several routine investigations that together make up what is often known as the 'coagulation (haemostatic) screen', which should detect most major defects, but which cannot be expected to identify rare or mild deficiencies.

A useful coagulation screen is made up of:

- Full blood count (including platelet count) and blood film.
- Prothrombin time (PT).
- Activated partial thromboplastin time (APTT).
- Thrombin clotting time (TT).
- Fibrinogen assay.

The bleeding time has never been a popular routine test in children because of associated trauma and potential scaring. The recent introduction of in vitro bleeding time using the PFA 100 apparatus may be useful.

It is important to remember that unexpected results may be artefactual; for example: low platelet counts in poorly taken finger-prick samples; under- or over-filled coagulation bottles; heparin contamination (e.g. samples taken from arterial lines); and delay in the separation and analysis of samples (low factor V and VIII levels).

The coagulation screen will not detect:

- Abnormalities of platelet function associated with a normal platelet count.
- Mild coagulation factor deficiencies.
- A proportion of cases of von Willebrand's disease.
- A minority of lupus anticoagulants.
- Factor XIII deficiency.
- Hypercoagulable states.
- Small vessel dysfunction.

There are differences in haemostasis in infancy and childhood compared with adults. This is because coagulation factors do not cross the placenta to any significant degree. As a result, many coagulation factors and natural coagulation inhibitor levels are lower (when compared to adults) in healthy term infants and particularly in premature infants. Sick infants may have particularly low levels.

Inherited deficiencies that cannot be diagnosed with confidence in infancy include:

- Mild factor IX deficiency (factor IX level normally low).
- Most cases of von Willebrand's disease (von Willebrand factor normally high).
- Heterozygous deficiency of coagulation inhibitors (protein C, protein S and antithrombin III levels normally low).

Prothrombin time (PT)

The PT provides a measure of both the extrinsic and common coagulation pathways. The assay is per-

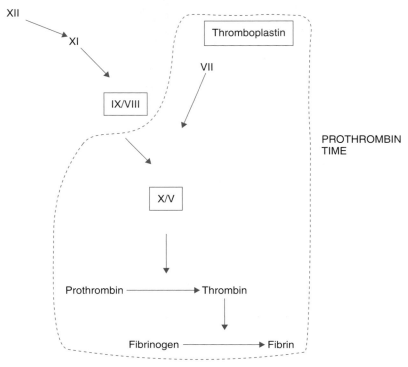

Fig 27.1   Prothrombin time (measures pathway within dotted line).

formed by adding calcium and brain thromboplastin, which provides a very strong stimulus to the activation of factor VII (Fig. 27.1).

Compared to the APTT, the PT is more sensitive to multiple deficiencies of the vitamin K-dependent liver factors. As a screening test for any single coagulation factor deficiency, the PT is most sensitive to a reduced level of factor VII. When the PT is twice the control value, factor levels are likely to be less than 10% of normal.

The PT may also be prolonged with:

- Warfarin therapy (probably the commonest cause of a prolonged PT, even in children).
- Large amounts of heparin.
- Hypofibrinogenaemia.
- Abnormal fibrinogen or fibrinogen fragments.

Activated partial thromboplastin time (APTT)

The APTT measures both the intrinsic and common pathways (factors XII, XI, IX, VIII, X and V). For this

assay, plasma is activated with a contact surface material such as kaolin, together with calcium and phospholipid (Fig. 27.2).

The APPT may be prolonged by a deficiency of any of the factors present in the common pathway, by the presence of a circulating inhibitor or because of a fibrinogen abnormality. Although the APTT is less sensitive than the PT to reduced vitamin K-dependent factors, it is more sensitive to the pressure of circulating heparin and the lupus anticoagulant.

Thrombin time (TT)

The thrombin time measures the last step in the coagulation pathway: the conversion of fibrinogen to insoluble fibrin. It is performed by adding a dilute solution of bovine thrombin to the test plasma. Prolonged TTs are seen in patients with reduced or abnormal fibrinogens or high levels of fibrin degradation products. It is therefore an indicator of disseminated intravascular coagulation (DIC) and

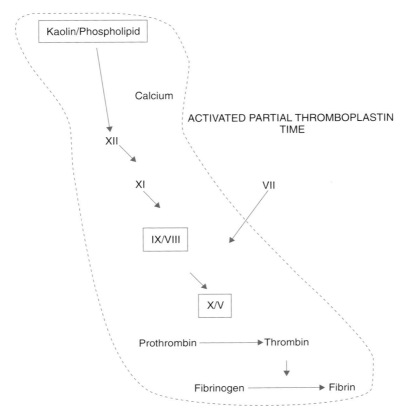

Fig 27.2 Activated partial thromboplastin time (measures pathway within dotted line).

liver disease. Very small amounts of heparin in the circulation can dramatically prolong the TT. The addition of the snake venom reptilase (reptilase time) can help in diagnosing heparin contamination. A prolonged APTT and TT in the context of a normal reptilase time is almost certainly due to heparin contamination.

Interpretation of PT and APTT results

Isolated prolongation of the PT

- Inherited:
  - Factor VII deficiency.
  - Hereditary disorders of bilirubin metabolism.
- Acquired:
  - Mild vitamin K/prothrombin complex deficiency.

Isolated prolongation of the APTT

Table 27.1 lists the more common causes of a prolonged APTT in the order they are most frequently seen.

Once an isolated prolonged APTT is detected, the following investigations should be considered.

Exclude heparin contamination if relevant:

- Reptilase time normal.
- Re-collect sample from a non-contaminated vein.

Further tests:

- Mixing tests:
  - No or only partial correction by normal plasma:
    - Specific factor inhibitor.
    - Lupus anticoagulant.
  - Correction by normal plasma.
    - Factor deficiency. Specific factor assays: F VIII, F IX, F XI, F XII.

Table 27.1 Common causes of prolonged APTT

Defect	Comment
Factor VIII deficiency (classical haemophilia)	The longer the APPT the lower the F VIII/IX level. Mildly affected patients may be missed.
Factor IX deficiency (Christmas disease)	Diagnosis of mild F IX deficiency in infancy because F IX normally low
Von Willebrand's disease	APTT prolonged in only about a third of cases
Heparin	TT usually also prolonged.
Factor XI deficiency	
Factor XII deficiency	Not usually associated with bleeding.
Other rare causes	E.g. pre-kallikrein, high-molecular-weight kininogen deficiency

Specific comments on von Willebrand's disease (vWD)

Von Willebrand's disease is the commonest inherited coagulation disorder and is due to either a quantitative (mild type 1 and severe type 3) or qualitative (type 2) deficiency of von Willebrand factor (vWF).

Severe cases can usually be detected by a prolonged APTT with follow-up investigations of factor VIII and vWF (vWF:antigen and vWF:activity (ristocetin cofactor).

Diagnosis of less severe cases can be a problem:

- Abnormal results (bleeding time, F VIII:coagulant, vWF:Ag, vWF:Act) are seen in only about 60% of cases.
- Mild cases cannot be diagnosed in infancy because vWF levels are usually high up to 6 months of age.
- vWF is an acute-phase reactant and levels rise due to stress, fright, exercise, trauma, inflammation, pregnancy and ovulation.
- Results may vary unpredictably over time and within a kindred. Symptoms may improve spontaneously in late childhood and during puberty.

Prolongation of both the PT and APTT

In terms of specific coagulation deficiency, reduced prothrombin complex (factors II, VII, IX and X) is probably the commonest cause of a combined PT and APTT prolongation. This may be seen in haemorrhagic disease of the newborn, vitamin K deficiency, malabsorption, liver disease and warfarin therapy. Excessive or iatrogenic heparin therapy is also a common association.

Disseminated intravascular coagulation (DIC) is also a cause of a combined prolongation of the PT and APTT but is usually associated with a different and more severe clinical presentation, together with other abnormal tests including raised fibrin monomers/degradation products, reduced fibrinogen, thrombocytopenia and red cell abnormalities on the blood film.

Thrombocytopenia and platelet disorders
(Table 27.2)

Comments

- A bone marrow examination should be performed if there is:
  - Suspicion of infiltrative disease, e.g. leukaemia, childhood malignancy, storage disorder, abnormal marrow function.
  - Suspicion of marrow hypoplasia, e.g. aplastic anaemia.
- Look for other clinical features, e.g. thrombocytopenia and absent radii, stigmata of Fanconi anaemia, eczema and X-linked inheritance in Wiskott–Aldrich syndrome, deafness and nephritis in Alport's syndrome.
- Abnormal sized platelets e.g. large platelets in Bernard–Soulier disease, small platelets in Wiskott–Aldrich syndrome.
- Abnormal platelet function tests and platelet membrane glycoproteins in Bernard–Soulier disease, Glanzmann's disease (thrombasthaenia).
- ITP is essentially a diagnosis of exclusion (i.e. normal clinical examination except for the clinical

Table 27.2   Differential diagnosis of thrombocytopenia

Reduced production	Abnormal distribution	Increased destruction
Marrow damage	Splenomegaly	Non-immune
Hypoplasia	Liver disease	DIC
Hepatitis	Myelofibrosis	HUS
Drugs		TTP
Malignancy		
Congenital defects		Immune
Fanconi anaemia		Drugs
TAR syndrome		Secondary to SLE, AIDS etc.
Wiskott–Aldrich syndrome		

features of thrombocytopenia), with a normal blood film (except for thrombocytopenia).

■ Do not forget neonatal (alloimmune) thrombocytopenia – a potentially lethal condition.

■ A prolonged bleeding time is seen in cases of thrombocytopenia (but is not usually performed!), platelet function disorders, and more severe cases of von Willebrand's disease.

Clinical problem 1

A 3-month-old baby girl presents with a history of purpura and easy bruising with some epistaxes since birth. There are no dysmorphic features on examination.

Hb 10.5 g/dL
MCV 80 fL

WBC 6.8 × 10 per litre
Platelets 275 × 10 per litre
Blood film normal
Coagulation screen normal
Bleeding time greater than 20 min

Discussion

The history, clinical examination and normal platelet count are suggestive of a congenital platelet functional abnormality. The normal platelet count and lack of large platelets on the blood film make a diagnosis of Bernard–Soulier syndrome less likely. Platelet function tests and the absence of platelet membrane glycoproteins IIb and IIIa on specific analysis confirm the diagnosis of Glanzmann's disease (thrombasthenia).

Clinical problem 2

A 4-year-old girl of Pakistani background presents with a long history of easy bruising and repeated severe nosebleeds. She has had a swollen painful knee on two occasions.

Hb 9.4 g/dL
Platelets 310 × 10 per litre
Blood film normal

Bleeding time greater than 20 min
PT 12 s (control 12 s)
APTT 95 s (control 32 s)
Factor VIII 0.05 iu/mL (5%)
vWF antigen < 10%
vWF activity (RiCof) < 10%

Discussion

The history is very suggestive of a congenital bleeding disorder possibly associated with haemarthroses. However, the sex of the child and the prolonged bleeding time make haemophilia most unlikely. The prolonged APTT, low factor VIII and von Willebrand factor assays are highly suggestive of severe (type 3) von Willebrand's disease. The ethnic background of the child raises the possibility of familial consanguinity, with both parents being mildly affected (heterozygous).

Clinical problem 3

A 3-year-old boy presents with a history of vomiting and diarrhoea. On examination he has periorbital swelling and marked pallor.

Hb 5.3 g/dL
Platelets 65 × 10 per litre

Blood film shows polychromasia, fragmented red cells and moderate thrombocytopenia
PT 16 s (control 12 s)
APTT 56 s (control 32 s)

Discussion

The history and examination are very suggestive of the haemolytic uraemic syndrome (HUS). This will need confirmation with renal function tests, stool analysis etc. The blood film changes suggest a reticulocytosis (which will need confirmation with a reticulocyte count) and a microangiopathic haemolytic anaemia as often seen in HUS. The thrombocytopenia and abnormal coagulation screen are often present and disseminated intravascular coagulation should be excluded.

ANAEMIA
Richard Stevens

Introduction

The signs and symptoms of anaemia in paediatric practice are a function of:

- Severity.
- Rapidity of onset.
- Age of child.

Mild anaemias at any age may be relatively asymptomatic. This is because changes in the haemoglobin–oxygen dissociation curve are able to compensate for modest falls in the haemoglobin level.

In older children progressive anaemia is associated with:

- Increasing pallor.
- Loss of exercise capacity.
- Tachycardia.
- Breathlessness.

In infants and young children reduced exercise performance will be less apparent but features of cardiac decompensation (e.g. peripheral oedema and hepatomegaly) may be more evident.

The rapidity of onset of anaemia is important. Changes in the haemoglobin–oxygen dissociation curve may occur rapidly but cardiovascular compensation for severe anaemia takes longer. Children with acute blood loss are at risk for signs and symptoms of both tissue hypoxia and cardiovascular collapse, whereas long-standing anaemia may be associated with expansion of the child's blood volume, increased cardiac output and localized changes in blood flow.

Examination

The clinical signs of anaemia depend very much on the rapidity of onset. Acute blood loss is associated with signs of hypovolaemic shock with distress, air hunger, tachycardia and hypotension. When anaemia develops more gradually there may be signs of

Table 28.1 Probable diagnoses associated with signs of anaemia

Sign	Differential diagnosis
Pallor with jaundice	Haemolytic anaemia
Pallor with bruising and purpura	Hypoplastic anaemia
Pallor, bruising, purpura, lymphadenopathy Hepatosplenomegaly (± bone tenderness)	Acute leukaemia
Bruising and purpura without pallor, lymphadenopathy or hepatosplenomegaly	Isolated thrombocytopenia (e.g. ITP) or abnormal platelet function

increased cardiac output with tachycardia, increased cardiac impulse, tachypnoea and cardiac flow murmurs.

Anaemia may also be apparent from the child's general appearance. Pallor of the skin, mucous membranes and conjunctivae are more evident in fair-skinned patients than those who are heavily pigmented.

If the child has significant pallor it is important to look for other clinical features. Table 28.1 may be helpful.

Investigations

The history and examination may go some way to suggest a cause for the child's anaemia. Nevertheless, a thorough laboratory evaluation is essential to enable a definitive diagnosis.

Table 28.2 lists the more routine tests relevant to anaemia diagnosis. A larger number of more specific tests come into play when confirming the diagnosis of a specific condition.

It is important to remember when diagnosing anaemia in a child that paediatric normal values may be different from those of an adult and are age dependent (see Table 28.3).

Classification and investigation of childhood anaemia

Anaemia in children may be classified on a physiological or morphological basis. A combination of both approaches is often used.

Table 28.4 lists the anaemias most commonly seen in infancy and childhood and classifies them

Table 28.2 Routine laboratory tests in anaemia diagnosis

Full blood count
Red cell number: RBC count, haemoglobin, haematocrit (PCV)
Red cell indices: mean corpuscular volume (MCV), mean corpuscular haemoglobin (MCH), mean corpuscular haemoglobin concentration (MCHC)
White cell count, white cell differential
Platelet count
Blood film morphology: cell size, haemoglobinization, anisocytosis (differences in size), poikilocytosis (differences in shape), polychromasia (differences in colour)
Reticulocyte count

Bone marrow examination
Marrow aspiration: cellular morphology, extramedullary infiltration, iron stain
Marrow trephine biopsy: cellularity, morphology, infiltration

Iron studies
Serum ferritin
Zinc protoporphyrin
Marrow iron stain

into three categories based on disturbance of function. The list is not intended to be totally comprehensive.

Anaemia can also be considered on the basis of red cell size, i.e. microcytic, macrocytic or normocytic (Table 28.5).

Table 28.3   Childhood haematology values

Age	Hb (g/dL) Mean (range)	PCV Mean (range)	MCV (fL) Mean (range)
Birth (cord)	16.5 (13.5–19.5)	0.51 (0.42–0.62)	108 (98–118)
1 day (cap)	18.5 (14.5–21.5)	0.56 (0.45–0.66)	108 (95–116)
1 week	17.5 (13.5–20.5)	0.54 (0.42–0.62)	107 (88–115)
1 month	14.0 (10.0–16.5)	0.43 (0.31–0.51)	104 (85–108)
6 months	11.5 (9.5–13.5)	0.35 (0.29–0.45)	91 (74–96)
1 year	12.0 (10.5–13.5)	0.36 (0.33–0.42)	78 (70–86)
5 years	12.5 (11.5–14.0)	0.37 (0.34–0.41)	81 (75–88)
10 years	13.5 (11.5–14.5)	0.40 (0.35–0.45)	86 (77–94)
15 years:			
Female	14.0 (12.0–15.5)	0.41 (0.36–0.46)	88 (78–96)
Male	14.5 (13.0–16.0)	0.43 (0.37–0.50)	90 (78–98)

Table 28.4   Classification of anaemias of infancy and childhood by disturbance of function

Red cell production less than for the level of anaemia

Marrow failure

Aplastic anaemia: congenital and acquired

Pure red cell aplasia: Diamond–Blackfan anaemia, transient erythroblastopenia of childhood (TEC)

Marrow infiltrative disease: e.g. leukaemia, neuroblastoma, osteopetrosis

Marrow hypoplasia with pancreatic insufficiency: Shwachmann's syndrome

Reduced erythropoietin production

Chronic renal disease

Hypothyroidism, hypopituitarism

Chronic inflammation, e.g. cystic fibrosis

Reduced oxygen affinity haemoglobinopathies

Disorders of erythroid maturation and ineffective erythropoiesis

Cytoplasmic defects, e.g. iron deficiency, thalassaemia

Nuclear maturation defects: vitamin B_{12} and folic acid deficiency. Hereditary abnormalities of folate metabolism and orotic aciduria

Refractory and dyserythropoietic anaemia

Haemolytic anaemias

Defects of haemoglobin:

a) structural, e.g. sickle-cell disease

b) synthetic, e.g. thalassaemia

Defects of red cell membrane, e.g. hereditary spherocytosis

Defects of red cell metabolism, e.g. G6PD deficiency

Antibody mediated, e.g. auto-immune haemolytic anaemia

Microangiopathic haemolytic anaemia, e.g. secondary to DIC or haemolytic uraemic syndrome

Table 28.5   Classification of childhood anaemia by red cell size

Microcytic anaemia

Iron deficiency, e.g. nutritional, chronic blood loss

Thalassaemia syndromes

Chronic inflammation

Other rare causes, e.g. sideroblastic anaemia, chronic lead poisoning

Macrocytic anaemia

With a megaloblastic marrow: vitamin B_{12} or folate deficiency, orotic aciduria

Without a megaloblastic marrow: aplastic anaemia, Diamond–Blackfan anaemia, hypothyroidism, liver disease, dyserythropoietic anaemia

Normocytic anaemia

Congenital haemolytic anaemias:

a) Abnormal haemoglobins, e.g. sickle cell

b) Red cell enzyme defects, e.g. G6PD deficiency, pyruvate kinase deficiency

c) Red cell membrane defects, e.g. hereditary spherocytosis

Acquired haemolytic anaemia:

a) Antibody mediated (Coombs positive)

b) Microangiopathic

Acute blood loss

Splenic pooling

Chronic disease, e.g. real failure, cystic fibrosis

The following considerations may be of some assistance in evaluating the history of children with anaemia.

Age

Anaemia below the age of 6 months is never caused by nutritional deficiency in term infants and rare in preterm babies until they have doubled their birth weight.

Anaemia in the neonatal period is usually the result of blood loss, isoimmunization, congenital haemolytic anaemia or congenital infection.

Anaemia between the ages of 3 and 9 months is suggestive of a congenital disorder of haemoglobin synthesis (e.g. beta-thalassaemia) or haemoglobin structure (e.g. sickle-cell disease).

Gender

Consider X-linked disorders in males (e.g. glucose 6-phosphate dehydrogenase (G6PD) deficiency).

Race

Haemoglobins S and C are more common in blacks; beta-thalassaemia is more common in whites; and alpha-thalassaemia is more common in black and yellow races.

Ethnicity

Thalassaemia syndromes are more common amongst Mediterranean people and those from the Asian sub-continent. G6PD deficiency is seen more often in Greeks, Sardinians, Kurds, Filipinos and Sephardic Jews.

Neonatal

Neonatal jaundice may be suggestive of hereditary spherocytosis or G6PD deficiency. Prematurity predisposes to early iron deficiency.

Drugs

- Oxidant-induced haemolytic anaemia (G6PD deficiency).
- Phenytoin-induced megaloblastic anaemia.
- Drug-induced aplasia.

Infection

- Hepatitis-induced hypoplastic anaemia.
- Viral-associated transient erythroblastopenia of childhood.
- Infection-associated haemolytic anaemia.

Inheritance

- Family history of anaemia, jaundice, gallstones or splenomegaly.

Diarrhoea

- Small bowel disease with malabsorption of folate or vitamin B_{12}.
- Inflammatory bowel disease with blood loss.

Clinical problem 1

An 8-year-old boy is admitted for routine tonsillectomy. His father is of Pakistani origin.

Hb 10.1 g/dL
MCV 65 fL

RBC 6.1 × 10/dL
Blood film: microcytosis, hypochromia and a few target cells

Discussion

These results are suggestive of thalassaemia minor (trait), most likely beta-thalassaemia minor. The haemoglobin A2 level will almost certainly be raised and possibly also the haemoglobin F level. Haemoglobin electrophoresis may show the raised Hb A2 band. Coexisting iron deficiency may lower the Hb A2 level to normal levels. A similar blood picture but with normal Hb A2 and Hb F levels may suggest alpha-thalassaemia (particularly if the child comes from South East Asia).

Haemoglobin electrophoresis is particularly important in suspected cases of structurally abnormal haemoglobins such as Hb SS (sickle-cell disease), Hb AS (sickle-cell trait), Hb SC etc.

Clinical problem 2

A 6-month-old child presents with severe pallor and failure to thrive.

Hb 3.5 g/dL
MCV 95 fL

Discussion

The most likely diagnosis is congenital red cell aplasia (Diamond–Blackfan anaemia). Most children present before the age of 6 months. Macrocytosis (for age) and raised Hb F levels are common. Bone marrow examination shows markedly reduced (although not totally absent) red cell precursor cells.

The main differential diagnosis is that of transient erythroblastopenia of childhood (TEC). These children are usually older, do not have a macrocytosis and may have a history of a preceding viral infection. The bone marrow may be normal if the child is already in the recovery phase.

Clinical problem 3

A 2-week-old baby is found to be pale and jaundiced.

Hb 9.3 g/dL
MCV 108 fL

Direct Coombs test: negative
Reticulocytes 15%
Blood film shows numerous spherocytes
Mother and baby are of the same ABO blood type

Discussion

This baby almost certainly has a congenital haemolytic anaemia, with hereditary spherocytosis being the most likely.

The negative Coombs test makes a significant iso-immune haemolytic anaemia (such as haemolytic disease of the newborn due to anti-D or anti-Kell) most unlikely. The fact that the mother and baby are of the same ABO blood group excludes ABO haemolytic disease.

The presence of a significant number of spherocytes on the blood film raises the possibility of hereditary spherocytosis. If there is a positive family history or haematological abnormality in either parent then the diagnosis is confirmed. However, a quarter of children have no positive evidence of parental involvement.

The red cell osmotic fragility is a test of the past and almost impossible to interpret in babies. More specific tests of red cell structural proteins are becoming available. If in doubt, arrange regular follow-up. If the child has hereditary spherocytosis then the blood spherocytes will persist and tests can be repeated at a later date.

HAEMATURIA

Peter Houtman

Introduction

Haematuria in childhood is associated with a very large number of conditions, the breadth of which can be quite daunting, encompassing the spectrum of both medical and surgical disorders.

Macroscopic or microscopic?

Visible blood in the urine will usually cause considerable alarm and prompt medical attention. At the other end of the spectrum the haematuria will only be apparent when sought by the use of dipsticks, confirmed by the presence of red cells on microscopy.

The incidental finding of urinary blood on dipstick or microscopy is probably normal. Fever, illness, trauma and rigorous exercise can all precipitate microscopic haematuria. It is found in at least 2% of the population at any one time. However, as the number of measurements increases over time, the incidental finding of haematuria in the general population decreases. It should be emphasized that, particularly regarding 'renal' causes, the degree of haematuria is poorly related to the likely severity of the underlying condition. The presence and degree of proteinuria is much more likely to be a prognostic factor.

Aetiology

The range of conditions that need to be considered in the child presenting with haematuria are listed in the Table 29.1.

In terms of the proportion of all cases of haematuria in childhood, urinary tract infection is clearly an important diagnosis but this is discussed elsewhere (see Ch. 30). A number of other conditions merit further comment:

Table 29.1   Causes of haematuria

Renal
Acute nephritis:
a) Post-streptococcal
b) Henoch–Schönlein purpura
c) Haemolytic uraemic syndrome
d) Others: systemic lupus erythematosus, polyarteritis, other vasculitides
e) Of unknown cause
Renal vascular thrombosis: venous or arterial
Trauma
Sickle cell anaemia
Tumours (particularly Wilms' tumour)
Polycystic kidney disease (infantile and adult type)
Recurrent causes:
a) IgA nephropathy
b) Benign recurrent haematuria
c) Henoch–Schönlein purpura, SLE, other vasculitides

Urinary tract
Urinary tract infection, including tuberculosis, schistosomiasis, viruses
Hypercalciuria and stones
Tumours (e.g. rhabdomyosarcoma of bladder)
Cytotoxic drugs (i.e. chemical cystitis, including cyclophosphamide)
Ulceration (e.g. meatal ulcer)

3. Generalized
Coagulation disorders
Haemolytic uraemic syndrome

4. Factitious
Factitious illness by proxy

Acute nephritis

The classical features of visible haematuria, oliguria, hypertension and other signs of fluid overload are the hallmarks of acute nephritis. Sometimes the process is severe, with significant hypertension, heart failure and major oedema, often with complicating features of acute renal impairment such as hyperkalaemia. Usually, however, the disease is much milder, with haematuria for just 2 or 3 days, and subtle features of fluid overload; mildly increased blood pressure and minimal oedema. Note that the oedema of nephritis is pathophysiologically completely different from that in nephrotic syndrome: the former is due to fluid retention, the latter a secondary effect of hypoalbuminaemia.

The most common cause of acute nephritis is an immunogenic response to infection with 'nephritogenic' strains of group A beta-haemolytic streptococcus. The primary site of infection is usually pharyngeal or, worldwide, the skin. It is commonest in school-age children, and typically occurs 1–2 weeks following pharyngitis and often longer following a skin infection. In most cases, the clinical features subside after a few weeks, and the long-term prognosis is very good. This is in contrast to adults, where the prognosis may not be so favourable.

The differential diagnosis of post-streptococcal disease includes post-infectious nephritis from other causes (e.g. staphylococcus, herpes viruses, parvovirus B19). The prognosis is similar here. However, other diseases that may present in a similar fashion with very different prognoses include:

- *IgA nephropathy*. The initial presentation of this chronic or relapsing condition can be identical to that in post-infectious nephritis. However, usually the development of haematuria follows only a day or two after a viral respiratory illness. Other presentations are with recurrent microscopic haematuria, and also with a nephrotic as well as nephritic component (nephritic–nephrotic picture). There is a close relationship with Henoch–Schönlein syndrome, the renal manifestations of which present in a similar fashion. Renal biopsy shows diffuse mesangial deposits of IgA on immunofluorescence. A proportion of these children will suffer long-term renal insufficiency as adults.
- *Membranoproliferative glomerulonephritis*. This is also known as mesangiocapillary. It is commoner in older children and adults, and often presents as acute nephritis or nephrotic syndrome. However, the features persist and in particular the complement C3 fraction does not return to normal. Prognosis is poor, with progression to chronic renal failure in at least 50% of cases within 10 years of diagnosis.
- *Acute vasculitides*. Apart from HSP (see above), other vasculitides (including ANCA-positive nephritis) and systemic lupus erythematosus (SLE) can present in older children, but usually there will be suggestive systemic features apart from nephritis.

Hypercalciuria

In most cases this is 'idiopathic', and is relatively common in the general population. It is often found in ex-premature children. Most are completely asymptomatic, but it can cause haematuria (usually microscopic only), dysuria, and nephrocalcinosis or renal stones. It is the commonest metabolic disorder associated with renal calculi in children.

Recurrent haematuria

This term is usually applied to macroscopic haematuria, but can also apply to microscopic haematuria which may be persistent between visible episodes. The list of causes includes many of those in Table 29.1, and IgA nephropathy is particularly important.

Familial conditions are also important to consider in this context:

- *Alport's syndrome*. Most cases are X-linked dominant. Features include sensorineural deafness, ocular defects and a hereditary nephritis characterized on biopsy by ultrastructural abnormalities of the glomerular basement membrane. The majority of males affected are deaf and in end-stage renal failure by 30 years of age. Females are usually more mildly affected, but the disease is quite variable.
- *Benign familial haematuria*. By definition, this refers to cases without proteinuria, deafness or progression to renal failure. If renal biopsy is undertaken (as is often the case particularly in adults) it may be normal, or may show attenuation of glomerular basement membranes. Inheritance is often autosomal dominant.
- *Thin basement membrane nephropathy*. This term is usually applied to a benign condition with thin glomerular basement membranes on biopsy. However, the situation is complicated, and there is an overlap both clinically and pathologically on biopsy with certain pedigrees of Alport's syndrome.

History

When a patient presents with red or smoky urine, it is important to establish whether or not this is true haematuria. Rifampicin causes pink discoloration of urine, tears and saliva; beetroot ingestion may also result in pink or red urine. Urate crystals can give an orange-pink tinge to the urine and in neonates pink staining of the nappy is commonly caused by urate crystals or occasionally due to bleeding from the umbilicus, but rarely due to haematuria.

In true haematuria, the nature of the blood in the urine will help characterize the likely type of condition. Usually blood passing through the glomeruli will be altered, and is often 'cola-' or tea-coloured. It will be mixed completely with the urine. Blood produced lower down the renal tract may be fresher, and more distally will not be completely mixed with the urine. Thus, blood from the bladder neck may well be 'terminal' to the urinary stream or even independent. A meatal urethral ulcer can cause a 'blob' of blood followed by clear urine.

Associated clinical symptoms may include:

- *Local pain*. This may help localize the source. However, the classic presentation of severe renal or ureteric colicky pain with stones is unlikely to be apparent until later childhood. Also nephritis, although usually painless, can be associated with renal pain in some cases. Dysuria usually accompanies urinary tract infection, but if there is visible haematuria other causes, particularly urethritis, should be considered.
- *Nephritic features*. Oliguria (but the absence of this symptom is not reliable), weight gain, body swelling, usually on the legs first, and tiredness on exertion. If blood pressure is severely raised, particularly acutely, the child may present with confusion or fits. It should also be noted that microscopic haematuria is common in the initial presentation of *nephrotic* syndrome.
- *Preceding infection*. A preceding upper respiratory tract infection may suggest Henoch–Schönlein purpura, whereas a sore throat or skin infection may herald post-streptococcal nephritis. An upper respiratory infection is a frequent antecedent of episodes of haematuria in recurrent benign haematuria and IgA nephropathy.
- *Vasculitic features*. In Henoch–Schönlein disease the features may be obvious, but it is also possible that the rash may have been mild and unrecognized as HSP, and in any case may have presented some time previously.
- *Chronic renal failure*. Poor growth and anaemia if the haematuria is associated with a chronic nephropathy.

■ *Tumours.* It is unusual for tumours of the renal tract to present with haematuria alone. Other features (e.g. a large mass in the flank detected by the parents) are more common presenting features.

A history of trauma may be relevant, particularly when there is a congenital renal anomaly of which horseshoe kidney is the classic example. Generalized coagulation disorders can present with haematuria and, although there are generally other indications, such as purpura in thrombocytopenia or a history of bleeding in haemophilia, haematuria may rarely be the initial presentation. Sickle-cell anaemia causes either microscopic or macroscopic haematuria in up to 20% of affected individuals.

Haematuria is one of the better-recognized presentations of factitious illness by proxy. Under these circumstances, the blood is generally of maternal origin and may be shown to be such by determining the blood groups of the child, mother and the blood present in the urine. A history of recurrent unexplained illnesses, such as haemoptysis, bullous skin eruptions or convulsions, should arouse suspicion of this diagnosis.

It is important to know whether this is the first episode or if there has been recurrent haematuria (see above). Assessment of the family is important here. A family history of recurrent haematuria (usually microscopic) and deafness is not always found in Alport's syndrome but should be sought since a history of deafness will not usually be volunteered. However, a family history is more often associated with relatively more benign forms of familial haematuria.

Examination

Physical examination is usually unrewarding in cases of simple haematuria. However, depending on the history, the features of acute nephritis should be sought. Oedema is not always obvious: press on the lower shin for at least 10 seconds to demonstrate mild pitting oedema. Assess the cardiovascular status for fluid overload, including pulmonary oedema. Blood pressure measurement is mandatory, and results should be checked with the normal range for age. Look for evidence of systemic disease: rash and arthritis, as in HSP, anaemia as in some cases of nephritis and more chronic diseases. Examine the abdomen (may reveal a palpable kidney or ascites) and the genitalia for causes of local bleeding.

Investigations

Urine dipstick testing	For blood: particularly useful for monitoring at home in cases of possible recurrent or persistent haematuria. Also for testing of the whole family
	For protein: more quantitative measures are better (see below)
	For infection: see Chapter 30
Urine microscopy	This is simply performed and can be very helpful. Normal urine does not contain more than 5 red cells/μL. Red-cell casts indicate glomerular bleeding. White cells are common in any illness. White cell casts, however, indicate glomerular inflammation. Calcium phosphate and oxalate crystals are found in normal urine
Bacteriology	Urine culture is obligatory to exclude UTI (see Ch. 30)
	Throat swab, ASO and anti-DNase B titres should be performed in acute nephritis
Urine biochemistry	Proteinuria is a valuable predictor of significant glomerular involvement in chronic glomerulonephritis. Quantitative protein estimation is best measured in children in terms of protein/creatinine (or albumin/creatinine) ratio of the first urine passed following overnight sleep. This obviates the need for a 24-hour urine collection
	The same principle applies, and normal ranges exist, for calcium/creatinine ratio (for hypercalciuria). In the investigation of stone urinary oxalate, purines and cystine may be relevant

Blood chemistry	In acute conditions, electrolytes, particularly sodium and potassium, should be measured. Plasma creatinine is helpful both acutely and to monitor chronic renal impairment. Blood urea is too inaccurate a marker to be useful in renal failure except when very high (over 40 mmol/L), when it indicates a risk of fits. Hypercalcaemia is a rare cause of hypercalciuria. Acid–base status should be measured if renal tubular acidosis is suspected or significant renal impairment is present Plasma proteins help distinguish nephrotic syndrome from other diagnoses
Haematology	Thrombocytopenia may suggest a diagnosis of haemolytic–uraemic syndrome (HUS). Anaemia is also present in HUS, but is seen in other nephritides, and in chronic renal failure. There may often be a mixed picture of iron deficiency and anaemia of chronic disease. Coagulation studies should be performed if the overall presentation is suggestive
Immunology	Complement C3 fraction is almost always markedly depressed in typical cases of post-infectious nephritis, and recovers within 6–8 weeks. Failure to recover is a poor prognostic sign, usually indicating a more chronic glomerulonephritis. In contrast, C4 levels are usually normal throughout; and if depressed may indicate SLE, membranoproliferative GN or endocarditis with renal involvement Auto-antibodies, particularly antinuclear antibodies (ANA), anti-double-stranded DNA and anti-neutrophil cytoplasmic antibodies (ANCA), can be helpful in selected cases by indicating an autoimmune process
Imaging	Renal tract ultrasound, including the bladder, should be performed in most situations, as it is non-invasive and informative. Other imaging should proceed after discussion with the paediatric radiologist and urologist. The use of a plain abdominal X-ray is controversial except when stones are suspected (see Ch. 30)
Renal biopsy	The definitive investigation in cases of suspected glomerulonephritis, except acute post-infectious nephritis. The decision to recommend renal biopsy in individual cases is often difficult, and is affected by the expected prognosis and the ability to actively treat likely underlying conditions. The presence of ongoing proteinuria (see above) is often an important deciding factor When undertaken, light-microscopy, immuno-histochemistry and electron microscopy should be performed
Others	EUA and cystoscopy for urological cases. Audiology in suspected cases of Alport's syndrome. Assessment of glomerular filtration rate (usually with radioisotope) in chronic renal impairment

Clinical problem

A 7-year-old boy presents with blood in the urine for the past 2 days. It is completely mixed in with the urinary stream, which is a dirty brown colour. It is now clearing. There have been no other urinary symptoms. He has had upper respiratory tract symptoms within the last 5 days. Otherwise the child has been well but has had previous episodes of 'tonsillitis' over the years. There have been no known previous episodes of haematuria.

On examination he looks well. There is no anaemia and no oedema. Cardiovascular examination is normal. Blood pressure is 120/80. Abdomen and genitalia are normal.

Urine dipstick testing shows large amounts of blood and protein. Urine microscopy confirms haematuria (over 100 red cells/μL). Urine culture is sterile. Blood chemistry is normal, as is haematology. Complement C3 is normal. Renal tract ultrasound and plain abdominal X-ray are normal.

Questions

1. Is acute post-infectious nephritis the most likely diagnosis?

2. What is the relevance of the blood pressure reading in this case?

3. What would be the indications for renal biopsy in this case?

Answers

1. Although some of the features are compatible with a mild case of post-streptococcal nephritis, the story of an upper respiratory infection just prior to the onset of haematuria is not typical. This is rather more compatible with a different form of glomerulonephritis such as IgA nephropathy. Also, it is very uncommon for complement C3 to be normal in the acute phase of post-infectious nephritis (except sometimes very early in the course of the illness).

2. We are not told how the blood pressure was measured but, assuming it was verified to be 120/80, this is high (systolic approximately on the 95th percentile, diastolic above 95th percentile). This could be relevant and, although at this level does not need treatment acutely, it should be actively monitored.

3. Clinically, there is no indication of a rapidly progressive process. However, if there were to be a deterioration in blood pressure or features of renal impairment the situation would be different. The normal complement C3 level is concerning, and this should also be monitored as well as complement C4 and autoantibodies. However, the most important indicator in this type of case is proteinuria. Casual testing with sticks is not sufficient here, and this should be monitored with early-morning urines (as above). Heavy proteinuria or the persistence of proteinuria is a strong indication to consider renal biopsy. It would also be important in this case to consider a possible family history of haematuria, which could clearly influence the relative need for biopsy.

URINARY TRACT INFECTION
Peter Houtman

Urinary tract infection (UTI) includes infection anywhere from the kidney to the urethral orifice. However, unlike in adults, distinction is not made routinely between upper and lower urinary tract infection, particularly in younger children.

In children UTI is important for several reasons:

- It is a cause of serious sepsis in babies and is often difficult to diagnose.
- It may indicate major structural defects of the renal tract.
- It may be associated with renal scarring, a potential cause of hypertension and chronic renal failure.

Incidence

UTI is a common bacterial infection of childhood. An accurate incidence is difficult to assess, but by 10 years of age, at least 3% of girls and 1–2% of boys can be expected to have had a symptomatic UTI. The incidence is greatest in the first year of life, and this is particularly the case in boys. Circumcision significantly reduces the incidence of UTIs in males.

Asymptomatic bacteriuria is a special case, and should be considered separately from those with clinical symptoms. On its own, it is not a cause of renal scarring and need not be treated. However, many cases of asymptomatic bacteriuria are in fact associated with symptoms of bladder dysfunction (urgency etc.) and therefore 'covert' bacteriuria may be a better term. A significant proportion of these patients will be found to have renal scarring.

Factors predisposing to urinary tract infection

Vesico-ureteric reflux (VUR)

Reflux of urine from the bladder up one or both ureters predisposes to UTI by providing a pool of stagnant urine in which organisms can multiply. Any reflux bypasses the washout mechanism that normally clears bacteria rapidly from the bladder. The grading of reflux was standardized by the International Reflux Study, and is defined on cystography.

- *Grade I* fills the ureter only.
- *Grade II* fills the ureter and collecting system without dilatation.
- *Grade III* or moderate reflux causes mild blunting of the calyces.
- *Grade IV* has more than 50% of calyces blunted with more distorted appearances.
- *Grade V* has all calyces blunted and papillary impressions lost.

With each grade, ureteric dilatation becomes more severe, and in grades IV and V the ureter is also tortuous.

While an understanding of the grade of reflux is relevant in an individual child to help predict the likelihood of recurrent urinary infections, it is controversial as to whether the grade of reflux should influence management of the reflux. It is now most common practice in the UK to treat VUR, even the higher grades, conservatively unless there are problems with recurrent infection despite prophylactic antibiotics. Most cases are self-limiting in any case, but it is not standard practice to repeat investigations to check for the resolution of reflux.

Mechanical obstruction

In the neonatal period, UTI is associated with structural abnormalities more than at any other time. Posterior urethral valves in boys will cause bilateral hydronephrosis and hydroureter, and stasis of the urine predisposes to infection. A duplex system with ureteric obstruction, vesico-ureteric junction (VUJ) or pelvi-ureteric junction (PUJ) obstruction will cause urinary stasis and increased risk of infection.

VUJ or PUJ obstruction may not become clinically apparent until later in childhood, when infection is one possible presentation. Other less common causes of obstruction to urine flow in children are post-infective or postoperative urethral stricture, bladder diverticulae and constipation.

Neurological

The neuropathic bladder, which contains stagnant urine for much of the day, is particularly susceptible to infection and the management of UTIs, and their prevention in children with spina bifida is of great importance. Other children appear to have no neurological deficit even on investigation, but their bladders behave as if there is a neuropathic problem with voiding dysfunction, urinary infection and acquired renal tract damage (Hinman syndrome). Many of these children may have psychological factors leading to these problems.

Sexual abuse

Some children with recurrent UTIs have been sexually abused. The clinician should be vigilant for such cases in both history taking and examination.

Pathophysiology of renal scarring and dysplasia

'Renal scarring' is the term used for the spectrum of radiological abnormalities in the kidney associated with focal or diffuse areas of irreversible parenchymal damage. Vesico-ureteric reflux and infection are important factors in the development of renal scarring. Experimental evidence suggests that intrarenal reflux, perhaps into compound papillae allowing backflow of urine into the renal parenchyma, is particularly likely to lead to scarring, although only in the presence of infection. This is particularly likely to affect the developing kidney and is much less likely to cause new scarring after infancy. Also, as primary VUR is self-limiting, this mechanism becomes less likely with age. It also means that the absence of documented VUR in an older child does not mean that a renal scar has not been caused by previous reflux.

However, recent experimental work and clinical observations, particularly through follow-up of antenatally diagnosed renal tract abnormalities, has complicated the issue of renal damage associated with renal tract abnormalities in early childhood. In particular, it is now known that 'renal scarring' can occur without infection, and it is by no means clear whether scarring is the direct consequence of abnormalities such as vesico-ureteric reflux, or rather merely an association with a more fundamental primary cause. The term 'congenital renal dysplasia' is often more appropriate in cases where it is more likely that the 'scarring' has occurred prenatally in the embryo. In many cases it is likely that a primary abnormality in early renal tract development is associated with both bladder and ureteric dysfunction, including susceptibility to vesico-ureteric reflux, and renal dysplasia.

Differential diagnosis

The most common differential diagnosis is trivial viral illness or, in young children and infants, other generalized sepsis.

Acute onset of local bladder-related symptoms may indicate primary neurological abnormality in the presence or absence of UTI. Constipation may cause a similar picture.

Vulvo-vaginitis and balanitis are different conditions from UTI. However vulvo-vaginitis in particular is not always easy to distinguish either on history or examination, and the two conditions may exist together. The principle of microbiological confirmation of UTI is particularly relevant here, as is the appropriate management of vulvo-vaginitis with, in most cases, simple local hygiene measures and avoidance of local antibiotic creams.

History

A clinical history suggestive of a UTI is important at any age. Obviously the older the child the more specific the symptoms are likely to be, and include:

- *Change in pattern of micturition*. Sudden onset of frequency, urgency or wetting in an otherwise continent child. But note that in a younger child these symptoms, particularly frequency, can be brought on simply by an acute viral illness.
- *'Dysuria'*. Often difficult to assess in a young child, and again may be non-specific for any acute illness.
- *'Smelly urine'*. Unlikely to be helpful as a symptom, and usually merely an indication of concentrated urine.
- *Symptoms suggesting 'pyelonephritis'*. Unilateral loin pain with high fever and traditionally 'rigors'. Remember that in the absence of these symptoms in childhood UTI is still likely to involve the upper renal tracts.

In babies, these specific symptoms are of course less obvious. UTI is considered part of the differential diagnosis of an infant with fever, and the younger the child the more important to suspect UTI with non-specific symptoms. These include vomiting, lethargy and jaundice of the newborn.

The past medical history includes an attempt to define any previous UTIs, particularly those not previously diagnosed as such. It is just as important to document what was not in fact a UTI – children will often have been treated for UTI without proper evidence (see below) and it is appropriate to ask questions as to whether previous infections were confirmed when the urine results came back 'after a few days', thus distinguishing the results from dipstick testing.

Even in older children, ask about unexplained fevers and illnesses in infancy. It is these early infections which are more likely to have caused renal scarring.

Most children in the UK will have had antenatal ultrasound screening as a routine. Enquire as to whether there was any follow-up of potential renal tract abnormalities.

Family history is important for two distinct reasons: first, to help define any added risk to the individual patient – for example, with one parent with scarring ('reflux') nephropathy there is approximately a 40% chance of children being similarly affected; second, to identify other children at risk if abnormalities are found in the index case (see below).

Examination

Acute urinary infection as such does not usually cause specific clinical signs. However, in the older child, renal angle tenderness indicates pyelonephritis, but, as in the history lack of abdominal pain or tenderness does not correlate well with lack of renal involvement. The bladder should be assessed clinically as lower renal tract inflammation may be associated with urinary retention.

However, the greater part of possible clinical signs is associated with predisposing factors for UTI, rather than UTI itself, and should be assessed in the follow-up evaluation, if not acutely. Examine the lower spine and pelvis, although the lack of clinical abnormalities does not exclude neurological involvement of the bladder. Examine the genitalia: acutely for soreness, as in vulvo-vaginitis or balanitis; also for congenital abnormalities such as hypospadias.

Blood pressure measurement is mandatory, in view of the risk of pre-existing renal scarring.

Investigations

Urine collection

Collection type	Advantages	Disadvantages
'Bag urine'	Minimal expertise. Non-invasive	Very likely to be contaminated, but less so if performed diligently
Various 'pad' methods	Non-invasive	Requires some expertise and familiarity
Clean catch	Likely to be clean. Non-invasive	Time-consuming. Requires patience
'MSU'	Growth of over 10^5 colony-forming units per mL urine is standard confirmation of UTI	This standard developed from adult data, and applicability to children unconfirmed.
Catheter specimen	Clean. Guarantees a successful sample	Invasive. Requires skill and resources. Can introduce infection
Suprapubic aspirate	Sterile. Suitable in a very sick patient	Invasive. Requires expertise

Urine investigation

Test	Advantages	Disadvantages
Dipstick tests	Near-patient testing: results immediately available. If both nitrite and leucocytes negative, UTI is unlikely	Detection of nitrites has a sensitivity of 50% for UTI and a specificity of 95%. Detection of leucocytes by dipstick has a sensitivity of 80% and specificity of 90%. If both positive UTI very likely but needs culture to confirm. Other tests (protein, blood) very non-specific (can be positive in any febrile illness)
Microscopy	Results quickly available. If no white cells, significant UTI unlikely.	Labour-intensive. Pyuria very common in any febrile illness. Presence of bacteria does not confirm UTI
Culture	Standard for confirmation of UTI. Mandatory for definitive diagnosis. Gives antibiotic sensitivities.	Delay of days to result. May show 'mixed growth' in which case needs repeat although by this time usually impracticable

Radiological investigations

Test	Clinical indication	Function
Renal tract ultrasound	Any child with first UTI	Non-invasive screening of renal tract. Abnormalities detected in this way include: Hydronephrosis: can be due to obstruction or vesico-ureteric reflux (VUR) Hydro-ureter: as above, except not with pelviureteric junction obstruction Renal size: decreased in renal scarring/dysplasia Duplex kidneys: associated with both obstruction and reflux Bladder emptying: incomplete emptying associated with UTI and possibly neurological dysfunction
Micturating cysto-urethrogram (MCUG)	Infants with first UTI. Recurrent infections resistant to appropriate management. Relevant abnormalities of ultrasound.	Standard direct test for VUR. Standard test for posterior urethral valves
Static radioisotope scan (DMSA)	Infants and younger children with first UTI. Relevant abnormalities on ultrasound	Used to detect renal scarring, although some units now rely on ultrasound alone after infancy. (NB. The DMSA scan is usually temporarily abnormal for up to 3 months after an acute UTI due to reduced perfusion)
Dynamic radioisotope scan (MAG-3 or DTPA) a) With diuretic b) 'Indirect' cystogram	Significant hydronephrosis Concern for VUR/scarring. Less traumatic than MCUG	Delay in excretion of isotope especially after diuretic correlates with upper tract obstruction Less invasive test for VUR- but not very sensitive

Investigation of other family members

In view of the known familial risk of scarring nephropathy, children of parents with significant nephropathy and siblings of children with VUR, and particularly scarring, should be considered for investigation. The extent of investigation is controversial but an ultrasound scan is certainly reasonable. Also, subsequent newborn infants may be started on prophylactic antibiotics pending renal tract investigations.

Clinical problem

A 7-month-old girl is referred with lethargy and fever for 2 days. She has vomited twice in the last 24 hours. She has had a mild upper respiratory tract infection in the last few days but seemed to be recovering from this. She is passing urine but less than usual into the nappy. There are no respiratory symptoms.

Previously she has been well, with normal growth and development. Two months previously she was treated at home with antibiotics for a febrile illness with some minor respiratory symptoms. The illness was ill defined.

There is no known family history of renal problems. She has a 4-year-old sister, who is well.

On examination she is moderately unwell, and mildly dehydrated. Temperature is 37.8°C. She is well perfused. After paracetamol she looks better and is alert. Systemic examination was unremarkable.

A small quantity of urine is obtained from a urine bag. This shows positive for nitrite and leucocyte esterase, as well as protein.

Questions

1. What further initial investigations would you do?

2. What is the significance of the previous ill-defined febrile illness?

3. What investigations would you do if UTI was confirmed?

Answers

1. The bag urine is likely to be contaminated. A further clean urine sample should be obtained before starting antibiotics, probably by clean catch, or if not possible by catheter or suprapubic aspiration, and this sent for culture and antibiotic sensitivity. Meningitis should always be considered in such a case, and the case for possible lumbar puncture made on clinical grounds. Blood tests in this case are not mandatory, but if taken should include blood cultures.

2. Although this may well have been a 'viral' illness, it was treated 'blind' with antibiotics and may have been a previous UTI.

3. It is important to send a further urine specimen for culture after the initial antibiotic course, to confirm resolution of the infection.

   At this age, a renal tract ultrasound, micturating cysto-urethrogram (MCUG) and DMSA radioisotope scan are indicated. MCUG can be performed after the infection has cleared, but the DMSA scan should be delayed (probably for at least 6 months) to allow time for any renal inflammation to settle – the scan is looking for permanent renal scarring. Further investigations depend on the results of these tests.

CHAPTER 31

WETTING

Peter Houtman

Normal development of bladder control

Babies commonly empty their bowels and pass urine immediately after feeding. After 6–8 months the frequency of voiding decreases and volume increases, but it is rare to develop voluntary control of bladder function before 15–18 months. Usually the first indication of voluntary control is an interest in having just passed urine, but the child of 2 years of age will usually recognize the sensation of bladder fullness. Urinary urgency is common at this stage, but when this gradually lessens toilet training can start. In the next few months, the child is usually still wet at night, but the retention span gradually increases, so that by 30 months two-thirds of children are dry at night.

Urinary incontinence

The term 'enuresis' is usually defined as involuntary, but otherwise normal, voiding occurring at a socially unacceptable time or place, day or night. Different societies and families have diverse expectations of the age of acceptability of bladder control and so there are no specific age limits at which this term can start to be applied. Incontinence is not always synonymous with enuresis, and continual dribbling or dampness suggests lower urinary tract abnormalities, such as an ectopic ureter opening into the urethra, or a bladder diverticulum. Other conditions associated with incontinence include:

- *Urinary tract infection.* Apart from the obvious association with acute infection, it is common for children to continue to be wet for some months afterwards.
- *Neurological abnormalities* (e.g. spinal dysraphism).
- *Polyuric conditions.* Metabolic disorders such as diabetes mellitus and diabetes insipidus; chronic renal failure.

- *Chronic constipation.* As a result of compression of the lower renal tract by faeces.

Nocturnal enuresis

Approximately 15% of 5-year-old children are still wet at night. There is said to be a 15% resolution rate per year (without treatment) after this age. About 5% of 10-year-olds are wet, and about 1% post puberty. Boys are more likely to have nocturnal enuresis. Secondary enuresis (wetting that occurs after a period of normal bladder control) accounts for about 20% of cases. Whether primary or secondary, if the problem is compatible with the definition of involuntary but normal voiding, and is not associated with daytime symptoms, very few will be found to have an organic condition.

Aetiology is multifactorial in most cases, but includes genetic factors, and up to 75% of affected children will have a first-degree relative with the problem. Psychosocial factors have long been known to be associated, particularly adverse 'life events' occurring between 2 and 3 years. Physiological factors can also predispose to wetting: some children with enuresis have been shown to have relative nocturnal polyuria. Others may have a small functional bladder capacity, or unstable detrusor contractions. It is still controversial as to whether children with nocturnal enuresis have poor arousability from sleep as a causative factor.

Daytime wetting

The incidence is difficult to assess, because only severe cases seek medical attention. At least 10% of 11-year-old children have occasional daytime urinary accidents. There is no formal classification of types of daytime wetting, but certain patterns are recognized with different characteristics, and these include the following.

Dysfunctional voiding

Within this group several abnormal patterns of voiding emerge, all of which are probably the result of long-term learned voiding behaviour resulting from attempts to suppress bladder contractions by inappropriate use of the pelvic floor muscles and urinary sphincter complex.

- *Fractionated voiding.* Characterized by a low voiding frequency with micturition in small fractions. There is incomplete bladder emptying and large residual volumes. Detrusor contractions are unsustained and bladder capacity is large. Can be considered a form of 'overflow incontinence'.
- *Lazy bladder syndrome.* Often the end result of fractionated voiding. Detrusor contractions are virtually absent and abdominal pressure is the main influence on voiding. Recurrent urinary tract infections are common.
- *Staccato voiding.* Caused by bursts, often rhythmic, of pelvic floor activity during voiding, resulting in peaks of bladder pressure and interruptions of urine flow. Duration of micturition is increased and, as above, bladder emptying often incomplete.
- *The Hinman syndrome.* Otherwise known as 'non-neurogenic neurogenic bladder', because of the similarities in both clinical, urological and urodynamic features with children with spinal neurological problems. The aetiology is poorly understood, but such children are probably at the severe end of the spectrum of those with dysfunctional voiding, and psychological problems are often associated. The bladder wall is usually thick and trabeculated and there may be 'functional' upper renal obstruction and significant renal impairment.

Urge incontinence

The main problem here is urinary urgency, which usually gets worse during the day. Functional bladder capacity is usually relatively small, and voiding can be frequent. Micturition itself is typically normal, but urine flow may be stopped too soon by pelvic floor contraction, with incomplete emptying. These children may get extremely sudden urges to void and they will often attempt to stop the process by manoeuvres such as squatting on one heel to compress the urethra. This pattern of wetting is much commoner in girls.

Giggle incontinence

Hilarious laughing can produce occasional accidents in many people, but in some children laughing or suppressed giggling regularly provokes detrusor overactivity regardless of the state of bladder filling. It is commonest in girls of school age but can continue into adulthood.

Urinary frequency syndrome

Extraordinarily high daytime voiding frequencies (as often as every 5–10 minutes) are seen, usually in boys. The condition, although disturbing, is usually self-limiting over weeks or sometimes months.

History

A detailed history is at the centre of the approach to the wet child. In particular, information about the pattern of wetting will be very valuable in terms of the subsequent level of concern about the child. Much of the history is concerned with information about the child for direct management purposes rather than looking for specific causes.

Regarding daytime wetting:

- *Has the child always been wet?* A child who has never had a normal pattern of daytime voiding is much more likely to have a structural organic problem.
- *At what times is the child wet?* In particular, the relationship with going to the toilet can be informative. For example, a child who has problems prior to normal voiding, especially with urgency, is likely to have bladder instability. However, if the incontinence is after going to the toilet, structural problems such as vaginal reflux in an obese girl, or phimosis in a boy, should be considered.
- *What is the toileting pattern?* Ask about the pattern of toileting during the day. If the child does not pass urine in the morning before school, for example, there may well be a subsequent management problem during the morning. To compound the issue, the child may not want to go to the toilet at school, for various reasons. It is always worth asking about the school toilets specifically. There may be a difference in toileting pattern and wetting between different sorts of days (e.g. schooldays and weekends), so try to establish what it is about these different types of days that may be the relevant factor.
- *How wet is the child?* To get an idea of the quantity of urine passed, ask whether it has been necessary for the child to wear sanitary pads and the number of changes of these pads or underwear throughout the day.
- *Does the child try to avoid wetting?* A story of leg-crossing or asymmetrical squatting indicates the child is consciously trying to avoid passing urine despite bladder signals. On the other hand, many children do not seem to know when they are likely to be wet, making toileting management more of a problem.
- *Is the child constipated?* Significant chronic soiling may actually be directly related to urinary incontinence in terms of a common cause. More commonly, however, constipation is an exacerbating factor for bladder instability, and should always be actively managed, including by assessment of the diet.
- *What and how much does the child drink?* Many children drink very little during the day and then too much in the evening. This obviously can affect nocturnal wetting, but it is also important for the day, in that establishing a regular toileting pattern may not be possible without reasonable bladder filling. Some children even avoid drinking during the day to minimize the amount of their wetting. Most families will know to avoid caffeine-containing drinks (including cola), but there is little doubt that some children also have their bladder instability exacerbated by specific 'fizzy' drinks. Rarely there may be concerns about possible polyuria: children with genuine polyuria will seek to drink plain water rather than only 'juice' and the pattern is regular rather than intermittent.
- *Is the child getting urinary tract infections?* A clear history of acute urinary infections is relatively easy to put into context. More difficult, however, is the child who seems to have intermittent symptomatology or periods of exacerbation of wetting habits. Only careful clinical judgment, with urine culture at relevant times, will separate the two related problems.

The medical history more generally may yield important information. Chronic conditions such as epilepsy may disrupt toileting. The child's general level of maturity will also be relevant: a child with significantly delayed psychomotor development cannot be expected to achieve toileting skills beyond his other milestones. In cases of possible neuropathic bladder enquire specifically about a family history of any type of spina bifida, or anticonvulsant therapy in pregnancy.

The assessment should also include a treatment history, as various management strategies, including anticholinergic agents, may already have been tried.

Regarding nocturnal enuresis: the most important consideration is whether there is a daytime component (not necessarily incontinence, but urgency, frequency etc.). If so, then the questions above apply. However, if nocturnal enuresis is truly isolated, as is usually the case, the history is geared towards management. Often questions about home circumstances are enlightening, including relatively mundane factors such as the proximity of the bathroom. Although it is reasonable to ask about family dynamics, the approach to most cases of bed-wetting is pragmatic, without reference to psychological factors. Previous attempts at toilet training should be documented since the management of toilet training shows enormous variation and efforts may simply have been inappropriate. Many children will have already had professional input for their enuresis, particularly from community-based specifically trained nurses, and it is important to ask what management strategies have been tried, and their level of success.

A family history of bed-wetting into late childhood is not uncommon, and it is sometimes reassuring for the family to know that genetic factors may be related.

Examination

Children with simple enuresis do not require detailed examination. At the other end of the spectrum, a child with refractory daytime or diurnal wetting should not be investigated further without a full examination. This should include the spine, looking particularly for hairy patches, dimples, naevi, a sinus or lipoma, and also for partial absence of the sacrum (not always obvious: look for asymmetry of the buttocks). Neurological examination of the lower limbs should include observation of the child's gait and, if there are any further suspicions, formal examination for lumbrosacral nerve root problems should follow.

Palpate the abdomen for the bladder and also for constipation. The external genitalia should be examined in both sexes:

- For boys, look for phimosis, meatal stenosis or hypospadias.
- For girls, look for labial adhesions, and clitoral abnormalities which may be associated with urethral problems.

Obesity can be related to wetting, especially in girls, where it can act as a contributory factor for vaginal reflux. Look also for scarring, bruising and warts, and generally be aware of signs of abuse.

Investigations

The vast majority of children with isolated nocturnal enuresis require no investigation (apart from urinalysis). Those with daytime symptoms deserve fuller evaluation, but even these children will rarely merit major investigation once a detailed clinical assessment has been performed. In particular, formal urodynamic studies are reserved for only a very small proportion of cases and should not be considered until indirect means of assessing bladder function such as frequency–volume charts (see below) have been followed. In these circumstances a specialist nurse is invaluable, as the assessment process requires skill and patience.

Urinalysis	In particular, for glucose and for infection. Any child with daytime wetting should be evaluated in terms of a possible relationship with urinary infection. Often, it is helpful to issue urine sticks (for nitrite and leucocyte esterase) to the family for regular testing at home
Ultrasound	Can be used not only for renal tract anomalies, but also to assess bladder capacity and degree of emptying, so should be performed pre- and post-micturition
Other renal tract imaging	May be indicated depending on abnormalities of the renal tract found on ultrasound, but might include micturating cysto-urethrogram and radioisotope studies (see Ch. 30)
Spinal imaging	Plain X-rays are of limited value. In rare cases, when a neurological cause is suspected from the clinical assessment, an MRI scan is indicated
Biochemistry	Serum creatinine should be measured in children with abnormal upper renal tracts, particularly bilateral renal anomalies. Urinary concentrating ability should be assessed if polyuria is suspected

Frequency–volume charts and other records	These should be considered an investigation, as they are time-consuming. At their simplest they are a record of the number of voidings and episodes of wetting during the day and night. In practice they can also include voiding volumes, thus estimating 'functional bladder capacity'. Records of fluid intake and bowel actions can also be integrated. These charts are best done over a few days, and can be therapeutic as well as yielding valuable information
Urine flow studies	'Uroflow' studies are indicated for those children with suspected disordered micturition or large post-micturition residual volumes. Patterns such as 'staccato' or 'fractionated' voiding can be demonstrated. When used in conjunction with a portable ultrasound probe for the bladder these studies can be considered as 'non-invasive urodynamics'
Urodynamics	Formal, invasive assessment of bladder and urethral function to measure bladder and detrusor pressure in relation to bladder filling and urinary flow. Often combined with video to record the contrast cystography. Reserved for those in whom less invasive assessment has not been decisive, and clinical problems despite treatment are severe
EUA/cystoscopy	Reserved for those with suspected urethral or bladder anomalies (e.g. female epispadias). Vaginoscopy for girls with post-micturition wetting unresponsive to usual management

Clinical problem

An 8-year-old girl presents with a 2-year history of daytime wetting. She has urinary accidents almost every day of varying severity, mostly in the afternoon. She often suddenly feels the need to pass urine and is not always able to hold on until reaching the toilet. At other times she goes to the toilet normally, but probably more frequently than her friends at school. She is dry at night. She was toilet-trained by 3 years of age. There have been no medical problems, and she seems otherwise happy at home and at school. Examination is unremarkable.

Questions

1. What pattern of incontinence does she demonstrate?

2. What investigations would you perform?

3. What would be your approach to management?

Answers

1. This is urge incontinence. It is common for attacks of detrusor instability to start towards the end of the morning with peaks in the afternoon. Functionally, she probably has a relatively small bladder.

2. Apart from a urine sample for microbiological culture, investigations are not indicated routinely. However, a simple frequency of voiding chart is likely to be useful.

3. The mainstay of management is bladder retraining, consisting of simple education, positive reinforcement and scheduled regular toileting at predetermined intervals. This is in contrast to the usual response of parents, i.e. frequent questioning of the child as to whether he or she wants to go to the toilet! If the problem is persistent, an ultrasound looking particularly at bladder emptying may be performed, and anticholinergic therapy (oxybutynin) can be given as a trial. Bladder training should continue.

CHAPTER 32

RECURRENT INFECTIONS
David Isaacs, Meryta May

Introduction

In assessing a child for recurrent infections, there are two major considerations. The first is whether or not the child's pattern of infections is so abnormal that the child needs any investigations at all. It is normal, for example, for a child aged 1–3 years to have 6–10 viral upper respiratory tract infections a year. The second consideration is what tests should be done. Many doctors tend to regard 'immune deficiency' as an entity in itself and, when it is suspected, to send off a battery of tests without sufficient consideration of the different components of the immune system and exactly what the immune defect is likely to be. It is far better to consider the pattern of infections and what these suggest about the nature of the immune defects which could cause such infections.

Immunity to infection

The different areas of the immune system to consider are humoral immunity (B-cells and immunoglobulin production); cell-mediated immunity (T-cells); granulocytes (neutrophils, polymorphs); and the complement cascade. The type of infection and the nature of the organisms causing infections are a pointer to possible immune defects.

Invading organisms can be divided into intracellular and extracellular. Extracellular organisms are mainly bacteria, and are predominantly cleared by phagocytic cells, aided by opsonization with antibody (produced by B-cells) and complement. Pyogenic bacteria are extracellular organisms. Once infection is established, the most important defence mechanism is phagocytosis and killing by neutrophils, enhanced by specific antibody and complement (see Fig. 32.1). Immunological response to intracellular pathogens is predominantly mediated by cellular immunity. Organisms such as viruses, *Mycobacterium*

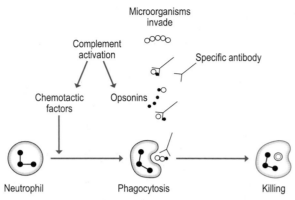

Fig 32.1   Host defences against infection with pyogenic bacteria. (Reproduced with permission from Isaacs D, Moxon ER 1999 Handbook of neonatal infections. WB Saunders, London.)

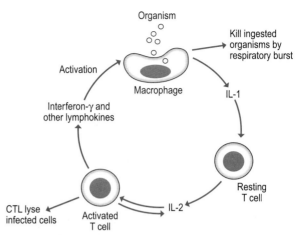

Fig 32.2   Host defences against intracellular pathogens. IL-1, IL-2, interleukins 1 and 2; CTL, cytotoxic T-lymphocytes. (Reproduced with permission from Isaacs D, Moxon ER 1999 Handbook of neonatal infections. WB Saunders, London.)

tuberculosis and *Listeria* are intracellular pathogens, and are hidden from extracellular defences.

Early mechanisms of defence are antibody-dependent cellular cytotoxicity, the production of interferons and natural killer cells. The production of interleukins and lymphokines by macrophages and T-cells, respectively, produces further activation of T-cells and macrophages, producing an amplification of the host response (see Fig. 32.2). T-cells also play a role in the activation of B-cells, and therefore antibody production. Hence, a severe T-cell deficiency will usually affect B-cell function as well.

Primary deficiencies of the immune system are rare, with an overall incidence of approximately 1:10 000–20 000. The exception is IgA deficiency, which occurs in approximately one per 500–700 in a Caucasian population, but is often asymptomatic or causes only mild symptoms.

Some diseases can cause recurrent infections through mechanisms other than primary impairment of immune cells. Cystic fibrosis, which has an incidence of one in 2500 in Caucasian populations, causes recurrent pneumonia, sinusitis and bronchiectasis. In populations of African origin, sickle-cell anaemia results in impaired splenic function and susceptibility to invasive infections with *Streptococcus pneumoniae* and *Salmonella* species. Significant causes of acquired immune deficiency in our society are diabetes mellitus, liver and renal dysfunction and, more recently, human immunodeficiency virus infection. Iatrogenic

immunodeficiency is seen in children on long-term immunosuppression following solid organ transplantation, and children receiving cytotoxic drugs for malignancy.

It is important to be aware of the clues that suggest primary immune deficiency. Depending on the severity of the immune deficit, symptoms may be quite non-specific, and these children do not uniformly fail to thrive. Defects in different parts of the immune system present in different ways (see Table 32.1).

Clinical approach to the child with recurrent infections

The most important initial step in evaluation of frequent infections in childhood is to determine whether the child falls outside recognized acceptable patterns of infection. Protection against infection and susceptibility to infection are affected by both extrinsic and intrinsic factors (see Table 32.2), which need to be considered in the assessment of a child with recurrent infection.

Normal children can have up to 10 viral upper respiratory tract infections and two episodes of gastroenteritis per year for the first 2–3 years of life,

Table 32.1   Presentations of different immune component deficits

Type of immune deficiency	Specific condition	Types of infections or presentation
Predominantly antibody deficiencies		
B-cell function	Agammaglobulinaemia (X-linked)	Sinopulmonary infections, arthritis, osteomyelitis, meningitis, urinary tract infections, chronic viral encephalitis
	Common variable immunodeficiency	Sinopulmonary infections, severe giardiasis. Autoimmune disease, e.g. arthritis, iridocyclitis, ITP
Control of antibody production	IgA deficiency	Recurrent respiratory tract infections, bronchitis, conjunctivitis, diarrhoea. May be asymptomatic
	IgG subclass deficiency	Recurrent respiratory tract infections, bronchitis. May be asymptomatic
Cellular immunity		
T-cell function (also affects B-cell function)	Severe combined immunodeficiency (SCID) (X-linked, AR)	Failure to thrive, diarrhoea, oral candidiasis, *Pneumocystis carinii* pneumonia (PCP)
	Human immunodeficiency virus infection	Resembles SCID clinically
	Wiskott–Aldrich syndrome (X-linked)	Eczema and purpura. *Pneumocystis carinii* pneumonia, recurrent bacterial infections
	Hyper-IgM syndrome (X-linked, AR)	Resembles SCID clinically
Defects of phagocytic function		
Granulocyte defect	Chronic granulomatous disease (X-linked, AR)	Superficial or deep abscesses, osteomyelitis, infections with *Staphylococcus aureus*, *Pseudomonas aeruginosa*, *Aspergillus* species
	Hyper-IgE syndrome (Job's syndrome)	Diffuse, unusual eczema. Deep abscesses. Very high IgE
	Cyclical neutropenia	Episodes of neutropenia every 3–4 weeks, with mouth ulcers, fevers and gingivitis at nadir of neutrophils
	Iatrogenic neutropenia (e.g. due to chemotherapy)	Septicaemia with Gram-negative organisms, *Staphylococcus aureus*, and opportunistic organisms such as fungi
	Leucocyte adhesion defect (AR)	Very rare. Severe gingivitis, delayed separation of umbilical cord

Table 32.1   Presentations of different immune component deficits – cont'd

Type of immune deficiency	Specific condition	Types of infections or presentation
Complement deficiencies		
Complement deficiency	Isolated deficiency of C1–4	Very rare. Pyogenic infections, SLE
	Isolated deficiency of C6–9	Very rare. Recurrent meningococcal or gonococcal infections
Hyposplenism		
Asplenia	Congenital (AR) or acquired (surgical removal)	Severe infections with encapsulated organisms, especially pneumococci
Splenic dysfunction	Haemoglobinopathies, e.g. sickle-cell anaemia	Infections with encapsulated organisms and *Salmonella* species

AR, autosomal recessive; SLE, systemic lupus erythematosus; ITP, idiopathic thrombocytopenic purpura

Table 32.2   Factors affecting susceptibility to infection in childhood

Extrinsic	Day-care attendance
	School-aged siblings
	Passive exposure to cigarette smoke
Intrinsic	Anatomical defects
	Immunodeficiency: congenital/ acquired
	Impaired mechanical defences: ciliary defects; impaired cough, gag, swallow; cystic fibrosis

Table 32.3   Clinical features which may indicate immune deficiency

Three or more episodes of acute otitis media in 6 months or four in a year
Persistent purulent ear discharge
Two or more serious sinus infections within 1 year
Two or more episodes of pneumonia within 1 year
Failure to thrive
Recurrent deep skin or organ abscesses
Persistent or recurrent candidiasis
Two or more 'deep' tissue or 'sterile site' infections: e.g. pneumonia, meningitis, osteomyelitis, deep abscesses
A family history of primary immunodeficiency

particularly if regularly exposed to other children. Clues that the child is otherwise normal are:

- The infections are mild.
- The infections are acute and short-lived.
- The child recovers without sequelae.
- There are no persistent symptoms.
- The growth pattern is normal.

Conversely, clues to suggest impaired or compromised immune defences are shown in Table 32.3.

Key point

Having decided that a child has an abnormal pattern of infections, the most important step is to work out which part of the immune system appears to be compromised (see Table 32.4).

History

The history of infections should include the following:

1. Recurrence at a particular site:
   a) If the infections only recur at one site, this implies either residual, partially treated infection, or a mechanical problem, which may be allowing continued proliferation of organisms, e.g. an inhaled foreign body, the presence of a

Table 32.4   Major patterns of organisms causing disease in immunodeficiency

Immune deficiency	Bacterial infections	Viral infections	Fungal infections	Protozoan infections
B-cell (antibody)	+++	+	−	+++
T-cell or combined B- and T-cell	+++	+++	+++	+++
Complement	+++	−	−	−
Phagocytic disorder	+++	−	+++	−

fistula or urinary tract abnormalities. (One exception is recurrent herpes simplex virus infections, which tend to recur in the same site due to infection of a particular nerve root.)

b) Generalized infections or multiple different sites imply a more global impairment.

2. Type and severity of infections:
   a) The type of infections, whether viral, bacterial, fungal or a combination, can help to pinpoint a particular cell line deficiency or dysfunction (see Tables 32.3 and 32.4).
   b) Children with immunodeficiency tend to have a more severe disease course, with little or no symptom-free interval between acute infections.

3. Age of onset:
   a) As a generalization, the younger the child when significant infections occur, the more severe the immune abnormality. Children with severe combined immunodeficiency (SCID), with deficient B- and T-cell lymphocyte function, present within the first few months of life with life-threatening and opportunistic infections and failure to thrive.
   b) For the first 6 months of life, children with defective antibody production, such as boys with X-linked agammaglobulinaemia, are passively protected by maternal IgG acquired transplacentally in utero. This masks an innate deficiency for these initial months.
   c) More restricted abnormalities of immune function may present later in life, and even go unrecognized until adulthood.

4. Growth:
   a) Children with frequent infections but normal immunity usually grow and develop normally.
   b) Immunodeficient children, particularly those with T-cell defects, may have chronic diarrhoea, or be small for their age.

5. Family history:
   a) *Autoimmune disease.* Check for a family history of autoimmune disease or lymphoma, which can occur in families with patients with common variable immunodeficiency (CVID), or IgA deficiency.
   b) *Immunodeficiency.* A positive family history of immunodeficiency is highly suggestive, but a negative history does not exclude an inherited immune disorder. Autosomal recessive disorders can affect males or females, but low carrier frequencies make it unlikely to find affected relatives other than the child's siblings.
   c) *Consanguinity.* Elicit any history of consanguinity, or infantile deaths in the extended family, especially of male babies on the maternal side. Many inherited disorders are X-linked, including agammaglobulinaemia, Wiskott–Aldrich syndrome, the majority of children with hyper-IgM syndrome or with chronic granulomatous disease (CGD), and some children with SCID.
   d) *Risk factors for HIV.* Question the parents about any risk factors for HIV acquisition, although again, a negative history does not exclude this diagnosis in the child.

6. Immunization history:
   a) Children with severe B-cell dysfunction can develop persistent asymptomatic excretion of poliovirus.
   b) Children with T-cell dysfunction may get severe disease from live virus vaccines, for example varicella, and can get disseminated BCG.
   c) Knowledge of a child's immunization status can be useful in investigation: a lack of serological response to previously administered vaccines can indicate impaired functional IgG production.

Examination

While a normal physical examination does not rule out immune deficiency, significant findings to be sought suggestive of an immune disorder are as follows.

Nutrition

- Failure to thrive suggests significant compromise in immune function, either congenital (e.g. SCID) or acquired (e.g. HIV).
- Children with agammaglobulinaemia are prone to recurrent *Giardia lamblia* infection, which may produce failure to thrive.

Skin rash

- Eczema:
  - Severe, atypical eczema, deep abscesses: hyper-IgE syndrome (Job's syndrome).
  - Eczema and purpura: Wiskott–Aldrich syndrome.
  - Eczema with failure to thrive and diarrhoea: SCID.
- Generalized molluscum contagiosum:
  - Most commonly occurs in normal children.
  - Rarely, however, associated with a T-cell defect, either congenital or acquired, e.g. HIV, iatrogenic.
- Persistent or recurrent oral and nail candidiasis: mucocutaneous candidiasis due to a specific T-cell defect to *Candida*.

Dysmorphic features

Certain rare syndromes have immunodeficiency as part of their phenotype. For example:

- Microdeletion at chromosome 22q11: unusual facies, with thin lips, long narrow philtrum, almond-shaped eyes, and cardiac anomalies, hypoparathyroidism, and aplastic or hypoplastic thymus tissue, resulting in aberrant T-cell function (Shprintzen's or velocardiofacial syndrome).

Mouth

- Children with granulocyte defects often have severe gingivitis or recurrent, large oral ulcers.

- Oral candidiasis beyond early infancy also suggests T-cell deficiency.

Ears

- Tympanosclerosis: white patches on the tympanic membrane due to recurrent ear infections.
- Purulent discharge: perforated drum or otitis externa.

Nose

- Mucopurulent discharge: common variant of normal (catarrhal child), representing recurrent mild viral upper respiratory tract infections.
- Unilateral discharge: suggests foreign body or choanal stenosis.
- Persistent mucopurulent discharge, associated with fever, tenderness, halitosis: suggests chronic sinusitis. Seen in children with cystic fibrosis, ciliary defects or hypogammaglobulinaemia. Usually associated with lower respiratory tract disease as well.

Clubbing

- Usually seen in older children rather than infants.
- Can be a sign of chronic undetected respiratory disease, such as bronchiectasis, or lymphoid interstitial pneumonitis, regarded as an AIDS-defining illness.

Lungs

- Bronchiectasis: chronic productive cough, coarse crepitations on auscultation. In severe cases, these crepitations may be audible without a stethoscope, simply by listening to the child breathe through an open mouth.
- *Pneumocystis carinii* pneumonia: increasing dry cough and dyspnoea, with or without fever, over 1–3 weeks. Auscultation characteristically normal. Chest X-ray shows interstitial pneumonitis, usually bilateral (see Fig. 32.3).

Heart

- Congenital heart disease: associated with deletions of chromosome 22q11, and asplenia.

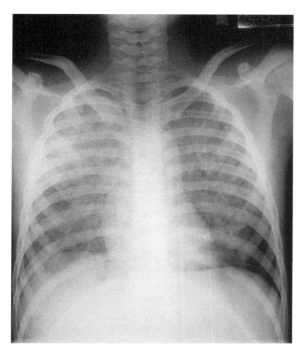

Fig 32.3 *Pneumocystis carinii* pneumonia. Diffuse, bilateral, interstitial pneumonitis, most marked in hilar regions.

- Dextrocardia: associated with Kartagener's syndrome (immotile cilia syndrome) – sinusitis, otitis media, bronchiectasis.

Lymphoid tissue

- Absence of palpable lymph nodes and no visible tonsils is seen in severe immunodeficiencies such as SCID, though is not a consistent finding.
- Persistently enlarged cervical adenopathy can be seen with B-cell deficiencies.

- Recurrent suppurative adenitis may be seen with chronic granulomatous disease (CGD).

Joints

- Pyogenic arthritis can occur in complement deficiencies or immunoglobulin deficiencies.
- A non-specific reactive arthritis can occur in hypogammaglobulinaemia, and also in CVID as one of the associated autoimmune phenomena.

Neurology

- Ataxia: associated with a rare syndrome, ataxia–telangiectasia – a progressive disorder in which ataxia, cutaneous telangiectasia and immune deficiency occur. The neurological symptoms may become apparent before the immune symptoms are manifest.

Investigations

Key points

- Be guided by information obtained on history and examination regarding pattern of infections, types of organisms and time of onset.
- Investigations need to be directed at the component of the immune system believed to be affected.
- May need both quantitative and qualitative evaluation of immune response to exclude immune dysfunction.

More specific tests for immune deficiency include qualitative assays of specific cell functions. Many different assays of specific immune component function are available, other than those listed below. These should not be performed routinely or as first-line investigations, owing to difficulties in interpreting the results, but only in consultation with an immunologist.

First-line investigations in recurrent infections

Blood

FBC

- Total white cell count and differential (lymphopenia suggests SCID; neutropenia in various conditions).
- Platelets (thrombocytopenia in HIV, SCID, Wiskott–Aldrich).
- Blood film (e.g. Howell–Jolly bodies in asplenia).

Serum immunoglobulin levels

- IgG, IgA, IgM, IgE (reduced or absent in congenital immunodeficiencies, usually high in HIV).

Radiology

- *Chest X-ray.* Looking for thymic shadow in infancy, and for evidence of bronchiectasis, dextrocardia, pneumonitis.

Sweat test

- Should be performed to diagnose or exclude cystic fibrosis in any child with recurrent sinopulmonary infections.

Second-line investigations in recurrent infections

Blood

- *Specific antibodies.* Ability to generate functional antibody against specific organisms post vaccination, e.g. diphtheria, tetanus, measles. This is a qualitative test of 'functional' IgG antibody production.
- *Isohaemagglutinins.* Presence of IgM antibodies to ABO blood group determinants. This is a qualitative test of IgM antibody production, only useful after 6–12 months old.
- *IgG subsets.* Children can have isolated IgG subset deficiencies despite a normal total serum IgG level.
- *NBT (nitroblue tetrazolium) test.* Test of neutrophil-mediated bacterial lysis; specific for chronic granulomatous disease (CGD).
- *CH50.* Screening test that evaluates the integrity of the complement cascade.
- *B- and T-cell subsets.* Quantifies numbers of B- and T-cells. Pinpoints specific deficits, e.g. low CD4 count in HIV infection.
- *T-cell function.* In vitro test of T-cell ability to react to antigenic stimuli.
- *HIV serology* (with consent). Positive result may be difficult to interpret in a child less than 12 months of age.

Cilia

- *Nasal brushings or biopsy and electron microscopy.* To diagnose ultrastructural and possibly functional ciliary defects (depending on availability of special laboratory to perform studies).

Clinical problem

A 3-month-old girl presented with fever, cough and rhinorrhoea for 2 days. She was the youngest of five children, and her parents were first cousins. Her second brother had a tetralogy of Fallot corrected in infancy and had since been well. She was born at term and was thriving. Her immunizations were up to date.

On admission she was febrile to 38.5°C, miserable and not feeding. She had a mild preseptal cellulitis involving her left eye. A full blood count showed haemoglobin 103 g/dL, white cell count 26.6×10^9/L with 72% neutrophils, and platelets 918×10^9/L. A chest X-ray showed ill-defined perihilar opacification and hyperinflation suggestive of bronchiolitis. She was treated initially with intravenous antibiotics, but blood cultures and an eye swab were sterile. Influenza A virus was isolated on viral culture of a nasopharyngeal aspirate (NPA). She made a successful recovery over 5 days.

She presented a month later with fever, cough and a papular erythematous rash. She was not unwell, but was febrile to 38°C. Her heart rate was 120 per minute and her respiratory rate was 50 breaths per minute with intercostal recession, and mild audible expiratory wheezing. Her oxygen saturation was 100% in 2 L/min of oxygen. Chest X-ray showed hyperinflation, bronchial wall thickening and hilar prominence, consistent with bronchiolitis. Respiratory syncytial virus was detected by immunofluorescence of an NPA. Her respiratory symptoms resolved over 6 days.

One week after discharge, she developed a fever, and became pale, unresponsive and tachypnoeic. She was pale, poorly responsive and mottled and clinically shocked. She required fluid resuscitation and intravenous antibiotics. Blood cultures and CSF grew *Streptococcus pneumoniae*. An echocardiogram showed trivial pulmonary stenosis.

Questions

1. What features, if any, in this history suggest immune deficiency?

2. If so, which component(s) might be affected?

3. What investigations, if any, would be indicated?

Answers

1. Children can have frequent viral respiratory tract infections, especially when there is increased exposure from multiple siblings. In children with normal T-cell function, these illnesses are usually self-resolving and not prolonged. The recurrent viral infections initially experienced by this child were felt to be within normal limits, and initially no investigations for immune deficiency were felt to be indicated.

■ The subsequent occurrence of *severe pneumococcal sepsis* made it far more likely that this child had significant immune deficiency. Occult pneumococcal bacteraemia is relatively common, and not usually associated with immune deficiency. This child, however, had severe sepsis and developed meningitis.

2. Immune deficiency states that predispose to severe pneumococcal sepsis include asplenia or hyposplenia, deficient antibody production and complement deficiency.

3. Investigations indicated in this child are an abdominal ultrasound, looking for the presence of a spleen, a full blood count including blood film examination, serum immunoglobulins and

CH50, a screening test of complement function. Investigation results:
- A blood film, sent with a request to exclude asplenia, was reported as showing multiple Howell–Jolly bodies.
- An abdominal ultrasound showed no demonstrable spleen.
- Serum immunoglobulins and CH50 were normal.

The diagnosis was felt to be *congenital asplenia*.

4. What is the significance, if any, of the echocardiogram findings?

4. Most congenital asplenia is associated with complex congenital cyanotic heart disease. Although this patient had trivial pulmonary stenosis, her brother had tetralogy of Fallot, raising the possibility of a link between congenital heart disease and asplenia in this family.

5. Do any of her siblings require investigation?

5. In children with isolated congenital asplenia, the possibility of autosomal recessive inheritance should be considered, and siblings screened for asplenia on blood film. *Consanguinity* increases the expression of autosomal recessive conditions, and this child's parents are first cousins.

- On further investigation, the child's brother with congenital heart disease was also found to have a blood film suggestive of asplenia and had no spleen demonstrable on abdominal ultrasound. The other three siblings had normal blood films.
- This finding had important implications for immunization of the two siblings with asplenia against pneumococcal and meningococcal infection, and warning the parents to bring the children straight to hospital if they developed an unremitting high fever.
- The variation in presentation of an immunodeficiency is illustrated here. Both this infant and her brother had a similar predisposition to infection, and yet his lack of splenic function had remained asymptomatic for several years.
- No evidence of failure to thrive and a normal physical examination do not exclude specific immune defects, although it makes severe generalized immune deficiency unlikely.

A final diagnosis of *familial congenital asplenia* was made.

CHAPTER 33

PERSISTENT OR RECURRENT FEVER

David Isaacs, Meryta May

Children presenting with persistent high fevers without a clear focus can present considerable diagnostic difficulties. The term *pyrexia of unknown origin* (PUO) or *fever of unknown origin* (FUO) is sometimes loosely used to refer to any child with unexplained fever of any duration. However, it is better reserved for children with fever that has persisted for at least 3 weeks, and remains unexplained despite appropriate investigations.

The list of possible causes of PUO is extensive, and about 25% of cases in children resolve without making a diagnosis. While infectious causes of PUO always need to be excluded, a significant proportion of the possible diagnoses are immunologically mediated, such as collagen vascular diseases. Malignancy in children may need to be excluded but, unlike the case in adults, PUO is a rare presentation of malignancy. Although the pattern of fever in different illnesses is very variable, some frequently recognized associations that may be helpful are listed in Table 33.1.

Investigation of the child with PUO

Investigation of the child with PUO should be as selective as possible. Some investigations, such as a full blood count, blood film and cultures of blood and urine, are mandatory. Most children have serology performed for EBV, CMV, *Mycoplasma pneumoniae* and any other organisms suggested by history or examination. Although the presence of acute-phase reactants such as CRP is non-specific, very high levels may suggest collagen vascular disease. Testing the serum for antinuclear antibodies is a good screen for SLE and related diseases, while anti-neutrophil cytoplasmic antibodies should also be sought when vasculitis is suspected. A chest X-ray and Mantoux test should usually be performed to exclude tuberculosis. Abdominal ultrasound may be helpful, especially if there is anything to indicate abdominal pathology. On the other hand, the yield from more extensive

Table 33.1   Association between fever type and disease

Type of fever	Associated diseases	Temperature graph
1. Sustained	Pneumococcal pneumonia Pneumococcal bacteraemia Rheumatic fever Typhoid	1
2. Intermittent (temperature normal once a day)	Abscesses Tuberculosis	2
3. Double quotidian (temperature normal twice a day)	Miliary tuberculosis Kala azar	3
4. Septic fever (hectic, unpredictable variation)	Tuberculosis Abscesses	4
5. Remittent (temperature returns towards normal, but is always elevated)	Empyema Systemic onset juvenile arthritis	5
6. Undulant or relapsing (bouts of fever and periods up to several days of normal temperature)	Infective endocarditis Brucellosis Q fever	6
7. Pel-Ebstein (step-wise rise in fever)	Hodgkin's disease	7

radiological or nuclear medicine investigations, such as computed tomographic scans, bone scans and magnetic resonance imaging, is low unless there is a clinical indication. Invasive investigations, such as bone marrow or liver biopsy, will also be dictated by clinical indications or by suggestive laboratory tests.

Recurrent fever syndromes in children

A number of unusual syndromes are characterized by periodic recurrent bouts of fever, sometimes associated with other symptoms, which have a remitting and relapsing course. They can be difficult to diagnose without a high index of clinical suspicion (see Table 33.2).

Familial fevers

Familial Mediterranean fever (FMF)

FMF is a disorder of inflammatory response that results in intermittent widespread serositis. Mutations in the 'Mediterranean fever gene' coding for a protein called pyrin or marenostrin are responsible for about 85% of cases. This protein, produced mainly by neutrophils, regulates inflammation by an unknown mechanism, and gene mutations allow recurrent episodes of serositis. FMF is autosomally recessively inherited, although a positive family history is absent in up to half of patients. It characteristically affects people of Italian, Jewish, Turkish, Arabic or Armenian ancestry, but can also occur in children with no documented Mediterranean background.

Symptoms that support a diagnosis of FMF are:

- The presence of fever with abdominal and/or chest and/or joint pain.
- The presence of at least three such attacks.
- A diagnosis of FMF or amyloidosis in a family member.

Attacks last from several hours up to 4 days, and consist of high fevers, marked abdominal pain from peritonitis, pleurisy, arthritis and headaches. A rash around the ankles can also be associated. There is a risk of developing amyloidosis later in life. There are reports of cases presenting in infancy, but symptoms usually start during childhood, with 80% having their first attack before the age of 20. Time between episodes varies between individuals. Treatment with colchicine reduces the incidence and severity of attacks and the risk of amyloid.

Hyperimmunoglobulin D

Hyper-IgD syndrome is a rare disorder, only recently defined, which is also familial. Symptoms include lymphadenopathy, abdominal pain and diarrhoea, hepatosplenomegaly, arthralgia, arthritis and a vasculitic rash. Typical attacks occur every 4–8 weeks. During the attacks, there is an intense acute-phase response. Serum immunoglobulin D (IgD) is characteristically elevated, both during and between attacks.

Autosomal dominant periodic fever syndromes (familial Hibernian fever)

A rare but important differential diagnosis, FHF is caused by a mutation in a tumour necrosis factor (TNF) receptor gene. It affects people of non-Mediterranean background, and is dominantly inherited. Abdominal pain is particularly prominent, the attacks tend to occur initially at an older age, and the fever bouts are more prolonged than in FMF. There is no response to colchicine, but steroids are effective.

Cyclical neutropenia

This is characterized by regular periods of high fever, often accompanied by mouth ulcers, pharyngitis or pyogenic infections. This cycle classically occurs every 3–4 weeks. Serial monitoring of white cell counts once weekly for 6–8 weeks shows a cyclical fall in neutrophils, with symptoms corresponding to the nadir.

Periodic fever, aphthous stomatitis, pharyngitis and adenitis (PFAPA syndrome)

The diagnosis of this clinically recognized syndrome is usually made by exclusion. There is no known aetiology. Periodicity and symptoms are similar to cyclical neutropenia, but there is no neutropenia. Throat cultures are negative, although tonsillectomy has been shown to be curative in up to 60% of affected children. The mean duration of attacks is 4–5 days, with the child healthy in between. The periodicity of attacks in PFAPA syndrome is usually almost exactly 4 weeks, although sometimes up to 4- to 6-weekly, and rarely every 3–4 months. Early treatment with prednisolone 2 mg/kg daily for 1–2 days characteristically aborts attacks and is highly effective in controlling symptoms, although spontaneous resolution occurs in some patients.

Juvenile idiopathic arthritis (JIA)

The systemic presentation of JIA is often non-specific. The child has high, spiking fevers, usually once or twice a day, which continue for many days. There is almost always an associated macular orange-pink or 'salmon'-coloured rash, which is often only evident with the fevers (evanescent). There can be associated splenomegaly and lymphadenopathy. Joint symptoms are not usually prominent, and arthritis may not develop for months to years after the onset of the fever.

Table 33.2 Comparative features of some periodic fever syndromes

Characteristics	PFAPA	Familial Mediterranean fever	Autosomal dominant periodic fever	Hyper-IgD syndrome	Systemic onset juvenile arthritis	Cyclical neutropenia
Onset <5 years old	Usual	Uncommon	Rare	Common	Common	Common
Mean length of episodes of fever	4 days	2 days	Days to weeks	4 days	>30 days	3 days
Interval between episodes	2–8 weeks	4–8 weeks	Not periodic	Not periodic	Hectic quotidian	3–4 weeks
Aphthous ulcers	Usual (two-thirds of cases)	No	No	No	No	Usual
Pharyngitis	Yes	Sometimes	No	No	No	Yes
Cervical adenitis	Tender	No	No	Yes	Yes	No
Abdominal pain	Sometimes	Yes	Rare	Yes	No	No
Joint symptoms	Arthralgia uncommon	Arthralgia	Arthritis	Arthritis or arthralgia	Arthritis	No
Splenomegaly	Sometimes	No	No	Yes	Often	No
Rash	No	Erysipeloid ankle rash	Yes	Yes	Yes	No
Ethnic origin	None specific	Mediterranean	Irish	Dutch, French or other European	None specific	None specific
Laboratory tests	None	Gene analysis	Gene analysis	Raised serum IgD, gene analysis	None specific	Cyclical neutropenia
Complications	None	Amyloidosis	None	None	Polyarthritis	Gingivitis

Clinical problem

A 5-year-old girl was referred because of recurrent episodes of high fevers to 40°C associated with exudative tonsillitis, mouth ulcers, bad breath, tender cervical adenopathy and, sometimes, abdominal pain with diarrhoea. The episodes started at 18 months of age, and initially occurred almost exactly once a month. The fever did not respond to paracetamol or naproxen, and she would remain febrile for 3–7 days. She was lethargic during the episodes but not particularly unwell, and described by her family doctor as 'viral-looking'. Between episodes she was a lively, active girl. She had one episode of peri-orbital cellulitis at 3 years of age. She never had joint pains or swelling. At the age of 4 years the episodes seemed to resolve spontaneously, then recurred with an interval of every 3 months.

On examination, when well, she was a pleasant, lively, well-looking child on the 75th centile for height and weight. She had flexural and truncal eczema, but examination was otherwise completely normal. Her tonsils were not enlarged or pitted, and she had no oral ulcers.

Questions

1. What is the likely diagnosis?

2. What investigations should be performed?

3. What advice would you give to the parents about her prognosis?

4. What major differential diagnosis needs to be excluded?

Discussion

The major clinical features in this child are periodic high fevers, aphthous stomatitis, pharyngitis and tender cervical adenitis. This combination of symptoms is strongly suggestive of PFAPA syndrome. PFAPA syndrome is an unusual condition of unknown aetiology with no diagnostic laboratory features. As such, the diagnosis is made clinically and by exclusion of other conditions. The most important differential to exclude is cyclical neutropenia, which can have a very similar presentation. Other possible diagnoses include recurrent bacterial tonsillitis, a humoral immune deficiency, hyperimmunoglobulin D syndrome and familial Mediterranean fever.

In excluding cyclical neutropenia as a diagnosis, it is obviously important to measure the neutrophil count during at least one episode, or to perform routine blood counts, weekly for 6 weeks.

Glucocorticoids are highly effective in controlling the symptoms of PFAPA. Symptoms resolve spontaneously in some patients but persist in others, although long-term sequelae are not described. It is possible that the tonsils are involved in an immune dysregulation. The success of one or two doses of prednisolone in treating PFAPA syndrome suggests immune dysregulation to be more likely than an infectious cause, although the two mechanisms are not mutually exclusive.

Investigations on our patient during episodes showed a normal neutrophil count, normal levels of complement C3 and C4 and moderately raised acute-phase reactants (ESR 50 mm/h). Antinuclear antibodies were not detected. Throat swabs taken during episodes did not grow beta-haemolytic streptococci or other potential bacterial pathogens, and viral swabs were negative for HSV. Serum immunoglobulins showed normal levels of serum IgG, A, M, D and E. A diagnosis of PFAPA syndrome was made, on the basis of her clinical features and exclusion of other diagnoses. Her attacks became much less troublesome when prednisolone was given at the start of each attack.

A final diagnosis of PFAPA was made.

CHAPTER 34

ACUTE FEVER

David Isaacs, Meryta May

Defining and measuring fever

- Fever is commonly defined as a rectal temperature >38°C, which is approximately two standard deviations above the mean. Normal body temperature varies with the time of day, but is generally less than 37.5°C centrally.
- In practice, rectal temperatures are rarely used, for practical reasons. Axillary temperature measurement is a reasonable alternative, recognizing that axillary temperatures have generally been shown to be about 0.9°C lower than rectal temperatures in children, although the difference is only about 0.2°C in neonates.
- In contrast to axillary measurement, oral temperature measurement has not been systematically compared to rectal measurement.
- Tympanic membrane temperature sensors are not reliable enough for accurate repeatable measuring, and are not recommended.

Aims

Most episodes of fever in childhood are caused by viruses, mainly respiratory viruses, and require no more than symptomatic management. It is important to be able to identify which children may have bacterial infections requiring antibiotics.

The main questions to address in evaluating a child with fever are:

1. Is the child obviously seriously unwell?
2. Is there a focus of infection?
3. Is the child at risk of occult bacteraemia or serious bacterial infection?
4. Does the child need empirical antibiotic treatment?

Children who are obviously critically ill require immediate resuscitation and treatment, in parallel with investigations. Sources of infection which could be detected on a physical examination are listed below, and should be sought:

- Meningitis.
- Pneumonia.
- Otitis media.
- Septic arthritis.
- Osteomyelitis.
- Cellulitis.
- Tonsillitis or pharyngitis.
- Upper respiratory tract infection.

If no causes are evident from examination and history, the risk of occult bacteraemia or serious bacterial infection (SBI) needs to be considered. In occult bacteraemia the child does not look unwell, and the urine and cerebrospinal fluid are by definition normal on microscopy, although the peripheral blood white cell count may be raised. Children with SBI, in contrast, may look unwell and may have an abnormal urine or CSF microscopy.

The incidence of occult bacteraemia in children under 3 years old presenting with high fever and no focus of infection is approximately 2–3%. *Streptococcus pneumoniae* is the commonest cause of occult bacteraemia, being responsible for around 80–90% of cases. Without treatment, only about 2% of children with occult pneumococcal bacteraemia will develop meningitis; the rest will recover spontaneously. The risk of meningitis is nearly 50% for children with the much rarer condition of occult meningococcal bacteraemia. Other organisms, such as *Salmonella*, may be important causes of occult bacteraemia in some countries.

Consideration will now be given to clinical indicators, which can assist in deciding on the management of febrile children.

Age

There is a higher risk of serious bacterial infection (e.g. urinary tract infection, pneumonia, meningitis) in febrile children less than 3 years of age than in older children, and a very high risk (13–25%) in neonates. The incidence of occult bacteraemia is also higher the younger the child.

Because of the high risk of serious infection, all febrile neonates (less than 4 weeks old) should have a full evaluation for sepsis, namely full blood count, blood culture, urine culture, chest X-ray and lumbar puncture, and then should receive parenteral antibiotics while awaiting investigation results. Older children can have a more selective evaluation and do not necessarily require empirical antibiotic treatment.

Key point

The younger the child, the lower should be the threshold for investigation and treatment.

Height of the fever

The rate of serious bacterial infection rises with the height of fever in neonates and young children. However, the sensitivity of even an extremely high fever (>40°C) to detect serious bacterial infection is low. Serious bacterial infection can still occur when the child has a low-grade fever or is afebrile. This particularly applies to neonates, who rarely generate a marked temperature response.

It should also be remembered that teething is *not* an accepted cause of high fever in young children. There is no objective data to support the widely accepted parental belief that teething is associated with pyrexia, and other causes should be sought.

Response to antipyretics

The response or lack of response of a fever to antipyretics is often quoted by parents as an important fact on history. This has *no* predictive value in deciding if the child has a serious infection or not.

Duration of fever

The duration of fever is also a poor predictor of whether or not a child has SBI or occult bacteraemia.

White blood cell count

A peripheral white blood cell count elevated to >15 × 10^9/L has a sensitivity of approximately 30–50% in predicting occult bacteraemia. While this test has limited usefulness in isolation, it can be helpful in the context of a febrile child who has a moderate risk of serious infection or bacteraemia, in deciding whether or not to give empirical therapy. Using a cut-off white cell count of $>15 \times 10^9$/L to decide empirical therapy correlates to treating approximately 65% of a highly febrile population in order to identify 96% of all bacteraemic children.

A low white cell count can occur in severe bacterial sepsis, but is much more common in viral infections, and is not as strong an indicator as a high white cell count of the need for investigation or antibiotics.

Appearance of the child

The clinician's impression of the child's well-being is an important guide for assessment. Factors that have been shown in studies to be significant in predicting risk of SBI include the following signs, which have been called signs of 'toxicity':

- **A** for alertness, arousal, activity.
- **B** for breathing difficulties, which may be dyspnoea or grunting due to pneumonia or tachypnoea due to acidosis or sometimes due to central stimulation in meningitis.
- **C** for colour (pallor) and circulation (capillary refill time greater than 2 seconds or cool peripheries).
- **D** for drowsiness and decreased feeding and decreased urine output.

Other useful signs include the quality of the child's cry (high-pitched, constant, irritable crying suggests a sick child) and the child's reaction to family members.

The Yale Observation Scale (Table 34.1) is one attempt to quantify these observations into a score to identify children at risk of serious bacterial infection. It is more often used in the USA than elsewhere. While scoring systems can be useful in assessing children, they are not foolproof, and a comprehensive assessment of the child and social circumstances is essential for good management.

Key points

- It is important to conduct repeated evaluation of children over time because their clinical state may change.
- Any child assessed as having a 'toxic appearance' should be admitted to hospital for parenteral antibiotics pending investigation results.

Use of empirical antibiotics

Because of the large numbers of febrile children with inconsequential illnesses, the use of empirical

Table 34.1   Yale Observation Scale

Observation item	Normal (1)	Moderate impairment (2)	Severe impairment (3)
Quality of cry	Strong, with normal tone, or content and not crying	Whimpering or sobbing	Weak or moaning or high-pitched
Reaction to parents	Cries briefly then stops, or content and not crying	Cries off and on	Continual crying or hardly responds
State variation	If awake, stays awake, or if asleep and stimulated, wakes up quickly	Eyes close briefly when awake, or awakes with prolonged stimulation	Falls asleep or cannot be roused
Colour	Pink	Pale extremities or acrocyanosis	Pale or cyanotic or mottled or ashen
Hydration	Skin normal, eyes normal and mucous membranes moist	Skin, eyes normal and mouth slightly dry	Skin doughy, dry mucous membranes and/or sunken eyes
Response (talk, smile) to social overtures	Smiles or becomes alert	Brief smile or becomes alert briefly	No smile, face anxious, dull, expressionless, does not become alert

The score given in parentheses for each description applies. The higher the score, the greater the risk of serious bacterial infection.

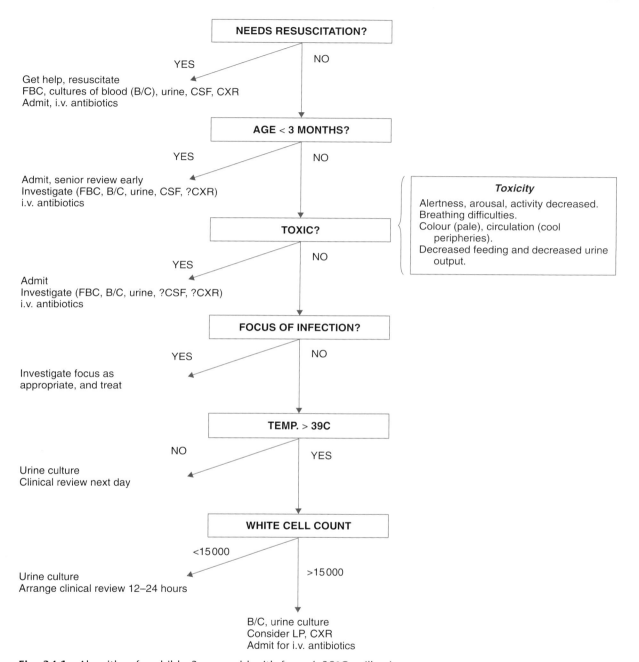

NEEDS RESUSCITATION?

YES → Get help, resuscitate
FBC, cultures of blood (B/C), urine, CSF, CXR
Admit, i.v. antibiotics

NO ↓

AGE < 3 MONTHS?

YES → Admit, senior review early
Investigate (FBC, B/C, urine, CSF, ?CXR)
i.v. antibiotics

NO ↓

TOXIC?

Toxicity
Alertness, arousal, activity decreased.
Breathing difficulties.
Colour (pale), circulation (cool
    peripheries).
Decreased feeding and decreased urine
    output.

YES → Admit
Investigate (FBC, B/C, urine, ?CSF, ?CXR)
i.v. antibiotics

NO ↓

FOCUS OF INFECTION?

YES → Investigate focus as
appropriate, and treat

NO ↓

TEMP. > 39C

NO → Urine culture
Clinical review next day

YES ↓

WHITE CELL COUNT

<15000 → Urine culture
Arrange clinical review 12–24 hours

>15000 ↓

B/C, urine culture
Consider LP, CXR
Admit for i.v. antibiotics

Fig. 34.1   Algorithm for child <3 years old with fever (>38°C axillary).

antibiotics for every child without a clear focus of infection is *not* recommended. Empirical therapy should be reserved for children identified as being toxic or at a high risk of bacterial infection, or where laboratory parameters (such as white cell count) suggest an increased likelihood of bacterial infection. See algorithm (Fig. 34.1) for a summary of a suggested approach.

Clinical problem

A 7-month-old child presented to the emergency department with an axillary temperature of 38.5°C. She had been a little miserable over the last 24 hours, and had refused one or two of her feeds. Her mother was not too concerned as she reported the child was in the process of teething, but she wanted her checked 'just to be sure'. On examination, the child was on the 50th percentile for weight, height and head circumference, and was appropriately interactive with both her mother and the examining doctor. Her heart rate was 110 per minute, respiratory rate 24 and she was well perfused. The child had no rash, no lymphadenopathy or organomegaly, and chest and abdominal examination were normal. There were no signs of an upper respiratory tract infection, no history of vomiting or diarrhoea, and the rest of the family was well. She had received all of her immunizations according to the schedule.

A bag urine sample was obtained. On urinalysis leucocytes were detected, but there were no other abnormalities. The sample was sent for culture. The child had breast-fed normally in the department and was now sleeping. She was sent home without starting antibiotics, with instructions to return for review after 24 hours, or earlier if she deteriorated or developed any new symptoms.

The child returned for review the following day as requested. On arrival she was febrile, with an axillary temperature of 39.2°C, and vomited once at triage. On examination, she was still interactive, but became easily irritable and was not as cooperative. Her throat and tympanic membranes were mildly red, although she was crying, but there was no cough, rhinorrhoea or lymphadenopathy. Her fontanelle was not bulging or tense. There were no other new findings. The urine result from the previous day showed 10–100 white cells, >100 epithelial cells and a mixed growth of three organisms. A full blood count was taken. which showed a white cell count of 17×10^9/L.

Questions

1. What investigations would you recommend for the child now?

Discussion

- The initial decision to send the child home without antibiotics, but with early review, because she appeared well and non-toxic, is in accordance with the algorithm given and seems reasonable.
- On her second presentation, however, the child has a high fever and appears less well. Although there are no clinical features that suggest she is toxic, as defined in the text and the algorithm, her high fever and high white blood cell count make it more likely that she is bacteraemic or has a serious bacterial infection. She should have a blood culture taken, a repeat urine sample and a chest X-ray.
- The algorithm does not say that a lumbar puncture (LP) should necessarily be performed in this clinical situation. Some would do an LP immediately, while others would delay, and only do an LP if she looked more unwell during her assessment and observation period in the department, or if blood cultures were subsequently positive. While awaiting the above investigations, apart from routine observations of her temperature, heart rate and respiration, she

should be reviewed at least every hour with regard to her behaviour, colour, alertness, feeding and interaction.

2. Does the child have a urinary tract infection?

■ The urine result is uninterpretable, and a more definitive sample should be obtained. While a negative bag urine result has a high negative predictive value, a result such as this most likely reflects contamination from the baby's perineum. In a child under 12 months of age, the most easily collected and reliable urine sample is a suprapubic aspirate, but a catheter sample is an acceptable alternative.

3. What treatment, if any, should the child have?

■ This child has a high fever and a high peripheral white blood cell count, and even if there is no evidence of pneumonia on chest X-ray, and urine microscopy is not suggestive of urinary tract infection, there is about a 10% risk that she has occult bacteraemia. According to the management algorithm given in this chapter she should be admitted for intravenous antibiotics awaiting blood and urine culture results.

4. Should the child be admitted to hospital?

■ The assessing doctor on repeated examination in emergency felt that the child did not have enough signs of clinical toxicity to suggest meningitis, and a lumbar puncture was not done. The child was admitted and given intravenous penicillin G. Twenty-four hours into the admission, she had become afebrile and was bright and alert. The chest X-ray was normal and a repeat urine sample contained no cells and showed no growth. *Streptococcus pneumoniae* was grown from her blood culture after 30 hours. A subsequent lumbar puncture was completely normal with no white cells, normal protein and sugar and no growth.

■ This child had occult pneumococcal bacteraemia, and received empiric antibiotic therapy, following a regime of repeated assessment and stratification according to clinical risk. It could be argued that antibiotics were not indicated, because there was a 98% chance that she would have recovered spontaneously without antibiotics, but many would accept the wisdom of treating 50 children with occult pneumococcal bacteraemia with parenteral antibiotics, to prevent one child developing pneumococcal meningitis.

A final diagnosis of pneumococcal bacteraemia was made.

RASH AND FEVER
David Isaacs, Meryta May

A rash is a visible lesion of the skin due to disease. The condition can be a primary skin disorder or a symptom of a systemic process. Rashes caused by infection can be limited to skin involvement or be part of a broader condition.

When considering the differential diagnosis of a rash, it is important to be able to describe its features. Ask the child's parents about the appearance, because rashes often change with time.

History

- Onset of the rash: sudden or gradual.
- Type of lesion: see Table 35.1.
- Distribution: whether central, peripheral or generalized.
- Progression: direction of spread, speed of progression.
- General well-being of the child, including prodromal illness or fever.
- Infectious contacts.
- Drug history: including over-the-counter preparations, topical treatments and drugs that have been ceased.
- Symptoms of the rash: itch, pain, burning.
- Travel history.
- Contact with pets and other animals.

Physical examination

Be sure to examine:

- The entire skin surface:
  - To determine the true extent of the rash.
  - Type of lesions.
  - Distribution.
  - Evolving lesions.
- The mucous membranes for involvement or ulceration.
- The conjunctivae for injection or episcleritis.

Table 35.1   Terminology of cutaneous lesions

Type of lesion	Description	Common causes
Vesicles	Small, fluid-filled blisters	Varicella zoster, herpes simplex, enteroviruses (particularly Coxsackie A)
Petechiae	Small, non-blanching spots	Vasculitis, meningococcaemia, thrombocytopenia
Pustules	Small blisters containing purulent fluid	Bacterial infection, e.g. *Staphylococcus aureus*. NB: not necessarily infective
Urticaria	Raised, itchy lesions	Drug eruptions, erythema marginatum, idiopathic
Macules	Flat spots, not palpable. Can form large sheets	Drug eruptions, viral exanthems
Papules	Elevated, palpable, small rounded lesions	Molluscum contagiosum, warts, enteroviruses
Plaques	Elevated, flat-topped lesions	Psoriasis, pityriasis rosea

- The scalp and hair for areas of inflammation, scaling or hair loss. Use of ultraviolet light (a Wood's light) can show fluorescence in some types of fungal infection.
- For lymphadenopathy.
- For hepatosplenomegaly.
- The joints for any associated arthritis.

Important rashes of infancy and childhood that are commonly seen in general paediatric practice will be discussed in the following section under descriptive headings, with a separate section for neonatal conditions.

Important rashes in the newborn

Erythema toxicum

This appears as red macules with overlying small yellow or white pustules. The condition is idiopathic and non-infective. It can be mistaken for infection: a Gram stain of the lesion shows multiple eosinophils. The rash often appears during the first few days of life and may persist up to a fortnight.

Staphylococcal skin infection

This can look similar to erythema toxicum: the skin may be indurated and pustules may be interspersed with vesicles and sometimes bullae. When bullous, it is referred to as bullous impetigo. In its most severe form, of staphylococcal scalded skin syndrome, there is extensive erythema in a clinically septic child, with widespread skin loss (Fig. 35.1). This condition is life threatening.

Localized herpes simplex virus (HSV) infection

Neonatal HSV infection may be localized, at least initially, to the skin, eyes and/or mouth, so-called skin–eye–mouth (SEM) disease. Vesicles are most often found on the scalp or around areas of minor trauma, e.g. scalp electrode sites. They can present as shallow ulcers only. Rapid diagnosis can be obtained, often within an hour or two, using specific immunofluorescent staining of cells swabbed from the base of a lesion. Polymerase chain reaction (PCR) for viral DNA is not usually helpful in this situation because of

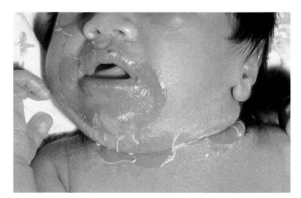

Fig 35.1   Staphylococcal scalded skin syndrome in a neonate. Skin desquamation with underlying erythema. (Courtesy of Dr Maureen Rogers.)

time constraints. Urgent early treatment of localized neonatal HSV infection with intravenous acyclovir is essential because, without treatment, 70% of affected babies will progress to disseminated HSV infection with encephalitis, hepatitis, DIC and an extremely poor prognosis.

Varicella zoster virus infection

Neonatal varicella is usually seen in the context of maternal chickenpox (or more rarely zoster) or of contact with an infected sibling. Rapid diagnosis can be obtained by specific immunofluorescence of vesicle fluid. Neonatal varicella resulting from perinatal transmission can be life threatening and, if severe, requires intravenous acyclovir.

Petechiae

The most common cause of neonatal petechiae is thrombocytopenia, either from platelet destruction by maternal antibodies, or from congenital infection such as CMV. Congenital rubella is extremely rare in most developed countries, because of immunization.

Rashes in infancy and childhood

Vesicular rashes

Varicella (chickenpox)

Chickenpox is caused by primary infection with varicella zoster virus (VZV). Classically, there is a short prodrome of about a day of sore throat and fever, after which varicella commences as crops of itchy, circumscribed, vesicular lesions on the scalp and trunk. These become pustular before becoming crusted and then resolve without scarring, if not superinfected. A range of lesions at different stages is usually seen at any one time. Mucous membranes may be involved. There is often only a mild prodromal illness of fever and mild lethargy. When varicella occurs in the context of significantly damaged skin, such as eczema, the risk of serious illness is much higher, and careful monitoring and treatment are indicated.

Herpes zoster (shingles)

Zoster is caused by the same virus as chickenpox – VZV – but occurs due to reactivation of VZV, which

has remained latent in nerve cells following earlier chickenpox. The rash is characteristic, with the eruption of crops of vesicles in a dermatomal distribution, although there are often one or two spots outside the dermatome. Confusion with herpes simplex stomatitis may occur when facial nerve dermatomes are involved. Pain is surprisingly rare in children, although older children may sometimes have painful lesions. Although zoster is common in immunocompromised children, it is not uncommon in normal children, and is virtually never the first presentation of underlying malignancy or immune compromise. Zoster in young children often results from having chickenpox in the neonatal period, or from intrauterine exposure due to maternal VZV in pregnancy.

Herpes simplex virus (HSV)

While HSV infection is often asymptomatic, the most common presentation during childhood is with gingivostomatitis. The child is febrile and develops ulcers of the gums, buccal mucosa and pharynx, and often on the cheek where saliva dribbles. There may be marked facial swelling and redness. Involvement of a finger can occur (herpetic whitlow), and may mimic paronychia. HSV infection of eczematous skin (eczema herpeticum) can spread rapidly (Fig. 35.2) and, if the vesicular nature of the lesions is overlooked, may be misdiagnosed as worsening eczema or bacterial superinfection. A clinical diagnosis of eczema herpeticum can be confirmed rapidly with specific

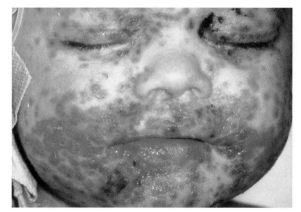

Fig 35.2 Eczema herpeticum. Widespread inflammation, but discrete vesicular lesions are distinguishable.

immunofluorescence, and affected children usually require intravenous acyclovir.

Enteroviruses

Non-polio enteroviruses are a common cause of vesicular rashes, especially in summer and autumn. Hand, foot and mouth disease is caused by different enteroviruses, most commonly Coxsackievirus type A16. It often occurs in epidemics in daycare centres or schools. It is associated with a papulovesicular eruption on the palms, soles, mucous membranes and sometimes the buttocks. There may be mild associated respiratory or gastrointestinal symptoms, but the clinical course is benign.

Enterovirus 71 can cause hand, foot and mouth disease, but differs from the other enteroviruses in that infections may be accompanied by significant neurological manifestations, such as aseptic meningitis, brainstem encephalitis with neurogenic pulmonary oedema, and acute flaccid paralysis.

Impetigo

Impetigo is the most common skin infection encountered in infants and school-aged children. It is caused by *Streptococcus pyogenes* or *Staphylococcus aureus*. The early lesion is an erythematous papule, which progresses to transient vesicles and then becomes a shallow ulcer with surrounding honey-coloured crusted exudate. The lesions are often found in an area of traumatized skin, and are commonly around the nose, mouth and extremities. It is spread among individuals through close physical contact.

Maculopapular rashes

Many virus infections, especially enteroviruses, produce maculopapular exanthems. These are often non-specific and generalized in distribution (Fig. 35.3). They can be difficult to differentiate from allergic drug reactions. Features that favour a viral aetiology are:

- Occurrence along scratch marks.
- Some lesions in straight lines.
- Exaggeration in areas of sunburn.
- Occurrence under hospital arm bands or on prior skin disease.
- Presence of lymphadenopathy.

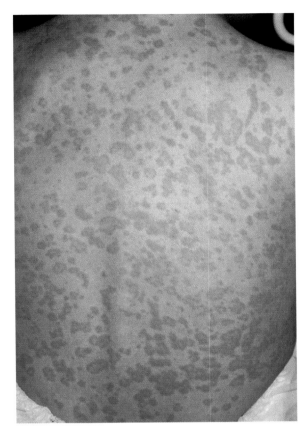

Fig 35.3 Viral exanthem. Widespread macules, some in a characteristically linear pattern.

Measles

Measles is rare in countries with high levels of immunization. While the diagnosis should be considered in a child with a blotchy, geographical, erythematous exanthem, other causes are usually more likely in an immunized child. Characteristic features of measles are:

- 3–5 days of prodromal features of fever, malaise, conjunctivitis, coryza and cough.
- High fever, which persists after the rash appears.
- Downward spread of the rash from the pre-auricular area and the face to involve the body.
- Tendency of the rash to become confluent on the trunk and remain discrete lower down.
- Tendency of the rash to become brown and then desquamate after 2–3 days.

Rubella

Rubella virus infection results in an erythematous, discrete exanthem that is often faint but may be morbilliform (measles-like) and spreads down from the face. Occipital and/or post-auricular lymphadenopathy is typically (but not exclusively) associated, and arthritis and conjunctivitis can occur. There are relatively few systemic symptoms in children. It is important to trace and investigate pregnant contacts of a case.

Kawasaki disease

This is an important differential diagnosis of a child with rash and fever. Clinical features include persistent high fever with characteristic marked irritability, rash, cervical lymphadenopathy (sometimes unilateral resembling abscess), non-exudative conjunctivitis, stomatitis, and swelling or redness of hands and feet. The rash is not specific and can take many forms. It may resemble erythema multiforme, scarlet fever, measles, urticaria or a drug reaction. It is usually non-pruritic, and may be transient or evanescent (comes and goes).

Erythema infectiosum (slapped cheek disease, fifth disease)

Parvovirus B19 infection produces a rash that develops in two stages. The initial appearance is of 'slapped cheeks': an intense erythema of the malar areas resembling sunburn in a child who may be well, or have mild systemic symptoms of malaise and fever. The patient then develops a reticulated macular erythema over the limbs (Fig. 35.4). This is often asymptomatic or may be associated with arthralgias. This form of the rash may wax and wane for weeks after the initial illness. Children are no longer infectious once the rash has appeared.

Roseola infantum

Roseola is a condition that affects infants and young children. Children initially have 3–5 days of high fever and mild systemic symptoms, before the rash then appears with simultaneous defervescence. The rash consists of small rose-pink macules or papules, which may be morbilliform and are most prominent on the trunk and face. The most common aetiological agent is human herpesvirus 6 (HHV-6). Children with measles are febrile and miserable when the rash is present; in contrast, the child with roseola becomes afebrile and well as the rash appears.

Meningococcal infection

A transient macular rash, mimicking an enteroviral rash, can occur early in infection with *Neisseria meningitidis* in up to 20% of cases. It typically disappears in less than a day, and purpura may then appear.

Petechial and purpuric rashes (Table 35.2)

Meningococcal infection

In a febrile child without an infectious focus, a localized petechial or purpuric rash can be the first sign of *N. meningitidis* septicaemia (Fig. 35.5). The lesions may be very subtle early in the course. Purpuric lesions

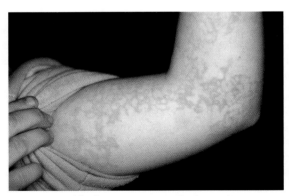

Fig. 35.4   Fifth disease. Lacy, reticular rash. (Courtesy of Dr Maureen Rogers.)

Table 35.2 Differential diagnosis of child with purpura or petechiae	
Bacterial infections	**Other causes**
Neisseria meningitidis infection	Viral illnesses, e.g. enteroviruses,
Staphylococcus aureus sepsis	EBV, CMV
Streptococcus pneumoniae sepsis	Rickettsial infections
Listeria monocytogenes sepsis	Henoch–Schönlein purpura
Group A streptococcal pharyngitis	Thrombocytopenia (ITP, malignancy)

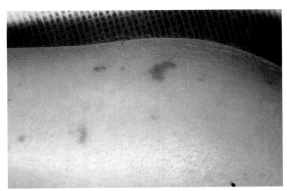

Fig 35.5 Purpura. Discrete purple lesions > 2 mm in diameter, which will not blanch on pressure.

do not blanch with pressure. A simple test is to press a glass slide or a drinking glass on the lesions and observe through the glass whether the lesions stay purple or go white (blanch).

Henoch–Schönlein purpura (HSP)

HSP is an immunologically mediated vasculitis, thought to be a reaction to an infectious agent, although no single organism has been implicated. It is usually preceded by an upper respiratory tract infection. It is the most common cause of non-thrombocytopenic purpura in children. The rash characteristically involves the buttocks and extensor surfaces, starting off as pink, blanching maculopapules, which progress to palpable non-blanching purpura that evolves from red to purple and then brown, before fading over 2–3 days. The lesions occur in crops and may recur at intervals over days to months after the initial episode. Fever is uncommon.

Idiopathic thrombocytopenic purpura (ITP)

ITP is an immunologically mediated disease, in which platelet destruction by auto-antibodies leads to petechiae, and occasionally a purpuric rash with frank bleeding. Many different viral infections can sometimes be triggers for the occurrence of ITP (which is not really idiopathic in those cases). Children are not usually febrile at the time of onset of the rash of ITP.

Leukaemia

Children with marrow infiltration by malignant cells, particularly leukaemia, may present with a petechial rash. This is usually accompanied by a history of easy bruising, malaise or fatigue, bone pain, and often pallor caused by the associated anaemia. Fever may also be present due to infection.

Papular rashes

Molluscum contagiosum

Molluscum is a poxvirus infection, which causes multiple, 2–5 mm diameter, flesh-coloured papules with a central dimple (umbilication). Initially firm, the lesions become softer and waxier with time. Some lesions have a mildly erythematous base and lesions may become superinfected. The lesions can occur on all parts of the body, but are least common on the palms or soles. Auto-inoculation and spread to others via close contact can occur. In the vast majority of cases, the condition will resolve over some months without specific treatment. Immunodeficiency, e.g. HIV, predisposes to severe molluscum.

Acral papular viral exanthem

While classically attributed to the exanthem associated with hepatitis B (Gianotti–Crosti syndrome), acral papular exanthems can occur with a number of virus infections, especially enteroviruses. There are many terms used for this exanthem, including papular acrodermatitis of childhood and papulovesicular acrolocated syndrome (PALS). The appearance is of papular and occasionally vesicular lesions, restricted to the acral part of the limbs and occasionally the face (Fig. 35.6). There is often associated pruritus. The predominant age group affected is 2- to 4-year-olds. The reaction has a prolonged course and may take up to 10 weeks to resolve.

Erythema multiforme (EM)

EM is characterized by an abrupt eruption of erythematous macules or plaques, usually most prominent on the extensor surfaces of the upper limbs (Fig. 35.7). The diagnostic lesion is doughnut shaped, with an erythematous outer ring, and a pale inner ring around a dusky or necrotic centre (target lesions). The lesions are mostly asymptomatic, but may be mildly uncomfortable or pruritic. The lesions remain fixed in position, and are often characteristically symmetrical bilaterally. They fade after a week to 10 days. Oral lesions may occur (but other mucosal surfaces are not

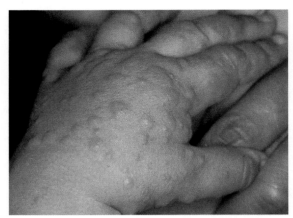

Fig 35.6   Acral papular viral exanthem. Raised papules on the hands of a child. (Courtesy of Dr Maureen Rogers.)

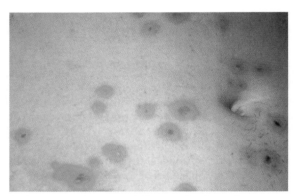

Fig 35.7   Erythema multiforme. Oval, erythematous 'target' lesions with dusky centres. (Courtesy of Dr Maureen Rogers.)

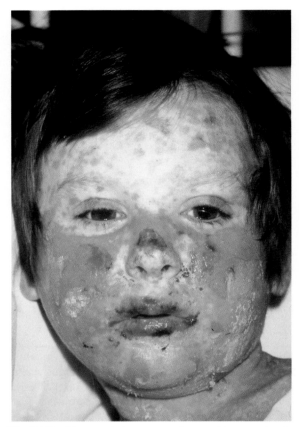

Fig 35.8   Stevens–Johnson syndrome. Haemorrhagic lesions, some bullous, plus severe mucosal involvement.

involved), and 25% of cases involve the oral mucosa alone. The most common infective cause is HSV.

Stevens–Johnson syndrome

An important differential of EM, this eruption differs in that two or more mucosal surfaces are involved, lesions are more widespread, and there is progression to bulla formation and haemorrhagic crusting (Fig. 35.8). Mucosal ulceration of the mouth and genitalia may occur and is severely painful. There is often significant internal organ involvement and a prodrome of flu-like upper respiratory tract illness. The most common infectious agent implicated is *Mycoplasma pneumoniae*; the other major causal agent is drugs.

Generalized erythroderma

Staphylococcal scalded skin syndrome

This manifestation of *S. aureus* infection is mostly seen in children under 5 years. Foci of infection include the nasopharynx, urinary tract, umbilicus and skin abrasions. The skin reaction is mediated by staphylococcal epidermolytic toxin A or B. It consists of a scarlatiniform, generalized erythroderma, accompanied in severe forms by internal organ involvement and severe systemic illness. The child may be irritable and unwell; the erythroderma is markedly tender and may progress to take on a wrinkled appearance, before forming sterile bullae and erosions, with extensive epidermal loss. The conjunctivae may be erythematous and purulent, and radial fissuring is common around the mouth, nose and eyes. Perioral erythema is prominent. Owing to skin loss, fluid and electrolyte imbalances and secondary infection are common complications. The split in the skin layers is superficial, so that with antibiotic treatment complete recovery occurs with no scarring.

Scarlet fever

Scarlet fever is a systemic manifestation of *Streptococcus pyogenes* infection, resulting from exotoxin production. It affects mainly children aged 3–12 years and is rare in infancy. Scarlatina is the name given to a milder illness in which streptococcal infection causes scarlatiniform rash alone, without the systemic features. True scarlet fever causes an erythematous, fine, punctate rash which characteristically has a sandpaper texture. It appears initially on the trunk and spreads rapidly. Petechiae may be found on major skin folds. Other distinctive features are glossal inflammation, with prominent papillae (a 'strawberry tongue') and circumoral pallor, with the rash sparing the skin around the mouth. There is often desquamation of fingers and toes on resolution.

Toxic shock syndrome (TSS)

Like scarlet fever, TSS is a severe, systemic, clinically defined reaction to bacterial toxin. By definition, clinical features must include high fever, rash with desquamation, hypotension and involvement of at least three organ systems. Organisms associated with this syndrome are *S. aureus* and *S. pyogenes*. While TSS is usually recognized by the combination of all symptoms, the rash is typically a diffuse erythroderma, and may be accompanied by conjunctival and other mucous membrane hyperaemia. Its distribution and intensity may alter from hour to hour during the course of the illness.

Urticaria

It is important to appreciate that, while classically associated with hypersensitivity reactions, urticaria in children under 5 years of age is most commonly caused by a viral illness. In this situation, there is often less associated pruritus than would be expected with an allergic reaction. Severe lesions may be associated with a purple discoloration due to bruising (purple urticaria; see Fig. 35.9). Viral urticaria differs from erythema multiforme because the position of the lesions changes, and the erythema disappears from individual lesions over a 24-hour period.

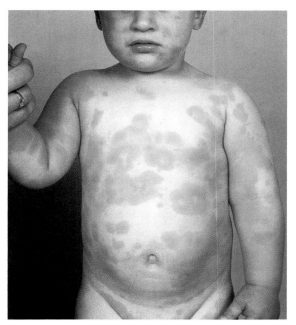

Fig 35.9 Purple urticaria. Blotchy truncal rash, purple in places. (Courtesy of Dr Maureen Rogers.)

Erythema marginatum

The rash associated with rheumatic fever (RF) is a form of urticaria. It manifests in around 10% of patients with RF, and is considered one of the major diagnostic criteria for RF when present. The rash has an erythematous macular component and a raised edge (Fig. 35.10). It is non-pruritic and non-painful, and the lesions coalesce to form a serpiginous pattern.

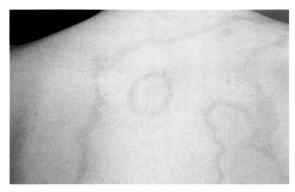

Fig 35.10 Erythema marginatum. Widespread urticarial rash with thin, pink margin. (Courtesy of Dr Maureen Rogers.)

The rash may be fleeting and may reappear intermittently over weeks.

Drug reactions

Cutaneous manifestations are the most common form of adverse drug reaction in children. While classically drug reactions are urticarial in nature, almost all morphological variants are possible. Angioedema related to drug ingestion is more significant, as it implies an IgE-mediated pathway for the reaction and hence possible risk of anaphylaxis on re-exposure.

Clinical problem

A 3-year-old girl was brought by ambulance to the emergency department after a seizure at home. On the day of presentation, she had been non-specifically unwell. In the afternoon she complained of a few non-specific aches and pains, and was anorexic. Her mother thought she felt hot. She had vomited once during the evening. She had no rhinorrhoea, cough or rash. Just after midnight she had a brief generalized tonic–clonic seizure and was brought to hospital.

Her only significant medical history was of a febrile convulsion at 18 months of age, from which she had recovered uneventfully. She had been born at term, with no perinatal complications. Her immunizations were up to date. She had no siblings.

On examination in the emergency department she was sleepy but easily rousable. Her temperature was 39.4°C, her heart rate was 130 beats per minute and respiratory rate 24 breaths per minute. Her throat was slightly red and there were a few petechiae around her left eye. The remainder of the examination was normal. Her blood sugar was 6.1 mmol/L. A diagnosis of febrile convulsion was made and she was observed overnight. The petechiae around her eye were considered to be secondary to her vomiting. She vomited several more times overnight.

On review the next morning she was sitting up in bed watching television, but her father was concerned that she did not seem well. On closer examination she had further petechiae around her face and a spreading purpuric rash was found over her legs and chest.

Questions

1. What is the likely diagnosis?

2. What is the differential diagnosis of a child with fever and petechiae?

Answers

1. The most likely diagnosis in this child is meningococcal septicaemia. The main clinical features of meningococcal disease at presentation are fever (88%), rash (68%), vomiting (67%) and drowsiness (55%). Early recognition of this condition is vital for successful treatment. The classic spreading purpuric rash discovered in this child is virtually pathognomonic. Earlier diagnosis based on the scattered petechiae around her eyes would have required a higher degree of clinical suspicion.
   - Meningococcal disease may present with a petechial rash alone, a maculopapular rash or no rash. Atypical presentations may lead to delayed diagnosis and a worse outcome.

2. There is a wide differential diagnosis to be considered in the child presenting with fever and petechiae. Only about 10% of children presenting to hospital with fever and petechiae in the USA and UK have meningococcal infection.
   - Risk factors for serious bacterial infection in these children include: appearing unwell or toxic, signs of meningism, lack of pharyngitis, numerous petechiae, the presence of purpura and high (>15 × 10^9/L) or low (<5 × 10^9/L) white cell counts. In the absence of these risk

factors, much diagnostic information can be obtained by a period of close observation, looking for progression of or appearance of a rash, the development or persistence of fever or any deterioration in general condition. It is important to periodically re-examine the skin closely to detect any new changes early.

3. What should be the immediate diagnostic and therapeutic steps?

3. Appropriate diagnostic procedures in this child would include a full blood count, blood cultures, throat swab for bacterial culture, culture of skin lesions for meningococcus, a lumbar puncture if there was any suspicion of meningitis and blood PCR for meningococcus if available. This latter test can be particularly valuable when antibiotics have been given prior to blood cultures being obtained.

- In this child, a full blood count showed an elevated white cell count of 15.1×10^9/L, with 13.3×10^9/L neutrophils. A Gram stain of the serosanguineous fluid expressed from one of the purpuric skin lesions showed Gram-negative diplococci. Lumbar puncture was not performed. She responded rapidly to intravenous penicillin G. Blood and throat swab cultures were negative, but blood PCR for *N. meningitidis* was positive.

4. Is there a rapid diagnostic procedure available?

4. Gram staining of films obtained from petechial lesions is an extremely useful diagnostic aid, with a sensitivity of up to 80%. It can be performed by pricking one of the purpuric spots and squeezing some fluid from the spot onto a slide for staining.

- Intravenous or intramuscular antibiotic should be given as soon as possible in suspected meningococcal disease. Diagnostic procedures (including lumbar punctures) should not delay giving antibiotics by any longer than 15–20 minutes. Children with meningococcal infection require close monitoring, generally in an intensive care setting, as they can deteriorate rapidly due to toxaemia and cardiomyopathy.

A final diagnosis of meningococcal infection was made.

THE ILL-LOOKING CHILD
Tina Sajjanhar

The ill-looking child may present with compromise of the respiratory, circulatory or neurological system, or a combination of these.

Initial management of the child must include a rapid early assessment and stabilization of the child's condition prior to progressing to full history and examination.

An understanding of the physiology relating to the response to serious illness can help with the early assessment and subsequent management.

Respiratory system

Airway

The function of the airway is:

- To conduct air to the alveoli for gas exchange.
- To warm and humidify the air.
- To filter harmful substances.

Obstruction of the upper airway by swelling or foreign body may result in stridor.

Stridor may be:

- *Inspiratory*. Obstruction at or above the vocal cords or in cervical trachea, caused by collapse of the pharyngeal tissue in an already narrowed airway, due to negative inspiratory pressure.
- *Expiratory*. Obstruction in the intrathoracic trachea, due to reduction of the airway diameter in expiration.
- *Biphasic*:
  - Obstruction in the subglottic area; there is less collapse here as the cricoid cartilage forms a complete ring.
  - Tracheal obstruction if severe, although there may be a predominantly prolonged inspiratory or expiratory phase depending on the site.

Obstruction above the level of the vocal cords produces pharyngeal symptoms with difficulty swallowing, but below this there are no swallowing problems, although the voice may be hoarse and a barking cough can occur.

Lower respiratory tract

The function of the respiratory system is

- *Oxygenation.* Ventilation–perfusion mismatch is the most common cause of hypoxia; it occurs in asthma or atelectasis.
- *Regulation of carbon dioxide in the blood and consequently maintenance of pH.* The partial pressure of carbon dioxide ($PaCO_2$) in the blood is derived by the formula:

$$PaCO_2 = VCO_2 / Va \times K$$

where VCO_2 is CO_2 production, Va is alveolar ventilation and K is a constant. Therefore if Va is halved, e.g. by low tidal volume or low respiratory rate, $PaCO_2$ is doubled. Hypoventilation due to any cause, e.g. respiratory muscle fatigue or suppression of respiratory drive, leads to hypercarbia.

Problems anywhere in the respiratory tract can interfere with final gas exchange, and result in hypoxia ± hypercarbia and acidosis; this expresses itself in symptoms of respiratory distress.

Cardiovascular system

The major function of the cardiovascular system is to deliver oxygen to cells.

- Maintenance of perfusion, i.e. blood pressure, is dependent on cardiac output (CO) and systemic vascular resistance (SVR). Cardiac output is defined by the following formula:

$$CO = stroke\ volume\ (SV) \times heart\ rate\ (HR)$$

Cardiac output can only be measured directly by invasive techniques, so is assumed to be adequate if heart rate and blood pressure are adequate.

- Shock occurs when cardiac output is inadequate to meet the body's oxygen needs. Tissue perfusion is inadequate in these circumstances and at the cellular level anaerobic respiration occurs, leading to lactic acidosis, cell dysfunction, and subsequently to cell damage and death.

Shock is a progressive pathophysiological state.

- *Compensated shock.* In the early phases there is increased sympathetic discharge with vasoconstriction, increased heart rate and increased contractility, to maintain BP and cardiac output. Hence early signs of tachycardia and evidence of peripheral vasoconstriction (pallor, cool peripheries, increased capillary refill time) occur. The patient should be carefully evaluated as signs may be few.
- *Decompensated shock.* As shock progresses, the intrinsic compensatory mechanisms fail and circulatory impairment is established. There is decreased myocardial perfusion and increased myocardial oxygen consumption. Cardiac output and blood pressure fall, leading to tissue ischaemia and reduced cell function.

Hypotension is a late sign and signals the loss of at least 25% of intravascular volume.

- *Irreversible shock.* Ongoing shock leads to cell death and damage to key organs, resulting in multi-organ failure.

Neurological dysfunction

Coma results from a reduction in neuronal function, following disruption of cortical or brainstem integrity.

Clinical dysfunction results in an altered state of consciousness combined with a reduced capacity for arousal.

There are distinct gradations, from a state of total alertness to total unresponsiveness, divided into four categories: lethargy, obtundation, stupor and coma (Plum and Posner 1980. Diagnosis of stupor and coma III. Davis, Philadelphia).

- *Lethargy.* State of minimally reduced wakefulness in which the primary defect is that of attention. Drowsiness is prominent, and may include delirium. The patient can communicate verbally.
- *Obtundation.* Mild–moderate blunting of alertness with a reduced response to the environment. Communication is partly preserved.
- *Stupor.* Deep sleep from which the patient can be temporarily roused with vigorous stimulation, and communication is significantly impaired.
- *Coma.* Unrousable unresponsiveness, no movement, no speech and closed eyes. The patient may respond to pain, but not localize.

In any impaired neurological state, maintenance of blood to the brain is vital to provide oxygen and glucose for maintenance of cerebral homeostasis.

Within 10 seconds of the brain being starved of oxygen, unconsciousness ensues, and within 4–6 minutes irreversible brainstem damage develops. In brain injury oxygen is even more important to sustain cells and minimize injury.

For this reason, the focus for resuscitation needs to be on the airway, respiratory and circulatory systems to maximize oxygenation and delivery of blood supply, and takes precedence over specific therapy for the neurological disorder.

Primary brain injury occurs due to the initial insult, whether this is trauma or overwhelming infection. This may be treatable and reversible if not too severe, although cell death usually occurs.

Secondary injury is, however, usually preventable and is due to secondary events such as hypoxia and hypotension. Lack of appropriate therapy adds to the primary brain injury.

Brain response to injury

Responses depend on the extent of the primary and the secondary injury and what effect this has had, as well as the location of the injury in the brain.

- There is altered function with an altered level of consciousness: reduced levels of consciousness imply significant brain injury, and formal methods of assessment such as Glasgow Coma Score (GCS) may be used.
- There may be seizures, which if prolonged can lead to further brain injury as metabolic needs of the brain increase, and there may be hypoxia.
- Transient hypoventilation and apnoea are the most common forms of altered respiratory function in children often after seizures and head injury, and need to be treated aggressively.
- There is loss of autoregulation of cerebral blood flow. Oxygen delivery therefore becomes dependent on cerebral perfusion pressure, which may be defined by the formula:

$$CPP = MAP - ICP$$

where CPP = cerebral perfusion pressure, MAP = mean arterial pressure, ICP = intracranial pressure. Normal ICP is about 10 mmHg.

To protect cerebral blood flow, there must be:

- Adequate respiratory function.
- Adequate cardiovascular function.
- Adequate CPP: it is unclear what the normal CPP in a child is, although it is about 50 mmHg in adults; however, as children have a lower MAP, CPP is presumably lower.

If MAP pressure drops then CPP drops, and maintenance of BP takes priority.

Cerebral blood flow (CBF) (see Fig. 36.1)

Cerebral blood flow usually remains constant over a wide range of blood pressure but this autoregulation is lost after brain injury. After brain injury too little CBF causes cerebral ischaemia and too much leads to cerebral oedema and raised ICP:

- As mean arterial flow falls below 60 mmHg, CBF falls.
- As pO_2 falls below 60 mmHg, vasodilatation occurs leading to increased CBF and raised ICP as well as continued hypoxia.
- As pCO_2 rises, usually due to hypoventilation, acidosis develops, with vasodilatation and increased CBF.
- However, therapeutically reducing the pCO_2 leads to vasoconstriction and reduces CBF very effectively within seconds.

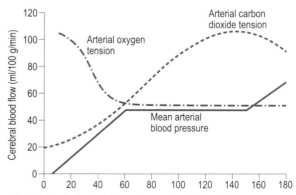

Fig 36.1 Relationship of cerebral blood flow to mean arterial blood pressure, arterial oxygen tension (pO_2) and arterial carbon dioxide tension (pCO_2). (From: Practical Paediatrics, 4th edn. Edited by Robinson, MJ and Roberton, DM. Churchill Livingstone, Edinburgh)

Initial assessment of the ill child

Airway

The following steps should be followed in the management of the airway:

- Position the airway.
- Clear the airway of any obstructions, e.g. secretions, which may require use of suction.
- If the airway is not maintained with position alone then an airway adjunct may be useful:
  - Presence of a gag reflex may cause the child to reject the airway, but the absence of a gag reflex indicates reduced neurological function, and this child may require airway support.
  - An unconscious child or one with a fluctuating conscious level is at risk of losing control of their airway and airway support should be considered in these cases.

Breathing

Look for evidence of respiratory distress:

- Stridor indicates an upper airway problem.
- Measure respiratory rate: as a child becomes exhausted the respiratory rate may fall.
- Heart rate increases due to increased work of breathing.
- Look for the presence of recession, use of accessory muscles, nasal flaring and grunting.
- Listen for wheeze.
- Look at chest expansion.
- Listen for air entry and the presence of crackles, bronchial breathing and reduced air entry in the presence of consolidation or a pleural effusion.
- Look for cyanosis and measure oxygen saturations by pulse oximetry.
- Evaluate the efficacy of end-organ perfusion, especially blood supply to the brain as evidenced by agitation or drowsiness.

Circulation

Circulatory insufficiency is indicated by the following:

- Increased heart rate.

- Reduced pulse volume.
- Prolonged capillary refill time.
- Reduced peripheral temperature.
- Core peripheral temperature gap of more than 2°C.
- Mottled pale skin colour.
- Raised respiratory rate.
- Poor end-organ perfusion.

Peripheral vasoconstriction occurs as a thermoregulatory response to fever, and this needs to be distinguished from shock.

Disability

An assessment of the child's conscious level is essential.

A quick assessment – the AVPU scale (see below) – can be used, although the more detailed GCS should be used for ongoing assessment (Table 36.1).

Pupils should be assessed for size and reactivity, and the child's posture noted.

A	Alert
V	Responds to voice
P	Responds to pain
U	Unresponsive

In addition to the above, a blood glucose measurement should be made as part of the initial assessment.

During the course of this assessment, acute treatment should be given where considered appropriate. This includes:

- Delivery of oxygen by face mask, or assisted ventilation if appropriate.
- Fluid may be required in cases of circulatory insufficiency.
- Glucose in cases of hypoglycaemia.

At this stage further history should be sought and a comprehensive examination carried out.

History

- Length of illness.
- Speed of onset.

Table 36.1 Glasgow Coma Score and Modified Glasgow Coma Score

Glasgow Coma Scale (adults and children > 4 years)

Eyes open:	Score
Spontaneously	4
To speech	3
To pain	2
Never	1

Best motor response:	
Obeys commands	6
Localizes pain	5
Flexion withdrawal	4
Decerebrate flexion	3
Decerebrate extension	2
No response	1

Best verbal response:	
Orientated	5
Confused	4
Inappropriate words	3
Incomprehensible sounds	2
Silent	1

Modification of Glasgow Coma Scale for children < 4

Best verbal response:	Score:
Appropriate words or social smiles, fixes on and follows objects	5
Cries, but is consolable	4
Persistent irritable	3
Restless, agitated	2
Silent	1

Eyes open:	As per adult scale
Motor response:	As per adult scale

- Preceding symptoms; for example:
  - URTI.
  - Trauma.
  - Prodrome to infectious disease.
  - Polyuria, polydipsia.

- Associated symptoms:
  - Cough.
  - Vomiting.
  - Fever.
  - Rash.
  - Anorexia.
  - Abdominal pain: may be referred from chest or be presentation of diabetic ketoacidosis.
- Exposure to herpetic infections; evidence of acute herpetic infections.
- Presence of fluctuating conscious level.
- Drug history:
  - Has the child been given aspirin?
  - Are there any drugs in the house, e.g. antidepressants, methadone?
  - Is the child on any medication, e.g. insulin?
- Immunization history: particularly HiB and Men C vaccines.
- Any known conditions, e.g. diabetes, history of previous collapse/coma, known neurological disease?
- History of foreign travel, particularly areas endemic for malaria; history of prophylaxis/appropriate precautions.
- Family history of epilepsy, diabetes, metabolic disease.

Examination

A detailed examination should be performed with the intention of picking up physical signs to allow a differential diagnosis to be made. Treatment of specific problems may need to be dealt with as they are found.

General examination

- *Pulse.* Pulse of greater than 220 may indicate supraventricular tachycardia.
- Examination of skin may reveal:
  - *Purpuric rash.* Suspect meningococcal sepsis, but may also occur in pneumococcal sepsis.
  - *Vesicular rash.* Suspect herpetic infection, also in chicken-pox.
  - *Maculopapular rash.* Non-specific, many infections including viral
  - jaundice, also apparent within sclera.
  - Presence of insect bites.

Fever may indicate:
- Infective cause.
- Hyperpyrexia associated with drug ingestion, e.g. Ecstasy.

Respiratory examination

- Look for evidence of respiratory distress which may point to the diagnosis.
- Respiratory pattern:
  - Tachypnoea in acidosis.
  - Deep Kussmaul's breathing in diabetic ketoacidosis (DKA).
  - Hyperventilation in aspirin overdose.

Cardiovascular examination

- Blood pressure may indicate a hypertensive state leading to encephalopathy.
- Presence of arrhythmia may indicate drug ingestion or be part of congenital heart disease.
- Presence of heart failure (gallop rhythm, hepatomegaly, basal crepitations) can occur in cardiomyopathy.

Abdominal examination

- Abdominal tenderness and peritonism in acute abdomen (remember DKA).
- Hepatomegaly.
- Splenomegaly: consider conditions leading to hepatic failure, infectious causes such as malaria and hepatitis, splenic sequestration.
- Ascites.
- Presence of bowel sounds.
- Presence of hernias.
- Examination of scrotum and testes in boys.

Neurological examination

- Evidence of trauma.
- Evidence of raised ICP: hypertension, bradycardia, deteriorating conscious level.
- Neck stiffness, Kernig's sign.

- Trends in GCS useful in monitoring potential deterioration.
- Pupillary size:
  - Small reactive in metabolic disease.
  - Constricted pupils in opiate overdose.
  - Dilated pupils with raised ICP: unilateral if lesion is one sided.
- Tone and reflexes in comatose child can reveal presence of underlying cortical lesion leading to hemiparesis or indicate post-ictal state.

Differential diagnosis of the 'ill-looking' child

- Respiratory:
  - Airway obstruction, e.g. foreign body, croup, epiglottitis, extrinsic compression, e.g. mediastinal mass, anaphylaxis.
  - Severe pneumonia.
  - Acute severe asthma.
  - Pneumothorax.
- Central nervous system:
  - Convulsion.
  - Meningitis.
  - Encephalitis.
  - Cerebral malaria.
  - Head injury.
  - Brain abscess.
  - Intracranial tumour.
- Sepsis; for example:
  - Meningococcal.
  - Pneumococcal.
  - Toxic shock syndrome.
- Metabolic/endocrine:
  - Reye's syndrome.
  - Diabetic ketoacidosis.
  - Hypoglycaemia.
  - Hyponatraemia.
  - Inborn error of metabolism.
  - Adrenocortical insufficiency.
  - Thyrotoxic crisis.
- Abdominal:
  - Acute peritonitis.
  - Acute hepatic failure.
  - Bowel obstruction.
- Poisoning – accidental/non-accidental:
  - Tricyclic antidepressants.
  - Aspirin.

- Non-steroidals.
- Substances of abuse.
- Methadone.
■ Cardiovascular:
- Hypovolaemic states, e.g. secondary to gastro-enteritis, haemorrhage.
- Heart failure.
- Congenital heart disease.
- Cardiomyopathy.
- Arrhythmias.
- Anaphylactic shock.
■ Renal:
- Hypertensive encephalopathy.
- Renal failure, e.g. haemolytic–uraemic syndrome.
■ Haematological/immunological:
- Sickle cell disease: splenic sequestration.
- Immunocompromised state with infection, e.g. HIV infection.

Investigation

The following may be helpful:

■ Full blood count:
- Neutrophilia in acute infection; may also occur post seizure.
- Neutropenia in severe infection, e.g. meningo-coccal sepsis.
- Anaemia indicates haemorrhage, haemolysis or bone marrow suppression in severe infection.
- Thrombocytopenia in sepsis, malaria.
■ Blood film:
- evidence of microangiopathic haemolysis.
■ Sickle screen.
■ Urea, electrolytes, creatinine:
- High creatinine in renal failure.
- High urea in dehydration.
- Low sodium as part of syndrome of inappropriate antidiuretic hormone (SIADH), sodium loss (renal failure, gastroenteritis).
- High potassium and low sodium may indicate adrenocortical insufficiency.
■ Blood sugar:
- May be raised in stress.
- Very high in DKA, with glycosuria and ketonuria.
- Low in severe infection, diabetic hypogly-caemia, inborn error of metabolism, cortisol deficiency.

■ Liver function tests:
- Raised transaminases in hepatic failure with hypoalbuminaemia, conjugated hyperbilirubi-naemia.
- Unconjugated hyperbilirubinaemia in haemoly-tic disease.
■ Ammonia:
- High levels alert to urea cycle defects.
■ Blood for serum amino acids.
■ Urine for organic and amino acids.
- If inborn error of metabolism suspected, should be taken at presentation.
■ Lactate:
- High in inborn error of metabolism but also in sepsis where there is poor perfusion.
■ Arterial blood gas:
- Points to metabolic or respiratory picture.
- Metabolic acidosis in inborn errors of metabo-lism, ingestion of salicylates, non-steroidal anti-inflammatory drugs and tricyclic antide-pressants.
■ Clotting:
- Deranged in sepsis, disseminated intravascular coagulation (DIC) and hepatic dysfunction.
■ Malaria screen.
■ Blood for toxicology screen including paracetamol and salicylate levels.
■ Thyroid function tests.
■ Blood culture.
■ Viral serology: specific viruses dictated by presentation.
■ Urine:
- Microscopy and culture.
- Electrolytes.
- Metabolic screen.
- Toxicology.
- Dipstick for substances of abuse.
■ Abdominal X-ray.
■ Chest X-ray.
■ Lumbar puncture:
- In stable patient with normal GCS and no evidence of raised ICP or clotting abnormalities.
■ CT scan/MRI scan:
- Intracranial lesion including bleeding.
- Raised ICP.
- Encephalitis.
■ EEG:
- Seizure activity.
- Encephalitis.
■ Echocardiogram.

Conclusion

The 'ill-looking child' presents a problem as any system may be involved. Initial assessment should concentrate on the acute management of any life-threatening problems, followed by a comprehensive history and examination, which will direct the clinician towards the appropriate investigations, and differential diagnosis.

Clinical problem

A 12-year-old boy is brought to hospital by his uncle, who speaks very little English. The boy arrived from China 1 week ago and had been unwell for 5 days. On the day of presentation, he was said to have 'collapsed' at home, and wet himself, although there was no history of jerking of his limbs. Since then he had been intermittently drowsy and was carried into the A&E department, semiconscious. There did not appear to be any significant past medical history, and his immunization status is unknown

On examination he was initially afebrile, although later he develops a temperature of 40°C, accompanied by an episode of sweating.

PR 90
RR 18
BP 110/60, capillary refill time 2 seconds
Oxygen saturations 98% in air
Responding to pain, GCS 9–11
No rash
No neck stiffness, Kernig's sign negative
No respiratory signs
No murmurs

Questions

1. What is the next important step in management of this child, and why:
   a) Load with anticonvulsants?
   b) Give i.v. vitamin K and platelets?
   c) Intubate and ventilate?
   d) Transfer immediately to an infectious diseases unit?

2. Two investigations were performed that helped to elucidate the cause of this child's symptoms and signs. What were they?

Examination of abdomen reveals 2 cm non-tender liver, no splenomegaly, or any other masses
Minimal jaundice
Pupils equal and reactive

Results

Hb	9.0	Urea	13.8
White cell count	11.0	Creatinine	89
Platelet count	17	Sodium	129
INR	1.0	Potassium	5.0
Blood gas	pH 7.34	Bilirubin	52
	pCO$_2$ 5.0		
	BE −3		
Blood sugar	5.0	Mildly raised transaminases	
Lactate	3.6	Albumin	24
Fibrinogen	Normal		
Urinalysis	NAD		
Chest/ abdominal X-ray	Normal		

Discussion

This child needs intubating and ventilating as he has evidence of fluctuating conscious level and a lowered GCS, indicative of an encephalopathy of unknown origin. He is at risk of developing raised intracranial pressure, and securing his airway enables him to be dealt with in a controlled fashion. There is no evidence of ongoing seizure activity, although if he did start to fit he would require anticonvulsant therapy. He is not acutely bleeding and does not need blood products at the current time, or vitamin K in the face of a normal INR. He should be stabilized before he is transferred anywhere.

He had a CT scan of his head performed, which ruled out an intracranial lesion and acute raised ICP. A malaria screen was positive for falciparum, consistent with a diagnosis of cerebral malaria.

CHAPTER 37

UNEXPECTED/UNEXPLAINED DEATH AND APPARENT LIFE-THREATENING EVENTS

Tina Sajjanhar

Introduction

- Sudden infant death syndrome (SIDS) may be defined as the 'sudden death of an infant or young child, which is unexpected by history, and in which a thorough post-mortem examination fails to demonstrate an adequate cause for death'.
- SIDS is responsible for the death of approximately seven babies each week in the UK.
- Epidemiological studies show a characteristic age distribution: SIDS is uncommon in the neonatal period, with a sharp rise in the second month of life and a peak around 3–4 months of age, with a gradual decrease in later months. 75% of cases occur in infants between 2 and 4 months of age, 89% are under 6 months of age and 95% under 9 months of age.
- The age distribution is related to gestational age rather than postnatal age.
- There is an increased incidence in the winter months, possibly associated with a higher incidence of respiratory infections.
- Maternal risk factors for SIDS include young age, maternal smoking, low social class, previous history of SIDS and postnatal depression.
- Major infant risk factors for SIDS include low birth weight (less than 1500 g), prematurity (less than 32 weeks) and history of apparent life-threatening events. Additional risk factors include prone sleeping position and overheating.
- Greater public awareness and prevention campaigns have contributed to a reduction in the incidence of SIDS by around 70% since 1991. There have been great attempts to understand the aetiology of SIDS in recent years, but no single cause has been identified; indeed, SIDS is likely to be multifactorial. Great emphasis has been placed particularly on the prone position and maternal smoking as significant preventable risk factors. The 'Back to Sleep' campaign (placing the baby in the supine position to sleep) has been credited with much of the reduction in the incidence of SIDS.

Pathophysiology of SIDS

- There are no post-mortem findings that adequately explain the reason for death in infants with SIDS.
- Review of the evidence shows that respiratory infections may play a significant role.
- Findings support the presence of prolonged hypoxaemia, but it is unclear if this is the result of upper airway obstruction, lower airway obstruction or asphyxic gasping.
- It may be that detailed studies of infants with ALTE will improve our understanding of the pathophysiology of SIDS.

Apparent life threatening episodes (ALTE)

Parents may seek advice over incidents they may feel are alarming and a possible prelude to SIDS. These were termed 'near-miss' cot death, but the term 'apparent life-threatening event' is preferable.

Definition

- An ALTE is an episode that is frightening to the observer and characterized by some combination of:
  - Apnoea.
  - Colour change (pallor or cyanosis).
  - Marked change in muscle tone.
  - Choking or gagging.
- There may be some attempt at vigorous stimulation or resuscitation of the infant.

History

- A good history may help to elicit a possible diagnosis and in deciding how to progress with investigation.
- The history of the event should be taken in some detail, including:
  - Skin colour.
  - Duration.
  - State of consciousness of the infant.
  - Mode of termination (spontaneous/requiring some form of resuscitation).
  - Coughing or choking.
  - Jerking movements.

The history should be expanded to include the following:

- Recent health: there may be a history of coryzal symptoms, fever, cough, vomiting, diarrhoea, abnormal sleepiness.
- Feeding history.
- Is the baby breast- or bottle-fed?
- How much feed does the baby take?
- Has the baby been feeding less than usual?
- Relationship of the event(s) to feeding.
- Cyanosis during feeding.
- Weight gain: has there been adequate weight gain since birth?
- Perinatal history.
- History of prematurity.
- Whether baby admitted to special care baby unit.
- Development.
- Medication.
- Family and social history.
- Any previous SIDS in family or relatives.
- History of consanguinity.
- Any previous ALTE in this or another baby.

Examination should include the following

- General health.
- Height.
- Weight.
- Head circumference.
- All these should be plotted on a growth chart and compared with any previous figures.
- Hydration state.
- Presence of pallor.
- Any signs of infection, including fever, rash.
- Respiratory system including evidence of respiratory distress, stridor, wheeze.
- Cardiovascular examination, listening for any murmurs.
- Any evidence of non-accidental injury (NAI): unexplained bruises, swelling of limbs, joints, retinal haemorrhage.
- Neurodevelopmental assessment, including muscle tone.

Investigation

- The extent of the investigations performed is a matter of clinical judgement, and all or any testing is not mandatory.
- Following history and examination it may be possible to exclude those infants who have a

straightforward reason for their collapse. This may be helped by directed investigation.

■ Where the diagnosis is less clear, further investigation may help.

ECG
CT/MRI brain

Sleep study: may be useful where the cause of the ALTE has not been elicited and is recurrent. Continuous measurements of oxygen saturations and heart rate are recorded, although breathing patterns may also be monitored

---

Possible investigations for ALTE

Blood analysis
Full blood count and film
CRP
Urea and creatinine
Sodium and potassium
pH
Glucose
Calcium
Liver function tests
Amino acids
Ammonia
Lactate
Thyroid function
Toxicology
Immune function

Urinalysis
Amino acids
Organic acids
Ketones
Toxicology
Osmolality
Electrolytes

Microbiology
Lumbar puncture
Urine for microscopy and culture
Blood culture
Stool for culture
Nasopharyngeal aspirate for respiratory syncytial
   virus
Pernasal swab for pertussis

Radiology
Chest X-ray
Upper gastrointestinal contrast study
Head ultrasound scan
Skeletal survey

Other investigations
pH study
Echocardiogram
EEG

Diagnosis

■ Following appropriate investigation, three groups of children may be identified:
  – Those in whom the history suggests a non-life-threatening episode, examination and investigation is normal, and no further action is required.
  – Those in whom a specific medical condition has been discovered sufficient to explain the presenting episode and requiring appropriate therapy.
  – Those in whom the presenting attack appeared significant and life threatening but in whom no clear pathology can be identified. Some of these infants may be incubating viruses such as RSV or pertussis and the nature of the illness may become clear in time. These infants may require further specialist investigations.

■ However, in many infants the cause of the ALTE may be ultimately unknown.

Conditions presenting as ALTE

Infection
Meningitis
Encephalitis
Septicaemia
Urinary tract infection (UTI)

Gastrointestinal
Gastro-oesophageal reflux
Gastroenteritis
Oesophageal dysfunction
Colic
Strangulated hernia

Central nervous system
Seizures

Febrile seizures
Central apnoea syndrome
Bulbar/pseudobulbar palsy
Degenerative conditions
Intracerebral haemorrhage
Spinal muscular atrophy

Respiratory
Pneumonia
Bronchiolitis
Pertussis
Upper respiratory tract infection (URTI)
Aspiration

ENT
Structural anomalies of the upper airway

Endocrine
Hypothyroidism
Hyperthyroidism
Congenital adrenal hyperplasia

Metabolic
Aminoacidurias
Organic acidaemia
Hypoglycaemia
Urea cycle defects
Hypocalcaemia
Hypo/hypernatraemia
Fatty acid oxidation defects

Cardiovascular
Cardiac arrhythmias
Structural congenital anomalies
Conduction anomalies (congenital or acquired)
  including long QT syndrome
Endocardial fibroelastosis
Acute myocarditis

Miscellaneous
Child abuse
Food allergy
Immune deficiency

Infection

Clinical signs include:

- Poor feeding.
- Floppy/lethargic.
- Apnoea.
- Pallor.

- Irritable.
- Vomiting.
- Lack of fever does not exclude infection, especially in younger infants.
- Infant will often still look unwell on presentation. Investigations include:
- *FBC*:
  - WCC may be high with neutrophilia or low in the presence of severe bacterial infection.
  - Hb may drop in severe infection.
  - Platelet count may drop in severe infection.
- *CRP*. May be high in the presence of infection; cannot differentiate bacterial and viral infection; normal CRP less likely to be associated with infection.
- *Biochemistry*. Helps to assess state of hydration (sodium, urea, creatinine).
- *pH*. Degree of acidosis may help with assessment of intravascular volume and severity of illness.
- *Lumbar puncture*. May be delayed if child is unwell or cardiovascular compromise as cerebrospinal fluid may be sent for polymerase chain reaction (PCR), and cell count should still be high if meningitis or encephalitis is present.
- *Urine*. Ideally suprapubic aspiration (SPA), catheter specimen or at the very least a clean catch (bag urine specimens are associated with a high incidence of contamination) for microscopy. Presence of leucocytes and organisms with no epithelial cells is highly suggestive of a UTI in SPA or catheter specimen.
- *Blood culture*. Adequate blood should be taken to obtain a reliable result; only 30–60% of blood cultures are positive in the presence of infection.

Gastro-oesophageal reflux (GOR)

- The temporal association of ALTE with GOR is unclear.
- Occurs due to incompetence of the cardiac sphincter.
- May lead to vagally induced disturbance of pulmonary gas exchange.

Clinical features

- Persistent vomiting.
- Apnoea.
- Excessive crying.
- Blue episodes.

- Failure to thrive in severe cases.
- Evidence of aspiration/unexplained lung collapse.

Investigation

- Diagnosis may be clear on history.
- Upper gastrointestinal contrast study – may not pick up all cases of reflux.
- pH study may only pick up acid reflux.

Apnoea

- Newborn infants continue to refine their respiratory control for several months after birth.
- Preterm infants show a significant tendency to develop both SIDS and ALTE.

Clinical features

- Defined as respiratory pause of 10–20 seconds.
- *Central*. Caused by absent neurological output from respiratory centre.
- *Obstructive*. Caused by closure of airway, usually upper airway.
- *Mixed*. An obstructive episode may induce an inappropriate response of central apnoea.

Investigation

- MRI may be useful to look for congenital brain anomalies that may lead to central apnoea, e.g. absence of corpus callosum.
- Nasopharyngeal aspirate (NPA) for RSV and pernasal swab for pertussis infections. Viral serology is usually unhelpful as the infants are too young to mount a significant IgG response.

Upper airway dysfunction

A number of upper airway anomalies have been recognized in association with ALTEs, including:

- Tracheomalacia.
- Laryngomalacia.
- Bronchomalacia.
- Cleft palate.
- Tracheo-oesophageal fistula.
- Laryngeal cleft.
- Pierre Robin's syndrome.
- Vascular ring.

- Paresis of the muscles of the palate, pharynx or larynx.

All produce symptoms in association with feeds. Some may produce symptoms in between acute episodes, e.g. stridor. If suspected, specialist investigation is warranted:

- Echocardiogram.
- Upper gastrointestinal contrast study.
- Flexible/rigid bronchoscopy by paediatric ENT specialist where possible.

A small group of infants in whom there is no structural anomaly will continue to experience intermittent obstructive apnoea. The management of this group is unclear but where symptoms persist tracheostomy may be indicated.

Inborn errors of metabolism

- Increasingly recognized as cause of SIDS or ALTE.
- Family history of unexplained infant death/ALTE.
- History of period of fasting prior to ALTE – medium-chain acyl-CoA dehydrogenase deficiency (MCAD).
- Fatty acid oxidation defects are most likely to be associated with SIDS; other metabolic conditions may cause some signs of illness in the infant.
- MCAD is the most common metabolic disorder associated with SIDS.
- Presence of metabolic acidosis may lead to clinical suspicion.

Investigation

- Blood gas to look for acidosis.
- Urine for presence of ketones.
- Blood glucose to look for hypoglycaemia.
- The presence of hypoketotic hypoglycaemia should lead to suggestion of fatty acid oxidation defect.
- Essential to send paired urine/blood samples taken at presentation (may be stored and sent later for organic and amino acids – the presence of dicarboxylic aciduria is characteristic of MCAD).
- Ammonia (ornithine transcarbamylase deficiency, glutaric aciduria type 2, carnitine deficiency).
- DNA analysis may be performed for common mutation of MCAD.
- Discussion with metabolic team at tertiary unit may be warranted.

Arrhythmias

- Despite extensive investigation, there is little supporting evidence to suggest a significant role for arrhythmias in the aetiology of SIDS.
- Specific abnormalities such as prolonged QT interval, R on T phenomenon and sick sinus syndrome may be sought on 12-lead ECG or 24-hour tape monitoring if appropriate.
- Some infants may have increased vagal tone, triggered by events such as reflux, to cause bradycardia.

Non-accidental injury

- Some infants who present with SIDS or ALTE may have been subject to child abuse.
- Every baby must be carefully examined for any evidence of NAI.
- In the presence of any suspicious features, the appropriate child protection procedures must be followed.

Key points in diagnosis

A complete history is essential

Decide if the child has had an ALTE

Admit the child for observation and further investigation

If the child is ill, perform a full septic screen

If the child shows evidence of respiratory disease, observe for further symptoms and perform the appropriate investigations

In a child with no obvious signs of illness, or where a septic screen is negative, and symptoms continue, the following should be performed:

- Metabolic screen including blood gas, ECG and cranial ultrasound scan

Secondary investigations include:

- EEG
- Echocardiogram
- pH study
- Upper GI contrast study

Third-line investigations include:

- MRI scan of head
- Sleep studies
- Referral to tertiary unit

Monitoring

Despite full investigation, a significant number of children will remain undiagnosed. The parents of these children are naturally very anxious and keen to obtain a respiratory or apnoea monitor for use at home. The ability of apnoea alarms to prevent cot death is unproven; generally the use of home alarms is medically indicated only in infants with a severe ALTE, i.e. one which received vigorous stimulation or resuscitation. However, in some cases, they may reduce parental anxiety.

The following points need to be considered during the use of an apnoea alarm:

- Most monitors detect respiratory movement alone and will therefore not detect obstructive episodes until the child's respiratory efforts stop.
- Many monitors show a high rate of false alarms, and also fail to alarm early enough in a number of ALTEs. This may be related to the fact that prolonged apnoeic or bradycardic episodes are not early features of sudden death in infants.
- The parent must understand the use and benefits of the monitor and be able to troubleshoot minor problems, or have access to appropriate information.
- Parents should be advised, if the alarm sounds, to check the baby is breathing first, since most alarms will be false. Parents must be trained in basic life support to be able to attempt resuscitation of a baby that is not breathing.

Post-mortem investigation of apparent SIDS

Where a child is brought to hospital having died suddenly at home, it may be worthwhile to perform some investigations to elicit cause of death, particularly to look for the presence of infection or metabolic disease. Some samples can be taken by hospital staff, although it may be difficult where the child has been dead for a significant length of time. Other samples and investigations can be performed at post-mortem; local policy may vary.

A thorough physical examination should be performed and documented, and discussion with the parents should take place.

Post-mortem examination should be carried out by a trained paediatric pathologist wherever possible.

Post-mortem investigations of SIDS

Blood tests
Full blood count
Urea and electrolytes
Liver function tests
Ammonia
Amino acids
Blood culture
Blood spots for DNA analysis

Urinalysis
Organic acids
Culture

Liver biopsy

Skin biopsy
Fibroblast culture for enzyme studies

Skeletal survey

Lumbar puncture
Bacterial and viral cultures

Swabs
Viral culture

Clinical problem

A 3-month-old boy was brought to the emergency department having apparently stopped breathing for approximately 15 seconds at home. His mother said that she had fed him half an hour prior to the event and was holding him when the episode occurred. He appeared to shudder and stop breathing, although she did not think he had changed colour. She blew into his face and gently shook him and he seemed to recover and behave normally after that. He had been well in the preceding 24 hours and fed normally. His 16-month-old sister has a cold but his parents are well. There is no relevant PMH, no previous episodes and no history of vomiting or 'colic'. There is no relevant family history.

While in the emergency department he had a further two episodes, half an hour apart. With the second episode the nurse thought he looked blue and applied oxygen by bag and mask for two breaths, at which point he picked up and cried. On examination he is pink, well perfused, but with slightly reduced tone, although he appears alert. He is afebrile, pulse rate 140, respiratory rate 60, capillary refill time 2 seconds. Anterior fontanelle is soft. He has no murmurs and his chest sounds clear. All pulses are present. His mother tries to feed him but he is not interested.

Questions

1. Of the following investigations, which three may be most useful in this child's management?
   a) Cranial ultrasound.
   b) EEG.
   c) Echocardiogram.
   d) Lumbar puncture.
   e) Nasopharyngeal aspirate for RSV.
   f) Pertussis swab.

2. What is the most likely diagnosis?
   a) RSV infection.
   b) Febrile convulsion.
   c) Meningitis.
   d) Whooping cough.
   e) Upper respiratory tract infection.

Answers

1. d, e, f. This child has had significant apnoeas, necessitating active intervention. Infection should come high on the list of differential diagnoses and would be easy to exclude by performing a full septic screen, despite the fact the child does not appear very ill. There are no cardiovascular signs, and, the story is not typical of seizure activity. Clinical signs of bronchiolitis or whooping cough may be delayed and it is important to send the appropriate swabs early in the illness. In illnesses where bronchiolitis is obvious, i.e. classical signs on examination, sending an NPA for confirmation is not mandatory.

2. a. Apnoeas are a common presentation of bronchiolitis, and as this child's sibling has a respiratory infection this child is likely to have contracted his illness from her. In this child, symptoms more typical of bronchiolitis appeared by the next day and the child became oxygen dependent, requiring nasogastric feeding for a short while. The NPA came back positive for RSV infection.

CHAPTER 38

ACCIDENTAL AND NON-ACCIDENTAL INJURIES

Elaine Carter

Introduction

Injuries due to genuine accidents

Accidents are the commonest cause of death in children over the age of 1 year. The incidence of accidental death has fallen over the last 50 years, but the relative importance has increased because of the decline in deaths from other causes such as infection.

Accidents are the commonest reason for children to attend the emergency department (about one in every five of the child population every year), but most are minor injuries.

Most accidents occur while out in a public place, followed by in the home. Only about 2% of accidents occur at school or during sporting activities. Only 2% occur on the road, but these cause the greatest morbidity and mortality. Accidents occur at the same rate at all ages, except they are less common under the age of 1 year. Boys have more accidents than girls and are far more likely to be involved in road traffic accidents. Twice as many accidents occur in summer as in winter.

The vast majority of accidents are soft-tissue injuries, the commonest being a sprain to the arm or leg. Fractures are less common. The head is often injured, but the skull is involved in only 1% of head injuries, which emphasizes the infrequency of serious trauma.

Many accidents are preventable. The main methods of accident prevention that have been employed are education of the public and environmental change. Efforts to prevent accidents by education, such as the UK Green Cross Code, have been shown to be minimally effective: they improve knowledge but do not change behaviour. However, changing the environment to reduce risk has been shown to be very effective in reducing accidents. Examples include child-resistant containers for drugs, legislation to make the wearing of seat belts compulsory, traffic-calming measures to lower vehicle speeds, teaching children to swim, pool fence legislation and ensuring supervision at swimming pools.

Injuries due to abuse

Injuries caused by abuse show some similarities in terms of their epidemiology. The importance of this problem has certainly grown in recent years as the extent of the problem has been recognized. Similarly, certain environmental factors increase the risk of particular children suffering abuse. For example, the socially isolated family under pressure financially with one or more young demanding children is known to represent a high-risk situation. Various strategies have been adopted to prospectively identify such families and offer support. Physical abuse, in which the child suffers injury, must always be differentiated from accidental injury. However, abuse is normally considered in five categories (see below) and children frequently present with more than one type of abuse. As a result, abused children may present with a combination of unexplained injuries and or symptoms. The five categories of child abuse are as follows.

Physical

The child may present with either soft-tissue or bony injury. Soft-tissue injuries include:

- Bruises, which may appear as fingertip marks, hand or grip marks and/or pinch marks.
- Bites or marks in the shape of an implement such as a belt or stick.
- Oral injuries from objects, such as a feeding bottle, forced into the mouth.
- Scalds and burns.

Some bony injuries are known to be commonly produced as a result of abuse. These include:

- Spiral or oblique fractures of the long bones.
- Subperiosteal bone formation.
- Multiple fractures of different ages.
- Rib fractures.
- Metaphyseal fractures.
- Skull fractures that involve the occiput, or which are multiple, branching or wide in nature.

As well as the type of injury, it is also important to consider the age of the child. For example, a young, immobile baby aged <9 months is unlikely to have accidental bruises on the face, while bruises on the forehead are commonly acquired accidentally around 18 months when the child is learning to walk.

Sexual

Up to 20% of adults claim they were sexually abused in some way as a child. The perpetrator is more often male, but can be female, and is usually known to the child. A child of any age and of either sex can be affected. The commonest form of presentation is an allegation made by a child. This must always be taken seriously.

Emotional

This is difficult to diagnose as there are no specific features, but clinicians should be alert to indicators of emotional abuse such as underachievement, substance abuse, overdose, hostile behaviour and self-harm.

Neglect

Neglect occurs when a child is not adequately cared for but can actually take many forms. For example, the child may not be provided with enough food, adequate clothes or warmth. Medical conditions may be neglected or school attendance may be poor. It is not always a parent's deliberate intent to neglect their child, and often the parents are doing their best under difficult circumstances, but are unable to cope with the needs of the child owing to external factors such as poverty or lack of education. It is important to recognize this, so that the family receives the help it requires rather than punitive intervention.

Factitious illness by proxy

This is a rare form of abuse, usually resulting in physical harm, and is defined as the creation of a false impression of illness in a healthy child, by a parent or carer. Repetitive medical examinations are sought which are in themselves abusive, as they are unnecessary. The parent refuses to be reassured and may go 'doctor shopping'. This type of abuse is most often carried out by the mother, who often has some medical knowledge. Examples include apnoea induced by smothering, recurrent drowsiness induced by drugs, falsifying evidence of a fever by warming the thermometer or inducing diarrhoea by laxative administration.

History

Accidental injury/harm

Typically in this situation there is a vivid account and this information should be documented. It is helpful to know how the accident happened. For example, in a road traffic accident:

- Was the child a passenger or a pedestrian?
- Was the child in the front seat or the back?
- Was the child wearing a seat belt?
- Were there fatalities during the accident?
- How fast were the cars travelling?
- How soon were paramedics at the scene of the accident?
- What resuscitation was given at the scene?
- Was there any loss of consciousness?
- What was the estimate of blood loss, if any?

In drowning:

- What was the length of time of immersion?
- What treatment was given at the scene?
- Was the water salt or fresh?

In relation to ingestion:

- What was taken? (The empty bottles are often useful in clarifying this.)
- How much was taken and how long ago?

In a fall injury:

- How far did the child fall and onto what type of surface?
- Was there a head injury and, if so, was there loss of consciousness?

These questions help provide a rapid picture both of what has happened to the child, what type of problems are likely to be encountered and what measures should be set in motion at an early stage. On some occasions incongruity between the story and the findings may raise the possibility that the incident was not accidental. It is important not to forget the child's past medical history and any medication the child is taking, so that ongoing care of other problems may be continued.

Non-accidental injury

The child usually presents with injuries for which there is no clear history. Alternatively, there is only a vague account or an accident is postulated that was not witnessed. The injuries may not fit the explanation given and the account of what has happened may change when repeated. There may have been a delay in seeking medical help. It is important to note the parents' affect during history taking: whether they are defensive, aggressive or inappropriately unconcerned. Parents may want to take the child home despite significant injuries. All these aspects should be carefully recorded.

The child may tell you what actually happened and their description must also be recorded. However, it is not advisable to subject the child to detailed questioning.

Enquires should be made about emotional indicators of abuse, such as school attendance and performance, soiling, bed-wetting and behavioural problems. All these problems occur in non-abused children but there is an increased incidence in abused children.

Family history is important, particularly who lives in the house with the child and who looks after the child besides the carers.

Examination

Serious injury of any cause

The first priority is resuscitation. Always call for extra help and ensure the child is safe before commencing resuscitation. The method follows the rules of 'ABCD'.

Primary survey and resuscitation

The respiratory, circulatory and central nervous systems are checked in a systematic manner, and any abnormality is treated as it is found before proceeding to the next part of the examination.

A: airway

Check the airway is patent and stabilize the cervical spine. Ensure the head is held manually in line until a hard collar is applied and sandbags and strapping to a hard board has been undertaken. Ensure the airway and spine are secure before proceeding to B.

B: breathing

Look, listen and feel for breathing, and if no breathing after 10 seconds commence artificial ventilation with a bag and mask and 100% oxygen. If there is spontaneous breathing, give oxygen by a high-flow mask and check the breathing is adequate by noting the following:

- Are there signs of respiratory distress, such as tachypnoea, recession, use of accessory muscles, flaring of nostrils, grunting?
- Is respiration adequate? Is there good chest expansion, is there good air entry, and is the child pink or blue?
- Are there differences in each side which may suggest a pneumothorax or haemothorax?

Any abnormality found with respiration must be treated before proceeding to C.

C: circulation

Feel the pulse. If absent after 10 seconds (or <60 bpm in an infant) commence external cardiac massage (ECM). If a pulse is present assess the adequacy of the circulation:

- Examine the peripheries: is the colour pink, blue, pale, mottled? Are the peripheries warm or cold? What is the capillary refill time? >2 seconds is too long.
- Measure the blood pressure, although hypotension is a late sign of shock.
- Measure the pulse rate and volume. If there are signs of shock, insert two wide cannulae and give rapid intravenous fluid, until the circulation is stable.

Then proceed to D.

D: disability

Check the central nervous system. Is the patient conscious? Use the AVPU score to describe their conscious level:

- A for 'Alert'.
- V for 'responds to Voice'.
- P for 'responds to Pain'.
- U for 'Unresponsive'.

Check also the pupil reactions and size, and the child's posture. Look for evidence of any focal neurological signs.

E: expose

Look all over for other areas of serious injury, such as a deformed femur which may indicate a fracture, and splint it to reduce blood loss.

If at any time there is deterioration, stop, return to 'A for airway' and repeat all of the resuscitation procedure.

After resuscitation, do the *secondary survey*. This means examining every part of the child from top to bottom, back and front. To examine the back and spine the child needs to be log rolled; the last part to be examined is the neck, while the collar is briefly removed.

Abusive injuries

A full physical and developmental examination is required: children who have been abused are more likely to have inadequately treated medical illnesses and are more likely to have developmental delay. Weigh the child and plot the value on the appropriate chart: abused children are at greater risk of failure to thrive. As part of the general examination observe and record what the child is wearing, i.e. is it clean clothing which is suitably warm for the weather? Note also the affect of the child: is he/she scared, quiet, watchful?

Bruises

Note bruises carefully and describe the shape, colour and distribution. These observations may help to determine how and when the bruising occurred and the likelihood of their being caused accidentally (the ear, buttocks and upper arms are common sites for abusive injuries). It is helpful to draw an accurate diagram or use a body map to record this information.

Burns

Again the site and nature of any burns can be helpful in suggesting whether they occurred accidentally. For example, small round burns with a depressed centre and rolled edges could be cigarette burns (these may be multiple); burns on the back of hand are suspicious, as a child who has reached for a hot object would normally burn themselves accidentally on the palm of the hand.

Scalds

Non-accidental scalds occur by the purposeful immersion of the child or part of the body in hot water. In this situation there is usually a clean cut-off along the line of the immersion, while in an accidental scald the edge is usually irregular and accompanied by splash marks. Accidental burns occur to the front of the child, and so burns that occur on the back should be considered suspicious.

Fractures

Any fractures should be carefully recorded and considered in relation to the explanation offered. Similarly, note if the fracture type is 'typical' of non-accidental injury, e.g. spiral fracture of a long bone. If multiple fractures are present consider whether they are different ages (and hence unlikely to be accidental).

Injuries to the mouth

These injuries will not be seen unless the mouth is specifically examined. Such injuries include:

- A torn frenulum, which may result from a blow to the mouth, or forced feeding.
- Burns from feeding with food that is too hot.

Subdural bleed

A shaking injury with or without a skull fracture causes the dura to shear away from the skull, causing tearing of the small vessels that cross the dural space, resulting in subdural haemorrhage. Children injured in this way may present acutely with reduced conscious level, enlarged pupils, fits and focal neurology, or more chronically in an otherwise well child with a rapidly expanding head circumference.

Sexual abuse

Where there is concern that the child has been subjected to sexual abuse the genitalia should be examined. However, this should only take place when a senior paediatrician and a police surgeon can see the child together, so that repeated examination is avoided and forensic material can be gathered.

Sexual abuse is difficult to diagnose on examination, because of the wide variation in normal appearances and 30% of sexually abused cases have no physical signs. There are some indicators of sexual abuse:

- The normal width of the hymenal opening should be <1.5 cm.
- Deep injuries involving the hymen are more likely to be abusive.
- Similarly central injuries to the genitalia are more likely to be abusive than lateral injuries, which can occur with accidental straddle injuries.
- The presence of some form of sexually transmitted disease provides unequivocal evidence.

Factitious illness by proxy (FIP)

FIP has a wide range of presentation, and examination depends on the illness fabricated.

Investigation

Serious accident

Test	Rationale
Blood tests: full blood count, urea and electrolytes, blood sugar and cross-match	These provide base line information although they may be useful in pointing to some early derangement. The need for cross match can be judged on an individual basis.
X rays	
Skull, cervical spine, chest and pelvis	These represent a 'minimum screen' after severe trauma
CT head scan	Essential if the child is unconscious
Abdominal X-ray and ultrasound	Should be performed if abdominal trauma is suspected
Bony X-rays	X-ray each individual suspected fracture

Non-accidental injury

In this situation, where the actual nature of the problem can show great variation, investigations must be tailored to the individual situation.

Situation	Test to be considered
Bruises	Full blood count, clotting screen and a skeletal survey in children under 2 years
Fracture(s)	X-ray of any suspected fracture, and skeletal survey if the child is under 2 years
Failure to thrive	Perform a basic screen to exclude malabsorption plus a full dietary assessment including, where appropriate, a brief admission to see if weight gain improves in hospital
Sexual abuse	Swabs for sexually transmitted diseases and forensic tests where appropriate (can only be performed by specifically trained individuals)
Factitious illness by proxy	Investigation in this situation has to be individualized, e.g. toxicology in suspected poisoning, serum and urine sodium in suspected salt poisoning. Admission and close observation as an inpatient may be needed

Clinical problem

A 6-month-old boy is admitted urgently with a 12-hour history of drowsiness, irritability, poor feeding and vomiting. He had been previously well. There is no fever and no history of trauma at the time of admission. He had an uneventful birth history. He is the first child of well parents and there is no family history of illnesses.

On examination he is drowsy, but responds to pain, cries irritably when disturbed and occasionally opens his eyes on stimulation. Estimated Glasgow Coma Score is 12. He is apyrexial but pale. He has a bulging fontanelle but no focal neurological signs.

Examination of heart, respiratory system and abdomen is unremarkable. There is a row of four small circular bruises vertically down his back.

Questions

1. What is your immediate management?

2. What immediate tests would you perform?

3. What are the two most likely diagnoses?

4. Would you do a lumbar puncture? Explain your answer.

Answers

1. The priority with this child is to stabilize his condition and therefore the initial priority is resuscitation using the ABCD approach.

2. The immediate tests need to provide baseline information and hence full blood count, urea and electrolytes, blood sugar, blood gas, blood culture and clotting screen are all indicated. His altered consciousness also mandates a CT brain scan.

3. Intracranial haemorrhage and meningitis. Meningitis is less likely because the child is afebrile.

4. Avoid lumbar puncture in this situation (i.e. reduced conscious level of unknown aetiology) as it can be hazardous. The change in pressure produced by the lumbar puncture may cause the child to cone. Lumbar puncture should be delayed until the scan results are available.

The patient's haemoglobin was 5 g/dL; his white blood cell count, platelets and clotting were normal. The CT scan showed a subdural haematoma, which was drained neurosurgically. Subsequent investigation showed both old fractures and retinal haemorrhages. A diagnosis of non-accidental injury was made, and the child was referred to the child protection team and notified to the child protection authorities.

CHAPTER 39

SLEEP DISORDERS
Elizabeth Sleight

Introduction

Few parents would say that their child had never had problems with sleeping. Most parents looking after infants and toddlers expect to suffer from chronic sleep disturbance, but when an older child suffers from chronically disordered sleep then the whole family can suffer; patient *and* family functioning is affected.

There is overlap with conditions that can cause sleep problems in the adult population, but certain conditions such as night terrors are a peculiarly paediatric problem.

What sorts of sleep disorders are there?

One way of categorizing childhood sleep disorders is to consider whether the problem is:

- A general medical or psychiatric condition.
- A true primary sleep disorder.
- A drug-induced sleep disorder.

Primary sleep disorders are further divided into dyssomnias and parasomnias.

The following are simplified examples of the different types:

- The child goes to bed and falls asleep without difficulty, but wakes up screaming in pain.
- Once the child is in bed, he/she does not fall asleep quickly and tosses and turns for hours.
- The child falls asleep at appropriate times, but then wakes regularly with nightmares.

The first case may be an example of a medical/psychiatric sleep disorder (e.g. gastro-oesophageal reflux), the second of a patient with a dyssomnia (i.e. difficulty of initiating or maintaining sleep) and the last of a parasomnia (a disruption of normal sleep).

Medical–psychiatric-associated sleep disorders

This term encompasses medical conditions that also may include sleep disturbance as part of the diagnosis, e.g. gastro-oesophageal reflux, nocturnal seizures, severe atopic dermatitis, substance-induced sleep disorders.

Remember that patients with major depressive symptoms suffer from difficulties in either initiating or maintaining sleep, as well as early-morning wakening. Hypersomnia can also be a feature of depression particularly in adolescence. However, disrupted or inadequate sleep can in its own right lead to behavioural, affective and cognitive dysfunction.

For a more complete list of possible differential diagnoses, please see below.

Parasomnias

These are sleep-related events that disrupt essentially normal sleep. The child often will not be tired or sleepy the next day. Examples include sleepwalking, nightmares, night terrors and primary nocturnal enuresis.

For a more complete list of possible differential diagnoses, see below.

Dyssomnias

These occur in individuals who have difficulties initiating and/or maintaining sleep. Thus they suffer from a disturbance in the quantity, quality and timing of sleep. They may also suffer from excessive daytime somnolence.

It is thought that such individuals may have an underlying abnormality in the part of the central nervous system that deals with sleep. Examples are narcolepsy and restless leg syndrome.

For a more complete list of possible differential diagnoses, see below.

Nightmares account for up to a third of reported sleep disturbances and up to 50% of 3- to 6-year-olds report nightmares that disturb the child's and their parents' sleep. Up to a third of children may have had one episode of *sleepwalking* during childhood. *Bedtime resistance* is an increasing problem and is reported as occurring in up to 15% of school children. *Night terrors* are estimated to affect 1–6% of children; onset is usually between 4 and 12 years and resolves during adolescence.

Narcolepsy is uncommon (1–20 per 10 000 children), whereas *obstructive sleep apnoea* is the commonest indication for a sleep laboratory referral in the USA and has been estimated to affect up to 2% of children (see Ch. 1 for details).

Kleine–Levin syndrome is a condition that may manifest with episodes of excessive somnolence, overeating and sexual disinhibition. It is three times more common in boys and often follows a febrile, flu-like illness or injury with associated loss of consciousness in a pre-adolescent child. Attacks may last for hours or weeks and may recur every few weeks or months. Spontaneous resolution is usual by late adolescence/early adulthood.

Pathophysiology

Sleep is divided physiologically into two types: rapid eye movement (REM) and non-REM sleep. REM and non-REM sleep cycle in 90- to 100-minute periods. As children grow older, more sleep is non-REM; the adult pattern is 75% non-REM. Most dreaming occurs in REM sleep; EEG patterns are very similar to an awake record.

Nightmares tend to occur in REM sleep, but usually have no physical correlates. Sometimes on waking from a nightmare there may be slight autonomic arousal.

Non-REM sleep is further divided into four categories; night terrors occur during the transition from stage 3 to 4. This tends to be a light sleep phase that occurs within 60–90 minutes of falling asleep. There will be evidence of autonomic activity, such as flushing and tachypnoea, and the child will appear agitated and inconsolable. Confusional arousal may occur even sooner after falling asleep, but the child tends to waken fully and there is less autonomic arousal than in night terrors.

Patients with narcolepsy have abnormalities of both REM and non-REM sleep.

Periodic limb movements in sleep (PLMS) are more likely to occur in non-REM stages 1 and 2. There are thoughts that this may occur secondary to dopaminergic dysfunction. Many people with PMLS also suffer from restless leg syndrome (RLS). There is an association with attention deficit hyperactivity disorder (ADHD), further strengthening the dopaminergic theory.

Rhythmic movement disorders such as head banging and body rocking tend to occur early after going to bed in stage 1–2 light, non-REM sleep.

Alcohol can affect sleep in several ways; acutely there may be decreased REM sleep and sleep disruption caused by increased stage 3/4 non-REM sleep. With habitual use, alcohol causes initial sedation followed by a pattern of disrupted sleep.

During alcohol withdrawal, there may be an increased amount of REM sleep.

Amphetamines and other stimulant drugs cause generalized sleep disruption along with reduced total sleep time, increased body movements and decreased REM sleep.

In Down's syndrome there may be upper airway hypotonia, which leads to obstructive apnoeas unrelated to obesity or congenital heart disease. Central apnoeas may also be a feature.

ADHD is associated with several sleep problems; hyperactivity per se can mean that it is generally more difficult to establish good sleep routines (called sleep hygiene). Sleep apnoea may also be a prime feature. Periodic limb movements in sleep and restless leg syndrome are also associated.

In Tourette's syndrome, up to 50% of children can have problems especially when tics persist into sleep. There is also a higher rate of enuresis.

Girls with Rett's syndrome have short and fragmented sleep patterns.

In Prader–Willi syndrome the associated obesity leads to obstructive sleep apnoea.

Differential diagnoses

Medical–psychiatric-associated sleep disorders	Parasomnias	Dyssomnias
Nocturnal epilepsies	Sleepwalking	Primary hypersomnia
Down's syndrome	Bruxism (teeth grinding)	Primary (idiopathic) insomnia
ADHD	Nightmares	Sleep-state misperception
Autism (pervasive developmental disorder)	Sleep/night terrors	Psychophysiological insomnia
Tourette's syndrome	Primary nocturnal enuresis	Narcolepsy
Rett's syndrome	Rhythmic movement	Obstructive sleep apnoea
Prader–Willi syndrome	disorders: head banging/	syndrome
Increased upper airway resistance	body rocking	Periodic limb movements in
Menstrual-associated periodic hypersomnia	Confusional arousals	sleep
GORD		Restless leg syndrome
Night time worsening of asthma		Limit-setting sleep disorder
Eczema		(may also be thought to fall
Separation anxiety		into the medical-behavioural
Acute/chronic stress: need to consider		list)
child abuse in this category		Insufficient sleep syndrome
Depression		Circadian sleep disorders
Psychotic disorders		
Substance abuse		
Withdrawal from substances of misuse		
Kleine–Levin syndrome		
Blindness with associated sleep disorder		
Daytime correlates:		
Daytime sleepiness/behavioural	Often no evidence of	Frequently there are associated
consequences dependent on severity of	daytime sleepiness/	daytime behavioural
night-time disturbance	behavioural	problems
	consequences despite	
	intrusion on sleep	

History: points to elucidate

Ideally, a sleep diary/record of events should be requested.

The following aspects of sleep need to be considered as well as taking a full general paediatric, social and developmental history:

- When did the problem begin?
- Is there a history of a relevant physical/psychological disorder in the child?
- Is there a positive family history of sleep disorders or related medical disease?
- What happens at home in the evening; what routines and rituals are there?
- Where does the child sleep: cot in same room as parents/shared room/heated or cold room, etc.?
- What sleeping position does the child adopt?
- Have the family noted any predisposing/perpetuating factors?
- How long does it take for the child to fall asleep?
- How often does the child awake from sleep? How does the child appear/behave during these periods and how easily does the child fall back to sleep?
- Establish total sleep time.
- Any nightmares, night terrors or sleepwalking?
- Time of waking: is the child well rested or tired and needs to take naps in the day?
- What is the impact on all other family members?
- Have the family or child tried any remedies/changes in behaviour?
- Is there any evidence of snoring, loud breathing, pauses in breathing?
- Incontinence: either urinary or faecal?
- Evidence of seizure activity: tongue biting, blood on bedclothes, incontinence.
- Document any deterioration of school performance or loss of skills.
- Take a full drug history including prescription or over-the-counter medications, as well as asking about whether the child could be taking illicit substances or has done so in the past. Include caffeine and herbal preparations in the list.

Examination points

Full physical examination including:

- Weight: indications of obesity or failure to thrive.
- Specific evidence of congenital abnormalities/syndromes such as features of Down's syndrome (see Ch. 13)/Rett's syndrome/Prader–Willi syndrome/Tourette's syndrome/ADHD (see Ch. 40).
- Evidence of seizure disorders: head circumference/general level of academic functioning/evidence of tooth injuries to tongue, mouth.
- Evidence of upper airway obstruction, e.g. mouth breathing/large tonsils/bad breath/neck circumference.
- Clubbing or cyanosis: as evidence of right heart failure.
- Full respiratory examination in children with severe/undertreated asthma.
- Signs of severe eczema.
- Any stigmata of chronic medical illnesses that might cause night-time pain, such as the juvenile arthritides or sickle cell disease.

Investigations

In general, investigations should rarely be needed as the vast majority of diagnoses can be made by discovering significant comorbid features and by taking a full history.

- An EEG is only indicated if there is any suspicion of nocturnal epilepsy.
- Contrast study/pH probe if considering dysmotility/gastro-oesophageal reflux disease.
- Overnight pulse oximetry will help exclude hypoxic episodes; depending on local service provision this can be done as an inpatient or at home.
- An ECG might be indicated if considering the presence of right heart strain in a child with evidence of nocturnal hypoxic episodes.
- An X-ray of the lateral postnasal space would be helpful when deciding whether to refer to ENT colleagues.
- Chromosome/genetics in a child with a previously undiagnosed syndrome.
- Lung function studies in children with severe/undertreated asthma.

Nocturnal epilepsies

There are some features common to both nocturnal epilepsies and parasomnias, namely recurrence during sleep, prominent fear and autonomic disturbances, evidence of autonomism and amnesia of the event.

Features that are more suggestive of complex partial seizures include that the event happens shortly after falling asleep (in stage 1–2 non-REM sleep) and an abnormal inter-ictal EEG.

Benign Rolandic epilepsy

This may initially present with brief nocturnal tonic–clonic seizures waking the child from sleep, although daytime seizures occur. Both are characterized by unilateral paraesthesiae, especially involving the face, with or without unilateral tonic, clonic or tonic–clonic convulsions affecting the face, lips, tongue, pharyngeal and laryngeal muscles, causing speech arrest, dysarrthria and drooling. Somatosensory aura may occur; eliciting this history may be difficult in young children!

The seizures occur between 2 and 12 years of age. There is a strong family history, physical examination is normal and the EEG has characteristic features of centrotemporal spikes and sharp waves. It is important to request a sleep EEG as 30% of children have a normal awake EEG. The seizures usually dramatically respond to carbamazepine, although the prognosis is excellent whether anticonvulsants are prescribed or not. Seizures always cease by 16 years of age.

Rett's syndrome

This condition usually affects girls and is quoted as having an incidence of 1 in 10 000. Most cases are sporadic and are thought to be caused by a mutation of the MECP2 gene on the X chromosome.

Presentation

- *Neonatal*. Placid and inactive with fall off in head growth. The child may reach a 9- to 12-month stage of development, but rarely progresses beyond this and regression may be a feature.

- *Childhood*. Strange finger movements develop and abnormal twisting hand movements become more obvious as purposeful hand use is lost. Muscle tone changes from low to high tone and joint contractures and scoliosis develop. Eye contact is maintained and the affected child is often said to have a lovely smile, and frequently has a pretty face. Stereotypically abnormal movements of the hands (wringing) and face are seen, along with episodes of severe agitation. Feeding difficulties may be profound, along with a disturbed breathing rhythm. Epilepsy may be a feature and is often nocturnal.

Tourette's syndrome

Ninety per cent of children found to have the disorder have a positive family history. It is thought that there is an autosomal dominant inheritance pattern with incomplete penetrance, although there is some thought that perinatal hypoxia may be implicated. The family history may be difficult to obtain, as the features may be barely noticeable in other relatives.

The condition is characterized by multiple tics. These might be facial (blinking, grimacing and nodding) or phonic (throat clearing, coughing, barking, clicking or spitting). Shoulder shrugging is common.

Echolalia (repetition of phrases or mimicking of gestures) and copropraxia (involuntary making of obscene gestures) are less common. Symptoms usually start between 5 and 11 years, and never after 21 years. There are associations with obsessive–compulsive disorders and ADHD. The EEG may be abnormal, showing focal dysrhythmias, which do not coincide with the tics.

Although the child may be able to control the tics for brief periods, he/she eventually has to give into the compulsion and afterwards feels a sensation of relief.

Clinical problem

A 5-year-old boy is referred to the paediatrician because his parents are concerned about his sleeping pattern. He is an only child, physically well, apparently enjoying his new school, and his parents feel that he seems generally happy. His parents are both 22; his mother is at home and his father is in full-time employment but often late home in the evening; the family does not always eat together. The boy usually watches television until his father arrives home at about 8 p.m., when he is made ready to go to bed.

Once ready for bed he becomes irritable, may have tantrums and if left alone in his room will continue to cry. He is often still awake when his parents go to bed at about 10.30 p.m. He does not usually seem sleepy the following day and his irritability has usually resolved.

What advice would you give his parents?

Discussion

This is a common pattern. There is no evidence of organic illness from the history. The parents are young and inexperienced; father's absence in the evening will interfere with a bedtime routine which is not only late in the evening but father's arrival may stimulate the child at a time when a 'settling down' routine is preferable.

Once a history excludes other concerns and family difficulties, advice should include the following:

- Establish a regular and consistent bedtime routine; bath, reading a story.
- Firmness in maintaining a regime.
- Avoid excitement, e.g. television or games after the evening meal.
- Explore ways of father being home earlier to share the routine.
- Ensure adequate lighting and removal of frightening objects from the bedroom.
- Discourage sleeping in parents' bed.
- Some children find favourite toys or blankets in bed particularly comforting.
- Avoid medication to encourage sleep.

CHAPTER 40

BEHAVIOURAL PROBLEMS
Adrian Brooke

Introduction

Behavioural problems represent a wide range of difficulties that span a spectrum of severity from the trivial through to life threatening. Although some children may exhibit well-recognized behavioural phenotypes that constitute explicit diagnoses, many problems are less well defined and may prove difficult to address and achieve positive behavioural and developmental outcomes. The very definition is imprecise as the determining characteristics of many problems rely on their divergence from normal patterns of behaviour; normality itself is a subjective term and may differ between individuals, families, communities and societies. For example, it is possible to see children with hyperactivity at levels consistent with a diagnosis of attention deficit hyperactivity disorder in families where the behaviour was not perceived as being problematic, in the same clinic as children with quite normal levels of attention and motor activity who are perceived to be pathologically hyperkinetic by their parents.

It is important to realize that some children are referred to paediatricians because of well-recognized behavioural difficulties, but that these are in fact secondary consequences of other developmental of cognitive difficulties. An example would be the child referred for school refusal who in fact exhibits this behaviour because of severe developmental coordination difficulties that are most starkly exposed in the academic environment of the school.

In some circumstances the behaviours may belie underlying conditions with well-recognized cause: for example, the pattern of motor restlessness, impulsivity and distractibility seen in attention deficit hyperactivity disorder; or the abnormal language development and lack of social reciprocity, social relatedness and behavioural restrictions present in autistic spectrum disorder; or the eating disorder seen in Prader–Willi syndrome. In other situations the behaviours exhibited only permit a descriptive label to be provided (e.g. oppositional defiant disorder) and causes may be harder to identify and address.

Some conditions may appear trivial to the clinician, for instance toddler tantrums or sleep problems. However, these children are often presented to the paediatrician as a last resort, after prolonged and desperate efforts to manage the conditions by the parents in the primary care setting. It is increasingly recognized that although many conditions are of low severity, they persist for very long periods of time, thereby increasing morbidity. Other behaviours may signify very serious pathologies either within the individual (e.g. abnormal eating behaviours of a child with anorexia nervosa which has a crude mortality rate of approximately 6%) or the family (e.g. sexualized behaviour in a child who is the victim of sexual abuse by the parent/carer).

The epidemiology of behavioural disorders is imprecise. Within healthcare settings more severe behavioural phenotypes will be labelled as psychiatric disorders, whereas within educational and social care settings they are usually referred to as emotional, attentional and behavioural difficulties. National studies suggest that 20–25% of children will at some point in their childhood suffer from a diagnosable behavioural disorder. Of this huge number, about 7% will present to a secondary care setting (often a paediatrician). Less than 2% will require the multidisciplinary or inpatient facilities. These figures consist of various conditions, some of which are relatively common (for example, feeding difficulties in 12–34% of preschool children; enuresis in 8% of 7-year-olds), while others are rarer (major depression 0.5–2.5% of children; 2–4% of adolescents).

With such a range of conditions and spectrum of severity, it is essential that a systematic approach is taken when evaluating children with behavioural problems. A suggested strategy is to delineate the exact description of the behaviour(s) causing concern, to assess its impact on the child's development, education, on others within the family, and try to identify obvious developmental or cognitive difficulties that may underlie or exacerbate the difficulties seen. Accurate description of the behaviours may allow the formulation of a specific diagnosis, which in turn may permit a specific line of investigation and ultimately inform approaches to management. An obvious example would be the behavioural phenotypes of ADHD and autism. This approach also allows the identification of complex or serious disorders that may require onward referral to colleagues in specialist child and adolescent mental health services.

Outline

The possible diagnoses that should be considered when assessing a child with behavioural problems are best broken down by age group, although some diagnoses cross more than one age group and others may operate across all age ranges in childhood.

Baby, toddler and preschool

- Sleep and settling difficulties at night and other separation anxieties.
- Eating problems: food faddism, food refusal.
- Toileting problems: constipation/stool withholding.
- Temper tantrums.
- Autistic spectrum disorders.

School age

- Phobias.
- Adjustment disorder.
- School refusal.
- Anxiety.
- Bullying.
- Parasomnias.
- Eating disorders.
- ADHD.
- Non-organic somatic symptoms.
- Language disorders, including autistic spectrum disorders and semantic pragmatic disorders.
- Obsessive–compulsive disorders.
- Specific learning difficulties (e.g. dyslexia, dysgraphia).

Adolescence

- Conduct disorder.
- Personality disorder.
- Truancy and delinquency.
- Depression.
- Self-harm and suicide.
- Psychosis: schizophrenia and affective disorders.
- Eating disorders.

History

The single most important part of the history is the exact qualification and quantification of the symptoms described. Thus it is identical to the mainstream clinical method. The behaviours described may appear vague and, for example, 'My child is hyperactive' is a common complaint of parents. However, the use of this (and other) term(s) needs to be interrogated to establish whether this is indeed the symptom being reported and also how frequently and in which situations the behaviour is exhibited by the child. Asking the question 'What is it you observe in his behaviour that makes you say that?' is often a useful qualifying question. While the recall and description of symptoms are necessarily subjective, behaviour can be described against an agreed diagnostic framework. This can in turn be useful for quantifying the significance of particular symptoms, for example the DSM IV criteria for motor restlessness (hyperactivity) as part of ADHD diagnostic criteria (Table 40.1).

Another example would be the child who 'lashes out'. This may represent impulsivity, seen in ADHD, or may be the result of frustration arising as a secondary phenomenon from specific learning difficulties. It may also represent the response of a child with semantic pragmatic disorder who interprets the banter of peers or adults literally.

The setting in which the behaviours are exhibited can be important. For example, motor restlessness seen only at home is not likely to represent ADHD because this is a pervasive disorder. Similarly, lack of spontaneous speech seen only in one situation is likely to represent elective mutism, whereas lack of speech in all situations may reflect language delay or an autistic spectrum disorder.

The length of time that the problems have been exhibited should be sought as this may give clues to the original precipitant to the behaviour: for example, secondary enuresis starting after an episode of bullying, or somatic symptoms which have only presented since a divorce or separation between the parents.

The trend in the behaviour may indicate whether there is a developmental dimension involved. For example, the diminishing motor restlessness seen in young boys who have just started school may contrast with the increasingly rigid food-based rituals observed in an older girl with an eating disorder.

The opinions of others or other agencies (e.g. school or nursery) should be noted and this should be followed up by direct contact after the consultation. This is very important in determining the pervasiveness of a problem and also in confirming the impression of the parent (who is usually the primary historian) and is a vital step in the diagnosis of conditions such as ADHD or autism.

As behaviour tends to fluctuate over time, it is often difficult to get a feel for exactly what problems are causing difficulty for the child, family or community. It is helpful to get the parent to describe what a typical behavioural pattern consists of, or to describe a typical behavioural episode or the child's behaviour over the course of a typical day. Any precipitating or relieving factors should be sought and any relationship of the symptoms to schooling should be established. For example, a child may be described as being particularly oppositional in school at the start of a particular lesson; this may point to the fact that the child has a specific learning difficulty. Another child may present with agitated behaviour or sleepwalking at roughly the same interval after achieving sleep, which may suggest the diagnosis of a parasomnia (night terrors).

The developmental status of children presenting with behavioural difficulties should be appreciated. In school-aged children enquiry as to their academic and cognitive progress should be made. Attention should be paid to the child's language attainments and degree of social skill. Specific enquiry should be made to determine the presence or absence of developmental coordination disorder (DCD), specific learning difficulties (e.g. dyslexia, dysgraphia, dyscalculia) or more generalized learning difficulties.

Diagnostic criteria can be used (see Table 40.1) when assessing children believed to have significant

---

Table 40.1   DSM IV criteria for ADHD; motor restlessness subset

Hyperactivity
Squirms in seat or fidgets
Inappropriately leaves seat
Inappropriately runs or climbs (in adolescents or adults, this may be only a subjective feeling of restlessness)
Has trouble quietly playing or engaging in leisure activity
Appears driven or 'on the go'
Talks excessively

inattentiveness, motor restlessness and/or impulsivity. It is important to realize that use of such instruments is only a tool and is no substitute for careful and comprehensive clinical evaluation.

The presence of psychiatric symptoms should be sought. Children presenting with aggression may in fact be suffering from depression; careful enquiry may reveal the sleep disturbance, low mood or other symptoms indicative of this.

Any neurological symptoms should be noted carefully. Parents will often describe sudden inexplicable tantrums or outburst of aggression. This may be interpreted by the clinician as representing the paroxysmal rage attacks that can be a feature of temporal lobe epilepsy. However, such a conclusion is only valid if the history excludes an identifiable trigger (however trivial). The presence of behavioural changes with changes in cognition (particularly loss of skills) or other change in neurological status should alert the clinician to the possibility of a neurodegenerative or structural cause for the child's presentation.

The carer's views of the cause of the child's problems are helpful to know as they allow some insight into the relationship between the parent and the child. For instance, a parent may ascribe a toddler's problems with establishing sleep to dietary causes, without appreciating the impact that the lack of a predictable bedtime routine has on this behaviour.

The involvement of any other agencies such as social services, the police, education or a voluntary group should be noted, as they may be able to provide further information pertinent to the child's presentation.

Any significant comorbidity should be recorded, including other behavioural difficulties or existing medical conditions. For example, in a child presenting with feeding difficulties or faddism the difficulties may relate to earlier adverse experiences with certain food textures or eating. Children have presented to the author with food avoidance and difficulties in eating who, on careful questioning, reveal a past history of choking or inhaling food.

Social history

The social history is very important in delineating a child's problems, as many components of a child's behavioural repertoire are reactions to the emotional environment. Thus, some children presenting with violent behavioural outbursts may do so as a response to witnessing episodes of domestic violence. This may have child protection implications. It is therefore vital to have a clear idea of the family set-up and to gauge the stability of the family unit. Attachment problems may arise in children where bonding has been problematic, e.g. maternal mental health problems, neglect or prematurity).

Knowledge of whether the child has ever been on the Child Protection Register can be useful if there are behavioural problems that may indicate prior or current exposure to abusive environments.

Family history

It is often worth taking a detailed family history with respect to behavioural problems in other siblings or relatives. This may reveal a pattern of difficulties that in turn may shed light on the emotional and behavioural environment of the child, or it may suggest a genetic component to the difficulties.

The doctor should ask about the academic level of the parents on leaving school and make a circumspect enquiry into whether there have been any learning or behavioural problems in the parents.

Finally, the presence or absence of any psychiatric or medical problems in parents should be established, as this may be material to the child's presentation. For example, some children presenting with somatic symptoms for which no physical cause can be found (e.g. abdominal pain) may reflect a somatizing disorder they have seen present in their parents. Equally, a child exhibiting chest pain may be echoing the concern that the family has about a relative with ischaemic heart disease.

Examination

The examination should start with general observation of the way the child conducts himself during the history-taking process. The child's demeanour and interaction with the clinician, siblings, parents or other relatives should be noted. This may, for instance, betray in a child presenting with 'hyperactivity' the lack of social relatedness present in an autistic spectrum disorder. Similarly it may reveal the poor coordination and fine motor development of a child with developmental coordination disorder who has presented with school refusal. It may show the child to be anxious, avoidant or over-familiar.

A general physical examination is mandatory and particular attention should be paid to the neurological system. The developmental assessment is crucial in determining the developmental and cognitive context of the child's presentation. The child's stature, OFC and weight should also be recorded. How the child attends to playing or listening should be noted; this may show the inattentiveness, distractibility and motor restlessness seen in ADHD, or may show the low mood and lack of engagement associated with depression. Talking to the child may allow the clinician to assess their understanding and use of language. Some children presenting with behavioural problems may have high-level language disorders that may only be apparent on testing the child's use and understanding of idiom or the social context of language.

The child should be asked to draw or write their name. The handiness, pen grip and (for school-aged children) the quality and speed of letter formation and meter of writing can be noted. This may shed light on possible developmental coordination disorder, or general or specific learning difficulties.

Investigation

Behavioural problem	Investigation	Possible diagnosis
General approach	Write to school/other agencies Diary (including food diary) Move assessment battery for children (screening tool for children with DCD) Conners questionnaire (screening tool for children with ADHD)	DCD; school phobia; interactional difficulties, oppositional behaviours; low self-esteem ADHD; hyperkinetic syndrome
Hyperactivity; learning difficulties	TFT	Hyper/hypothyroidism
Hyperactivity; learning difficulties	Serum lead	Lead poisoning
Hyperactivity; learning difficulties	FBC and ferritin	Low iron states; iron-deficient anaemia
Paroxysmal rage; night terrors occurring throughout the night	EEG	Localization-related epilepsy
Learning difficulties and behavioural problems, with suggestive dysmorphism present	Assess sex chromosomes	Klinefelter's, XYY syndrome
Learning difficulties and behavioural problems, when language disorder present	Cytogenetics studies for fragile X	Fragile X syndrome

Clinical problem

A 4-year-old boy presented to the clinic with a history of running out of the house, despite parental efforts to dissuade him. The family had resorted to locking all doors and windows in the house, resulting in the rest of the family feeling trapped and uncomfortable during periods of hot weather. He was unable to be taken out of the house without attempting to abscond, and he would attempt to escape from adult carers continually. This resulted in him never being taken out of the house, with his mother and father having to look after him in continual 'shifts', without respite. Further enquiry reveals that his interaction with the parents was quite variable; on some days he would converse with his parents, while on others he would not speak with or respond to them at all. Generally, behaviour was described as being quite troublesome in that he would only comply with his parents' wishes if it appeared to suit him, and would only communicate on his terms. He was described as child who was 'more interested in things than in people' and was said to have very little sense of danger. He was obsessed with trains and bridges and was able, despite his communication difficulties, to name every character in the 'Thomas the Tank Engine' books. He was described as a child who was fascinated with how toys work, rather than with playing with them imaginatively.

He had been born at term and had suffered from mild transient tachypnoea of the newborn but was not subject to neonatal intensive care. He had been noted to have a mild degree of plagiocephaly. Early motor milestones were achieved normally. He had presented earlier in life with speech and language delay as well as behavioural difficulties. These problems occurred in the face of normal attainments of motor development. At 18 months he was noted to have absent speech with no recognizable words. He started nursery soon after and was noted by nursery staff to be quiet and withdrawn. However, by the age of 2 years he was able to make a cup of tea, memorizing all the steps completely. By the age of 3 years he had one word expressively and continued to be quiet and isolated at nursery.

On examination he was noted to be a fair-haired male with a triangular face and slight prominence of the ears. However, on comparing him to his parents, he was noted to physically resemble his mother. Examination of the neurological, cardiovascular, respiratory and abdominal systems was unremarkable. During the consultation he was noted to exhibit very little interest in the people in the clinic and tried to open every door in the facility. He was observed to play with trains and light switches and was interested in being examined because he liked to play with the stethoscope and the ophthalmoscope. He only made very limited and fleeting eye contact with the examining paediatrician. When asked questions by the doctor, his answers were directed via his mother using whispered responses. When asking to dismount from the examination couch, he said 'Get down me'.

Questions

1. What is the likely diagnosis?

2. What is the significance of the speech he was observed to use?

Answers

The most likely diagnosis is that of autistic spectrum disorder. The history is punctuated with examples of strange behaviour (behavioural restriction), limited linguistic development and social interaction. These three aspects are the core 'triad of impairments' found in autistic spectrum disorders.

The mode of the speech used (indirect whispered response via the mother) indicates that the child has little regard for the needs of the listener and this betrays some of his communication difficulties. The content of the limited speech heard shows that, at age 4, he demonstrates disordered speech development, rather than merely just delayed speech development.

INDEX

Page numbers in italics refer to *tables* and *figures*.